Teaching Moments
For Interns to Students

B. Ellis Myers MD

Library of Congress Control Number: 2015914013
CreateSpace Independent Publishing Platform, North Charleston, SC

ISBN: 151700750X
ISBN-13: 978-1517007508

DEDICATION

Many people have helped me to get to this point in my life. My mother Margaret Ann McDonald. My siblings John Myers, Martin Myers, and Lana Moore. My nieces Jessica, Rosanna, Sierra, Nikki, and Erika; and my nephew Evan. My cousins Donnie & Janice Henderson, Gary Chapman, Terry Hays, Vickie Shannon. My closest friends Robert & Carson Bailey, Bryan & Alexandria Pierik, Sunit & Parul Mahajan, Tal Gafni, Bodil Bailey, and the whole Gardner clan: Phil, Preston, Sheri, Harris, Mary, Barrett, Lauren, Pierce, Sarah, Spencer, Janeth, and Lindsay. Special thanks for a warm bed, great food, and time away from studying during medical school goes to Edward, Donalda, and Dana Pierik; Kyle & Nicole Riggs, Zoogie, and the Becks (Mike, Kelly, Jennifer, and Michael). Special thanks to the best study partners ever Jason Douglas, Erik Bakken, Danith Ieng, Janki Chandarana, Robert Steele, Katrina Ramsey, and TC Vo.

Before getting accepted to medical school, a wonderful family medicine doctor Robert Knight, his wife Janet, and their two kids Chris and Greg opened their doors to me. They allowed me to stay in their home, eat their food, and shadow Bobby for a week. The way that I choose to mentor my students is firmly founded in this kindness.

Previous to leaving the corporate world and pursuing medicine, I was blessed to work with Bruce Covill, Tom Emerson, and one of my closest friends Scott Moore. If not for the allowances afforded me by Bruce and Scott, my transition from corporate life to lowly student would've been much worse. When you start something like the four of us started, you need great leadership and unmatched technical excellence. When you're winning awards, doubling, quadrupling, on your way to octupling, and one of your people is moving toward the door; that requires understanding. I got all of that and more. Thanks Bruce. Thanks Scott.

CONTENTS

B. Ellis Myers

ACKNOWLEDGMENTS

Special thanks to Scott Moore and Jack Sullivan for bringing this project to fruition and helping to establish other endeavors.

PEOPLE DON'T LEARN IN LARGE CHUNKS

People don't learn in 60 minute blocks. People learn in small chunks which they connect to other small chunks and order into traversable trees. In computer science, these are called tree data structures, but modern computers are a great deal simpler than our minds when it comes to storage. The size of a concept-chunk that is stored-easily varies depending on the material, the environment, and the current receptiveness of the learner. Generally, the more limited the scope, the more repetitive the important points, and the greater the number of memorable connections; the better a concept-chunk is stored.

People in general tend to remain focused for between 25 35 minutes. This period varies greatly, but one can be assured that it's almost never 60 minutes. Nor do we usually get 25 minutes of uninterrupted time per day in the hospital. Generally, if we can free up 5 to 15 minutes to hold a teaching moment, the day has been a success. Make the teaching moment appropriate for the setting and the time allowed.

Obviously, you aren't going to spend a lot of time covering pediatric renal impairment when doing a rotation in the adult psych ward. Nor should you pack a lesson on Fanconi Syndrome and other brush border related issues into 5 minutes. And, what's the value of covering every antibiotic in the history of mankind in a 25 minute lesson? Instead, spend 5 minutes on antibiotics that you can tie to a current patient and then have your med student review those drugs throughout the day. Save Fanconi Syndrome and other brush border related issues until you have 25 minutes, and really get into it. Ask questions. Hammer home important points. Brainstorm crazy mnemonics.

The more inappropriate a mnemonic is, the more likely you are to remember it.
Sadly, putting the great ones in print isn't a good career move.

ANCHORS
CONNECTIONS BETWEEN STORAGE LOCATIONS IN MEMORY

Learning something new is like trying to keep a boat from moving in a choppy lake. If you sit in the boat and don't drop an anchor, you might get thrown out from the waves. The more anchors you throw in the water, the more each anchor buries itself into the surrounding lake bed, the more directions your tethered rope goes off in, the more stable the boat.

So you just learned something new. Did you tie this new knowledge to anything? No, then try and access that knowledge later today. You'll find that it's gone.

Tie the new knowledge to some old knowledge. That's one anchor, but it may not be buried in the lake bed very well. Tying that knowledge to a patient helps a lot. Tying that knowledge to a patient, some old knowledge, the joke your group told, the fact that you forgot this same info 6 months ago, the smell of the room next door to the computer you were sharing, and the conversations you had about this exact topic three more times that day — that's a boat which holds steady in choppy water.

Second, you can not anchor an idea or review a thought too much. However, you need to come at it from as many different angles as you can think of.

Going back to the boat analogy — if you have 10 anchors and you throw all of them in on the east-side, a big wave coming from the west-side will flip your boat. You can't keep going over the same topic in the same books in the same way over and over again and expect to maximize your ROI (return on investment).

And let's stay with the boat for one more concept. Let us say you anchor your boat really well. Water laps against the side constantly, but the boat barely wiggles.

Every time the wave hits, the boat stays steady, but a few drops of water come over the side and into the boat. If you don't pump some of that water out occasionally, eventually the boat takes on too much water and sinks. Do you get the picture?

I had a great little picture about what happens in fetal development by day 10 that I drew. We joked and shared it all around. Test day came, we all nailed it. Step 1 came and I actually got a question about my picture, and I was able to dredge that picture up from my memory. I did my peds-rotation, and a neonatologist pimped me on the topic. I not only didn't remember the answer; I didn't remember ever covering the topic. I missed my chance to impress the attending, and four hours later the picture jumped back into my mind. In medicine, that experience is a regular occurrence. Everything you learn, you seem to forget. Learning, reviewing, reviewing, and learning is a constant process. Limit the times you get too cocky and fail to jump at an opportunity to learn or review. A friend of mine once joked that the difference between Step 2 and Step 3 was how much time had passed since she studied for Step 1.

The Poop Book - Medical Edition
(5-minutes on the toilet is the perfect time to learn)

PURPOSE OF THIS BOOK

The above is a book title suggestion from a friend. This isn't quite the purpose of this book.

My belief is that the practice of medicine should be an open dialog. Regardless of what medical school you attended, where you do your residency, and in what areas you decide to practice; we are stronger as a profession when our weakest members are still damn good. This is one of the last great mentor-apprentice professions. It's in our best interest to build concept-chunks and share them.

In 1956, George A. Miller formulated the idea of the "concept chunk" based upon his research into working memory. This is the strategy of breaking down information into bite-sized pieces so the brain can more easily digest them. Concept Chunks, and our product Teaching Moments, strive to make each chunk more readily understandable, storable, and retrievable than the last. To this end, we continue to build out a community dedicated to this common goal.

Misconceptions, misunderstandings, and plain ignorance of concepts and facts is not limited to one school or one hospital. We all rely on the same texts and study materials. Medical education has evolved very similarly across all areas of the country, and regular communication via conferences and shared publications results in shared areas of ignorance. Concept Chunks collects these points of misunderstanding and develops lesson plans around them. Lesson plans are not developed over the expanse of a topic, but instead are developed over the particular areas where the teaching of this expanse of topic failed.

Teaching Moments is not intended as reference material. Instead, this is an addendum to a quality medical education. It is a tool to overcome the common failings of our shared methods.

Much of education follows a policy of "we do it this way, because this is the way we've always done it". Today, we are a society becoming more connected. We are members of a profession which expects evidentiary-based practice. So, why aren't we developing evidentiary-based lesson plans which are shared, corrected, and expanded among our brethren?

Teaching Moments uses research into human learning and storage to develop lessons which facilitate long-term storage of information. The most important points are treated as such, and we do consider the storage effort required for all information. Data which requires more effort to store are delivered in smaller pieces with recommendations to repetitive use of the data to increase its permanence. Concepts which require less effort to store are accentuated by clearly casting a picture which develops the texture of the topic over a longer lesson.

Here, Teaching Moments works both as a guideline for interns to use in the instruction of their medical students, and also works as study material for medical students and interns to make notes upon.

Learn by teaching – Many evidentiary-based teaching concepts are used here. The idea is to learn by doing. Using Teaching Moments as a guideline in your lessons or as a medium from which to study will have you practicing some core concepts such as groupings, anchors, mnemonics, consolidation, summarization, repetition, repetition, turning it 90 degrees in your head and repeat. Consolidate.

It can't make all the presentations you receive better, but you can learn how to take another person's presentation, reformat it, and make it better for you.

With Teaching Moments, you will be taught using a presentation format similar to what you received regularly throughout medical school, but with the added dimension of a focus toward long-term storage.

1. Trouble-areas get covered more often, and important points get emphasized
2. Concepts are optimized for storage, and time is used efficiently
3. Teachers are refreshing/learning while instructing
4. Interaction is increased

SOMEONE ALWAYS HAS AN IMPROVEMENT

Everything could be a little better. Something is always missing. People learn differently. Students come in to every interaction with different levels of understanding.

While I do rely on the support of people purchasing this book to develop all future books and applications (and to eat and pay bills), I encourage you to share this material, but please make sure everyone knows where you got it. I encourage you to openly share with me your concept-chunks so that I may include them in future projects. I encourage you to kindly critique and correct all materials you find here. I encourage you to digest any research you come across that helps create a better teaching environment and let me know about it.

Over time, I want these lesson groups to become more integrated with other lessons. For instance, learning about von Gierke's while learning about RTA-2 is an excellent anchor for the knowledge on both sides.

To this end, Concept Chunks is developing a community for sharing ideas. If you have a correction to make, an innovation to suggest, or an idea for a lesson please contact us. The upcoming web site is http://www.conceptchunks.com. Until such time as the site is up, feel free to contact me directly at DrEllisMyers@gmail.com.

If you develop your own concept chunks, upload them to us. If your lesson is promoted to the site, you will be credited on the site; and if your lesson is published in upcoming books, you will be credited in the book.

USING THE BOOK

If you've made it this far, you've probably noticed that things aren't always linear in their presentation. Instead, emphasis is given to flow and separation of concepts. Flow helps with storage. Separation helps with delineation within memory. Here are some other points.

1. Black and white with predictable formatting is good.

2. Limited bolding or underlining is good when it's very limited.

    - Color is a distraction that can be used effectively once you understand its power.

3. Groupings. Use groupings. See lesson on groupings.

4. Writing is good. No, writing is GREAT! If all you do is buy this book and go lesson by lesson, writing everything out, you'll be better off.

    - Typing is not as good as writing. Fewer anchors.

    - When you take notes directly onto the pages of this book, use color.

        - This is an effective use of color.

        - eg. Different colors for stages or concepts or timeframes.

5. Talking is great. Talking back and forth during lessons is great. Going out of your way to talk about each lesson throughout the day increases permanence.

6. Don't cover similar lessons at the same time. A shift in time creates greater differentiation between the two topics.

    - ie. If you cover left-to-right shunts on Tuesday morning, don't also cover right-to-left shunts at that time. Cover right-to-left shunts tomorrow or next week.

7. Every time you read or write an abbreviation, say what it stands for out loud until the name comes to you effortlessly.

    - ie. If you read or write "MPGN", say "membranoproliferative glomerulonephritis" out loud until they are one and the same in your mind.

BEYOND THE BOOK

1. If a topic falls into one of two groups, become an expert at the first group, then whatever is left must be in the other group.

    - ie. If you get macrolides (ACE) and aminoglycosides (TAGS) mixed up, become an expert at macrolides. Whatever isn't a macrolide must be an aminoglycoside.

        i. *You can also do what I just did. Whenever I write "macrolides", I try to write "ACE". These are the most important macrolides: Azithromycin, Clarithromycin, Erythromycin*

        ii. *I do the same thing w/ X-linked diseases. I always write "X" somewhere. eg. WisXott-Aldrich or Wiskott-Aldrich XR*

2. Satiation of a question immediately is less effective than prolonging the wonder.

    - ie. If you're reading and come across Gaucher's disease, try and remember what it is. If you remember that it's an LSD, but you can't remember what substrate accumulates, don't google it now. Make yourself a note, and when you're done going over whatever your topic is, go through your notes and look it up then.

        i. *You can practice now. If you don't know what a "LSD" is, make a note and look it up later.*

3. Facebook, messaging, email, sports scores, and news updates are distractions. If you're using this book to study, turn off your electronics, close your laptop, pick up some colored pens, and get to work.

4. Sometimes just googling topics, reading Wikipedia, and confirming with Google Scholar is fun and educational. If the road you travel turns out to be informative and useful, make some notes, and send them to me.

    If you create a lesson and submit it, we'll credit you and possibly your organization.

CORE CONCEPTS

1. Groupings
2. Attaching to Memory Storage Areas From Many Different Paths
3. Separate Similarly Named Things With Time and Place
4. Repetition

GROUPINGS

Up to Five, Aim for Three or Four

The human mind as a general rule can only store 5 things in very-short-term memory. The sweet-spot is 3 or 4 things. This is why commonly used numbers are broken up as they are

- phone (ie. 333-333-4444)

- social security numbers (ie. 333-22-4444)

- zipcode (ie. 55555-4444)

- Note: most people have a harder time remembering their zipcode than their phone number. What's the last 4-digits of your zipcode?

Group of Two

When you are trying to relay numbers, store numbers in your brain long-term, or count items on a list rely on a group of 2.

Lets start with counting up a list. If you're counting items at the out-door of Costco, you will make more mistakes if you count each item on the list. You'll make fewer mistakes if you count every other item. ie. 17 items on the list should be counted 2-4-6-8-10-12-14-16-17. Try counting as many things as you can, and you'll find this to be true. Maybe count a bowl of beans, the number of socks, the number of stairs between floors.

In medicine, this is a handy bit of trivia to know. It helps you to accurately count the number of pills in a bottle, the number of patients on your list, the amount of supplies in your cabinet, etc.

But maybe counting things won't help you with your studies, but the group of 2 has another use. Your brain stores '22' the same way it stores '2'. That is, your brain stores "twenty-two" the same way it stores "two". Some people have been found to store "two-hundred-twenty-two" the same way as "two", but these are the exceptions. Don't expect that you're an exception. Just rely on the group of 2. How is this useful?

- Question: What's the ISBN of that book?
- Answer 1: 9-7-8-0-0-7-1-4-9-6-1-3-1
- Answer 2: 97-80-07-14-96-13-1
- Answer 1 required 13 storage locations in your very-short term memory to relay the information. The buffer you have to work with is generally a max of 5 spaces. After being told the fifth number, you better have cleared a memory spot, or you'll need to have the person repeat the sixth number
- Answer 2 required 7 storage locations in your short term memory to relay the information. You almost fit the entire ISBN into very short term memory. Much less chance that you will need to have numbers repeated, and also much less chance that you will make a mistake.

Get in the habit of reading and saying all numbers in groups of 2.

- Question: What's the number on your credit card?
- Answer: 12 34 56 78 12 34 56 78 (eight memory locations vs sixteen)
- Question: What's the number on your driver's license?
- Answer: 12 34 56 78 12 3 (six memory locations vs eleven)
- Question: What's the MRN of your patient?
  - MRN = medical record number
  - **You will ask this question a LOT!!!!**

How Does Learning Groupings Help With Studying & Learning

Concepts take up the same memory locations as numbers. Actually, numbers are concepts. So, when you go to store information in your brain, you need to store no more than 5 items at a time, preferably 3-4. The trick here is a concept takes up a memory spot, even if that concept is the concept of another grouping.

If you can take groupings of concepts and run a theme through them to tie them together, even better!

Example
Most commonly broken bones are

- clavicle
- radius
- humerus
- wrist
- ulna
- ankle
- hip

Obviously, "wrist" is already a grouping of little bones which, unless you're an orthopedic surgeon or plastic surgeon, you don't need to know. But grouping the items a little more, you can make this list even more memorable. Group the bones of the arm, and you now have a list of 4 items. One of the items is another list.

- clavicle
- arm: radius, humerus, wrist, ulna
- ankle
- hip

Now this is more memorable than the first list, but if we run a theme through it, we can make it even more memorable. The theme is head-to-toe. The clavicle is most cephalad, while the ankle is most caudal. The humerus is most proximal, while the wrist is most distal.

- clavicle

- arm: humerus, radius, ulna, wrist

- hip

- ankle

You have now taken a list of seven items, massaged them a bit, and increased their long-term storage.

Example

How do you take an HPI?

Ask about what brought the patient in today. Is she in pain? How long has she been in pain? What was she doing when the pain started? Has anything made it better or worse? Does the pain move or radiate? Where exactly is it? On a scale of 1-10? Is anything associated with the pain? Are you sick often? When was the last time you were sick? Surgeries? Are you on any meds? Do you have any allergies? How about existing medical conditions specific to this issue like bleeding difficulties? Any changes in urinary or bowel? Describe. Are you sleeping okay? Does your family suffer from anything? What's your OB and GYN history? Where do you live? Who do you live with? Are you safe? Do you have a support structure? Do you do any drugs/tobacco/alcohol? Are you sexually active, with which sexes, do you use protection, how many partners in the last year? …

You could've asked a hundred more questions and still missed something. How do you know that you covered the main points? You need a plan.

Lets start with grouping

- Group 1: What brought you in today?

- Group 2: What medical issues were you dealing with before this happened?

- Group 3: Have any of your main systems been effected?

- Group 4: Is your family predisposed to anything?

  o This also gives you a chance to establish a baseline.

- Group 5: Environmental factors.

That is your max of 5. Sure would be nice to get it to 3-4 groups instead of 5 groups. Also, can you tie a theme to how the groups follow each other. This would make remembering even easier. But now that you have the groups, how do you group the questions within each group? If you lose your place when taking an HPI, you sure would love to have something to refer back to.

Enter one of my favorite mnemonics of all-time ·

LIQOR-AAA PAM HUGS FOSS

That is 5 groups of groups. LIQOR is a group of 5. AAA and PAM are groups of 3. HUGS and FOSS are groups of 4.

LIQOR and AAA obviously go together, and PAM HUGS FOSS sounds like an action in itself, ie. a woman named "Pam" hugged a guy named "Foss". I think of it as "Pam hugged Foss at AAA Liquors". Whatever, I never forget it, and it does my entire basic-HPI for me.

LIQOR-AAA PAM HUGS FOSS

- **L**ocation of the pain
- **I**ntensity of the pain
- **Q**uality of the pain
- **O**nset
- **R**adiation
- **A**ggravating factors
- **A**lleviating factors
- **A**ssociated symptoms

- **P**MHx (ie. personal medical history)
- **A**llergies
- **M**eds

- **H**ITS - Hospitalization, Injuries, Trauma, Surgery
- **U**rinary problems
- **G**I problems
- **S**leep

- **F**Hx (ie. family medical history)
- **O**B/GYN
- **S**ocial Hx
- **S**exual Hx

Once you have this hammered into your memory, you can start attaching other concept-chunks to it.

- ie. When you do your oncology rotation, you'll learn to ask about bleeding and clotting issues during this process.
    - Do you have any bleeding disorders? Any family history of bleeding disorders? Do you have problems with bruising? Does anyone in your family have problems with bruising? Do you have any problems with healing? Any injuries that just wouldn't go away? Anyone in your family have problems with healing? Have you ever had a

stroke? Have you ever lost control of a part of your body or couldn't think/remember for a period of time? Does anyone in your family have problems with strokes?

- ie. When your dealing with people on long-term medication
  - How much of each med do you take and when do you take it? Do you eat or drink beforehand?
  - How many times a week do you miss a dose?
  - Did you bring your log book with you?
  - Who delivers your medications? Who prepares your meds? Where do you get your prescriptions filled? How many refills do you have left?

Did you catch the evolution of the skill here? You took one of the most important (and confusing) skills of being a clinician, turned it into a game plan, and organized it into a highly storable format. At the beginning of your clinical rotations, you can now write this at the top of a page to get you back on track when you lose your place. After the regular use of this game plan, it becomes second nature, and you now start adding on extensions to the original item.

Groupings, themes, repetition, and anchors.

LETS REVIEW BEFORE WE GET STARTED.

What to expect in the layout of the book.

1. Black and white with predictable formatting.

2. Limited bolding and underlining. No color.

   a. Color is for your imagination, not for my lessons.

3. Groupings: up to 5, aim for 3-4. Mnemonics are good.

How you should use the book

1. Make your own mnemonics.

   a. Inappropriate tends to work better.

2. Use different colored pens to write in the book and write on paper. Draw and write, don't type.

3. Talking is great. Interaction between people upon topics is fantastic.

4. Don't cover similar lessons at the same time. One today and one next week.

5. Every time you read or write an abbreviation, say what it stands for out loud until the name comes to you effortlessly.

Tips on studying

1. If a topic falls into one of two groups, become an expert at the first group, then whatever is left must be in the other group.

2. Looking up an answer to a question immediately is less effective than prolonging the wonder.

3. Turn off your electronics, close your laptop, pick up some colored pens, and get to work.

4. Create as many anchors from as many different directions as you can to each concept-chunk you store.

5. Consolidate. Repetition, repetition, teach, teach, repetition, teach, repetition, teach, teach, teach. Repeat.

1 RENAL CENTRIC

Ascending Loop and Bartters 1

Renal terminology is confusing

Whaaaaaaaat?

- Much of the trouble with understanding the kidney is the variation of terminology. It is actually very knowable, but when everyone who is teaching it can call everything by multiple names, the learner is easily confused.
- To learn the renal system, your terminology has to be as plastic as possible.
  - The kidney is not amorphous.

Do you know the definition of "plastic" and "amorphous"?

(then look it up)

Kidney = Renal

- **Nephron**: a functional unit in the kidney.
  - Consists of a **glomerulus** and its associated **tubule**.
  - A tubule has a <u>lumen</u> with urine inside it. The tubule itself is made of <u>epithelium</u>, and the epithelium is surrounded by <u>interstitium</u>, and the interstitium contains blood.
  - The tubule is a tube made of epithelial cells.
  - An interstitium is a space between cells in a tissue. In the case of the renal cortex and medulla, the interstitium is filled w/ **peritubular capillaries**. Inside the peritubular capillaries flows blood.
  - When something diffuses from the tubule lumen and into the interstitium, this means that this component has been "<u>reabsorbed</u>".
    - ie. something diffused from the urine and into the blood
    - ie. something diffused from the tubular lumen and into the interstitium
    - ie. something diffused from the tubular lumen and into the peritubular capillaries
  - When something diffuses from the interstitium and into the tubule, this means that it has been "<u>excreted</u>" into the urine.

Excretion, Resorption, Reabsorbed

- Excretion
  - Items moving into the tubule/lumen/urine
  - Items moving from the peritubular capillaries of the interstitium/through the epithelium/out of the blood
    - water, ions, drugs, ...
- Resorption
  - the process or action by which something is reabsorbed.
- Reabsorbed = tubular reabsorption
  - the flow of glomerular filtrate from the proximal tubule of the nephron into the peritubular capillaries, or from the urine into the blood.

Waste, Urine, Diffusion, Paracellular Reabsorption

- Waste is excreted into the lumen of the tubule.
- Urine is filtered blood components that are not reabsorbed PLUS what is excreted into the tubule and that is not later reabsorbed.
  - Some things excreted into the tubule are later reabsorbed
  - Diffusion happens along a gradient. One must know the gradient to know the direction of flow.
  - Paracellular reabsorption: movement of items from the tubular lumen, between the epithelial cells of the walls of the lumen, and into the interstitium/peritubular capillaries

Afferent, Efferent, Glomerular Filtrate

- Afferent renal blood flow: flow of blood into the glomerulus
- Efferent renal blood flow: flow of blood out of the glomerulus
- Glomerular filtrate: the afferent renal blood flow which filters through the glomerulus and into the tubule and not directly into the efferent renal blood flow
  - Only some of the blood that flows to the kidney is filtered through the glomerulus.
    - Filtration into the glomerulus is controlled by management of afferent (toward) and efferent (away) blood flows, as well as by the glomerulus itself
  - Glomerular filtrate passes through the nephron before emerging as urine.

Afferent != Efferent

- Afferent
  - Renal artery → segmental arteries → interlobar arteries (circulation of lobes of the kidney) → arcuate arteries (circulation between the cortex and medulla of the kidney) → interlobular arteries (circulation between lobes of the kidney) → afferent arteries to the renal corpuscles → Bowman's capsule → glomerulus
    - Don't worry too much about these names. Just realize that some of the blood that flows into the kidney supplies the metabolic needs of the kidney itself, and some of the blood that flows into the kidney is filtered by the kidney
    - Only the blood that flows into Bowman's capsule and filters across the glomerulus is filtered in the tubules

Turn It Around and Around In Your Head

- Kidney = Renal. Functional units of the kidney are called nephrons.
  - A nephron is made up of a glomerulus and its associated tubule.
    - A tubule has a lumen. The tubule walls are made of epithelium. The epithelium is surrounded by interstitium. Interstitium is a space between cells in a tissue.
    - In this case, the interstitium contain peritubular capillaries. Capillaries contain blood.
- The area between epithelial cells is called paracellular.
  - Things can be reabsorbed from the lumen of the tubule paracellularly down a diffusion gradient and into the peritubular capillaries.
- Things can be reabsorbed from the lumen of the tubule via ion channels, passive transport, or active transport; into the epithelial cells of the tubule wall, and then out through the epithelial cell via similar means and into the blood within the peritubular capillaries.
  - This is also referred to as resorption. (resorption is the act of resorbing)
- Excretion is the reverse of this and is used to deposit waste into the tubule. The final result of the tubule waste is urine. Urine flows through the tubule. Blood flows through the interstitium.

Keep Spinning and Turning

- Afferent means toward. Efferent mean away.
- A nephron is a renal functional unit consisting of a glomerulus and its tubule.
  - To enter the tubule, blood must filter through the glomerulus. Thus it is glomerular filtrate.
- Greater afferent flow increases the pressure at the glomerulus → increased glomerular filtrate.
- Decreased efferent flow increases the pressure at the glomerulus → increased glomerular filtrate
- Some of the contents of the glomerular filtrate within the tubule is reabsorbed. More is added to the tubule via excretion. Some things that are excreted are later reabsorbed.
  - What is left is urine/waste, and urinated out.

Ascending Loop and Bartters 2

Some Structure is Useful in Reference

How Blood Flows To/In

- Afferent
  - Renal artery → segmental arteries → interlobar arteries (circulation of lobes of the kidney) → arcuate arteries (circulation between the cortex and medulla of the kidney) → interlobular arteries (circulation between lobes of the kidney) → afferent arteries to the renal corpuscles → Bowman's capsule → glomerulus → tubule
    - tubule → peritubular capillaries or urine
- These names are rarely useful
  - Grasp the concept

Grasp The Concept

- The **cortex** is the outer region.
- The **medulla** is the inner region.
- The medulla feeds in to medullary **pyramids**
  - When you think pyramids, think <u>papillae</u>.
- A **pelvis** is a region where something comes together or is collected.
- Blood comes into the cortex, is filtered through the medulla, released from the pyramids, collected in the pelvis, and flows out through the **ureter**.

Grasp The Concept

- Blood comes from the renal artery → → → is filtered through the glomerulus and into the tubules → flows through the renal cortex → processed in the renal medulla
  - What is reabsorbed
    - Blood flows out through the peritubular capillaries → → renal vein
  - What is excreted
    - Urine feeds out through the renal pyramids → is collected in the renal pelvis → flows through the ureters and into the **urinary bladder** → and blows out the urethra

Picture the Problem Areas

- Renal arteries can stiffen or can get blocked.
  - Leading to decreased renal perfusion → acute renal failure
- Damage to the glomeruli can occur via
  - deposit build up: glucose, immune complexes, fibrin, proteins
  - damage and repair: sclerosis, hyalinosis, glycosylation
- Ion build up can occur in areas of urinary collection or transport
  - calcium, (ammonium, magnesium, phosphate), uric acid, cystine
  - picture where the occur, and how they build up
    - ie. Staghorn calculus build up around the pyramids w/in the renal pelvis
    - they all show up on x-ray except uric acid
- Ureters can clog
  - hydronephrosis

Ascending Loop and Bartters 3

Structure Teaches Impairment

Review: Picture the Problem Areas

- Renal arteries can stiffen or can get blocked.
  - Leading to decreased renal perfusion → acute renal failure
- Damage to the glomeruli can occur via
  - deposit build up: glucose, immune complexes, fibrin, proteins
  - damage and repair: sclerosis, hyalinosis, glycosylation
- Ion build up can occur in areas of urinary collection or transport
  - calcium, (ammonium, magnesium, phosphate), uric acid, cystine
  - picture where the occur, and how they build up
    - ie. Staghorn calculus build up around the pyramids w/in the renal pelvis
    - they all show up on xray except uric acid
- Ureters can clog
  - hydronephrosis

Disease Can Occur

- Acute: mostly cortical (cortex)
  - tender
- Chronic: corticomedullary scarring
  - vesicoureteral reflux is required to develop
    - backflow from the bladder (vesico), through the ureter
  - white cell casts
    - build up of WBC's

Acute Is Not That Simple

- Maybe a drug you gave affects beyond the tubules and leads to interstitial inflammation
  - Acute (Drug-induced) Interstitial Nephritis (**AIN**)
    - **pyuria**: WBCs and pus escape in urine
    - **azotemia**: nitrogen escapes in urine
- Maybe the epithelial cells of the tubules were killed
  - Acute Tubular Necrosis (**ATN**)
    - Early risk of hyperkalemia as can't get rid of K+
    - Later risk of hypokalemia as can't absorb enough K+
    - **Muddy brown casts**
    - From: crush injury, shock, or toxins

Acute Renal Failure

- Abrupt decline in renal function
  - Inc Creatinine + Inc BUN
- **Prerenal**
  - kidney failed due to lack of perfusion to the kidney
- **Intrinsic**
  - damage inside the kidney
- **Postrenal**
  - outflow obstruction from the kidney

Acute Renal Failure

- **Prerenal:**
  - inc BUN/Cr
    - dec RBF → dec GFR
    - Na+/H2O retained to maintain volume
- **Intrinsic**
  - dec BUN/Cr
  - Due to acute tubular necrosis (ATN) or ischemia
- **Postrenal**
  - Greatly inc urinary Na + inc BUN/Cr

Summary

- **AIN** = Acute Interstitial Nephritis
  - **pyuria + azotemia**
  - generally drug induced
    - contrast, diuretics, NSAIDs, PCN, sulfa
- **ATN** = Acute Tubular Necrosis
  - crush, shock, or toxins lead to tubular cell death
    - e.g. Antibiotics
  - **muddy brown casts**
  - hyperkalemia while epithelial cells are leaking too much
  - hypokalemia late when epithelial cells' transport mechanisms are being built

Summary: **ARF** (Acute Renal Failure)

- Abrupt decline in renal function: Inc Cr + Inc BUN
- **Prerenal** = lack of perfusion to kidney
  - inc BUN/Cr
- **Intrinsic** = damage inside the kidney
  - dec BUN/Cr
  - think ATN or ischemia
- **Postrenal** = outflow obstruction from the kidney
  - Greatly inc urinary Na + inc BUN/Cr

Ascending Loop and Bartters 4

<u>Loop</u> of Henle
This is the big day.
ie. <u>This</u> is why you gave the module such
a stupid title? Yeesh!

Loop of Henle

- Descending limb reabsorbs water
- The thick ascending limb is impermeable to water, but it reabsorbs ions.
  - Actively reabsorbs Na+, <u>K+</u>, and Cl-
    - Na+/K+/2Cl- cotransporter = **NKCC2**
  - K+ leak channels
    - The leaking of K+ back into the lumen increases the positive charge and leads to ...
  - Paracellular reabsorption of Mg2+, <u>Ca2+</u> (, and Na+)
  - Urine becomes less concentrated as it ascends

Ascending Limb

- In your medical practice, the ascending limb of the loop of Henle is more important
  - The descending limb is permeable to water thus concentrating the urine
    - Our drugs **don't** substantially effect an entire membrane.
  - The ascending limb is positively charged and impermeable to water
    - A problem here leads to electrolyte imbalances.
    - Our drugs **do** substantially effect specific ion transporters.
      - Na+, K+, Ca2+ are most important clinically.

Drugs and Gene Mutations

- Drugs target specific transporters. Drugs don't generally target specific membranes.
  - What are the major constituents of membranes?
    (Think about it)
- Gene mutations generally effect proteins. Transporters and ion channels are made of proteins.
  - Both in drugs and mutations, where are the proteins?
    (Think about it)

Animals Evolved Out of Salt Water

- Every evolutionary step was built on management of NaCl and water.
  - When wondering how a change will effect an organ system, expect Na+ and Cl- gradients to be compensated for by many other areas.
    - Na is usually not the issue. Cl is usually not the issue.
    - **K+ is the issue.** Ca2+ is the issue.

Water Follows Salt

- If sodium is lost, water follows.
  - If a drug blocks the NKCC2 cotransporter, neither Na+ or K+ are reabsorbed. (Neither is Cl-)
    - Na+ is lost, and water follows. This decreases fluid volume.
      - ie. decreases blood pressure
    - This occurs in the **Loop** of Henle, thus these are called **Loop Diuretics**.
      - ie. **Furosemide**
    - K+ is also lost.
      - Loss of K+ affects positive gradient → decreased resorption of Ca2+ and Mg2+
    - The lost water can be an issue, but like with salt, many areas compensate for changes in water balance

Loop SE Are Similar to Diseases

- Loop diuretics
  - **Furosemide**
    - -semide, -tanide, and ethacrynic acid
  - SE: hypokalemia (and increased urinary K+)
  - SE: dehydration and hypercalciuria
  - SE: hyperuricemia → gout
- **Bartter** Syndromes and Gitelman Syndrome (the milder form)
  - hypokalemia → heart/muscle issues & increased blood Ph
  - dehydration
  - hypercalciuria → nephrocalcinosis
    - kidney stones

Summary

- NKCC2 in the ascending limb
  - the **Na+/K+/2Cl-** cotransporter
- K+ leak channels allow potassium to leak back into lumen
  - **Ca2+**, Mg2+ paracellular reabsorption is driven by the K+ gradient
- Loop diuretics effect the NKCC2 cotransporter
  - Furosemide
- Bartters Syndrome is similar to furosemide SE
  - **hypoK**alemia (and increased urinary K+)
  - dehydration and **hyperCa**lciuria
    - not enough K+ in the lumen to drive the Ca2+ out of the lumen

Ascending Loop and Bartters 5

Loop of Henle

This is the big day.

ie. This is why you gave the module such a stupid title? Yeesh!

Review

- NKCC2 in the ascending limb
  - the $Na+/K+/2Cl-$ cotransporter
- K+ leak channels allow potassium to leak back into lumen
  - **Ca2+**, Mg2+ paracellular reabsorption is driven by the K+ gradient
- Loop diuretics effect the NKCC2 cotransporter
  - Furosemide
- Bartters Syndrome is similar to furosemide SE
  - **hypoK**alemia (and increased urinary K+)
  - dehydration and **hyperCa**lciuria
    - not enough K+ in the lumen to drive the Ca2+ out of the lumen

Hypokalemia

- K+ is needed for repolarization of muscle
  - abnormal heart rhythms
    - flattened or inverted T-waves
      - T wave: repolarization of the ventricles
    - **U wave**: a depression between S and T
      - U wave: repolarization of the papillary muscles and Purkinje fibers
      - QRS → u → T
        » By definition, U waves are always followed by a T wave
    - More widespread effects may appear as ST depression, wide PR, or prolonged QT

Severe Hypokalemia

- Severe (2.5 to 3 meq/L)
  - muscle weakness, myalgia, tremor, muscle cramps, constipation
- Very severe (< 2 meq/L)
  - rhabdomyolysis, respiratory depression

Hypercalcemia

- Stones
- Bones
- Groans
- Thrones
- Psychiatric overtones

- Usually you hear, "Stones, Bones, Groans, and Psychiatric overtones"

What Hurts

- **Stones** in the renal or biliary tract
  - Calcium nephrocalcinosis is the most common
- **Bones** hurt
  - Calcium is deposited in your bones and is also resorbed from them when PTH is high
- **Groans**
  - Calcium is absorbed in your gut.
    - Absorbed in the gut, and what tries to escape in urine is reabsorbed in the kidneys
  - Too much calcium interferes w/ Na channels → muscles can't depolarize → gut not moving → constipation

Thrones

- Some say **thrones** is about polyuria
  - Pt is peeing a lot because body is trying to get rid of the calcium
- Others say **thrones** is about Osborn waves

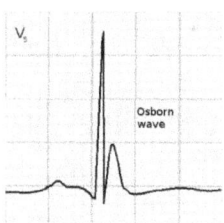

The Heart

- Ca interferes w/ Na channels and muscle is harder to depolarize

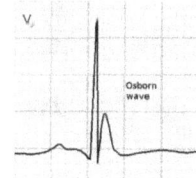

- Negative chronotropic effects
  - ie. dec heart rate
- Positive ionotropic effect
  - ie. inc contractility
  - possible short QT interval

The heart muscle has trouble depolarizing, but when it does, it really does!

- Osborn waves are also seen w/ hypothermia
  - *kinda for the same reason: too cold to depolarize, but when it finally does, it really does.*
- *Think of an Osborn wave being like when you try to push through something, and when you finally do, the force is disproportionally large and you get a little twitch immediately after.*

Psychiatric Overtones

- Remember, Ca2+ interferes w/ Na channels. This also makes nerves sluggish
- 40% are depressed.
- Pt may also be anxious, confused, insomnia
- Progresses to <u>coma</u>!

Hypercalcemia

Stones, Bones, Groans, Thrones,
and Psychiatric Overtones

- High: > 12 mg/dL
- Severe: > 15 mg/dL
  - Medical emergency: cardiac arrest, coma

Hypercalciuria and Dehydration

- Dec K+ transport into the epithelial cell of the tubule → dec paracellular Ca2+ reabsorption
  - **hypercalciuria & nephrocalcinosis**
  - **increased blood pH**
- **Furosemide + NS** (normal saline)
  - Tx: severe hypercalcemia
    - The loop diuretic causes loss of calcium reabsorption from the tubule, but we have to replace the water that is lost.
      - Keep an eye on the potassium.

Summary

- hypoKalemia
  - Problems repolarizing muscle
    - abnormal heart rhythms, esp. **U wave**
      - QRS → u → possibly flattened or inverted (or normal) T
    - Severe (2.5 to 3 meq/L); Very severe (< 2 meq/L)
- hyperCalcemia
  - Stones, Bones, Groans, Thrones, Psychiatric overtones
    - kidney stones, resorption from bones, constipation, Osborn waves & polyuria, depression/confusion/coma
    - High: > 12 mg/dL; Very severe: > 15 mg/dL
  - Tx: furosemide + NS
    - watch out for hypokalemia

Ascending Loop and Bartters 6

Loop of Henle
This is the big day.
ie. <u>This</u> is why you gave the module such
a stupid title? Yeesh!

Review

- hypoKalemia
  - problems repolarizing muscle
    - abnormal heart rhythms, esp. **U wave**
      - QRS → u → possibly flattened or inverted (or normal) T
    - Severe (2.5 to 3 meq/L); Very severe (< 2 meq/L)
- hyperCalcemia
  - Stones, Bones, Groans, Thrones, Psychiatric overtones
    - kidney stones, resorption from bones, constipation, Osborn waves & polyuria, depression/confusion/coma
    - High: > 12 mg/dL; Very severe: > 15 mg/dL
  - Tx: furosemide + NS
    - watch out for hypokalemia

Review:
Loop SE Are Similar to Diseases

- Loop diuretics
  - **Furosemide**
    - -semide, -tanide, and ethacrynic acid
  - SE: hypokalemia (and increased urinary K+)
  - SE: dehydration and hypercalciuria
  - SE: hyperuricemia → gout
- **Bartter** Syndromes and Gitelman Syndrome (the milder form)
  - hypokalemia → heart/muscle issues & increased blood Ph
  - dehydration
  - hypercalciuria → nephrocalcinosis
    - kidney stones

Bartter Syndrome

- Inherited defect in thick ascending limb
- Hypokalemia
  - muscle issues/arrhythmias, inc blood pH
  - normal to decreased blood pressure
    - remember others systems compensate
- Neonatal, Classic, or Gitelman
  - Neonatal: 24-30w
    - Classic: found in school age
  - Gitelman: mild form

Neonatal vs. Classic

- Neonatal (24-30w)
  - polyhydramnios (excess amniotic fluid) causes birth
  - life-threatening dehydration
    - polyuria, polydipsia
  - hypercalciuria → nephrocalcinosis → stones → ARF
- Classic
  - school age w/ less of the above, no stones, but may develop ESRD
  - chronic vomiting and growth retardation
  - Tests:
    - Urine: high urinary K+ and Cl- despite low serum values
      - must screen for diuretic abuse
    - Renal biopsy: hyperplasia of juxtaglomerular apparatus

Summary

- Bartter Syndrome
  - hypoK
    - muscle issues & arrythmias, inc serum pH
  - Neonatal: 24-30w
    - polyhydramnios → birth
    - polyuria, polydipsia → dehydration
    - hypercalciuria → nephrocalcinosis → stones → ARF
  - Classic
    - school age w/ no stones but possible ESRD
    - chronic vomiting and growth retardation
    - Tests:
      - Urine: high urinary K+ and Cl- despite low serum values
      - Renal biopsy: hyperplasia of juxtaglomerular apparatus

Glomerulus and Brush Border 1

The blood cometh, and the blood leaveth

Afferent, Efferent, Glomerular Filtrate

- Afferent renal blood flow:
  - flow of blood into the glomerulus
- Efferent renal blood flow:
  - flow of blood out of the glomerulus
- Glomerular filtrate:
  - the afferent renal blood flow which filters through the glomerulus and into the tubule and not directly into the efferent renal blood flow
- Only some of the blood that flows to the kidney is filtered through the glomerulus.
  - Filtration into the glomerulus is controlled by management of afferent (toward) and efferent (away) blood flows, as well as by the glomerulus itself
- Glomerular filtrate passes through the nephron before emerging as urine.

Afferent != Efferent

- Afferent
  - Renal artery → segmental arteries → interlobar arteries (circulation of lobes of the kidney) → arcuate arteries (circulation between the cortex and medulla of the kidney) → interlobular arteries (circulation between lobes of the kidney) → afferent arteries to the renal corpuscles → Bowman's capsule → glomerulus
    - Don't worry too much about these names. Just realize that some of the blood that flows into the kidney supplies the metabolic needs of the kidney itself, and some of the blood that flows into the kidney is filtered by the kidney
    - Only the blood that flows into Bowman's capsule and filters across the glomerulus is filtered in the tubules

Glomerular Filtration

1. **Size barrier:**
   - Fenestrated capillary endothelium
     - has to fit through the holes (fenestrations)

2. Negative **charge barrier:**
   - Fused basement membrane w/ heparin sulfate
     - this is what breaks down and allows protein to escape
     - Leads to **nephrOtic syndrome:**
       - the 'O' is where the protein go through
       - loss of protein —> generalized edema and hyperlipidemia

3. Podocyte foot processes make up the epithelial layer
   - The visceral layer

PAH = RBF (Renal Blood Flow)

- **Renal Blood Flow (RBF)**
  - aka. renal plasma flow (RPF)
  - the volume of blood delivered to the kidneys per unit time
  - PAH is freely filtered, not reabsorbed from the tubules, but is excreted into the tubules. PAH travels all the routes into the kidney and none of the ones out.

Filtration Values

- **GFR** = Glomerular Filtration Rate
  - estimated with creatinine
  - creatinine is freely filtered and not excreted
- **FF** = filtration fraction
  - normally 20% (or 1/5)
- Filtered load = GFR * plasma concentration

Drugs: Filtration Effectors

- **ANP** = Atrial Natriuretic Peptide
  - secreted by strained heart muscle
  - inc GFR
    - due to inc Na+ filtration at glomerulus
- Prostaglandins dilate the afferent arterioles
  - inc RBF and GFR
  - **NSAIDS** block prostaglandin synthesis
    - Results in prerenal-ARF if too effective.
- Angiotensin II constrict the efferent arterioles
  - dec RBF, inc GFR, FF increases
    - the decreased outflow results in greater pressure at the glomerulus (increasing GFR), but that same pressure reduces the inward flow thereby decreasing RBF
  - **ACE-Inhibitors** inhibit angiotensin II → dec BP

Angiotensin II

- Functions
  - <u>Constricts</u> vascular smooth muscle and <u>inactivate</u> the vasodilator **bradykinin.**
  - <u>Stimulates</u> the **Na+/H+ exchanger** in the proximal tubules
    - Greater reabsorption of Na+ and therefore water ("water follows salt")
    - Bicarb excretion is tied to H+ excretion, so the increased Na+ reabsorption also results in increased loss of bicarb → dec blood pH

- **ACE** = **A**ngiotensin-**C**onverting-**E**nzyme
  - Angiotensin I is converted to angiotensin II by ACE in the lungs
- Less angiotensin II means
  - less constriction of vascular smooth muscle
  - more bradykinin → inc vasodilation
  - less Na+ reabsorption → dec fluid
  - inc bicarb → inc blood pH

[renin is increased, but it doesn't really become an issue too often]

ACE-I = ACE Inhibitors

- **Captopril, Lisinopril, Enalapril**
  - and the rest of the –april's & -opril's
- ACE inhibitors first when treating **HTN** or **CHF**

- SE: **CAPTOPRIL** + hyperkalemia
  - **C**ough, **A**ngioedema, **P**roteinuria, **T**aste changes, hyp**O**tension, **P**regnancy issues (fetal renal damage), **R**ash, **I**ncreased renin, **L**ower angiotensin II
  - If pt gets **cough**, move them to **ARB**s (covered at another time)

- Contraindicated w/ bilateral renal artery stenosis
  - ACE-I decrease GFR due to preventing constriction of the efferent arterioles
  - The kidneys are already not getting enough RBF due to afferent-stenosis, and now the kidney can't constrict the efferent arterioles.
  - ➔ prerenal ARF

Summary: Pertinent Kidney Stats

- **Renal Blood Flow (RBF)** estimate by **PAH**
  - PAH is freely filtered, not reabsorbed, but is excreted.

- **GFR** estimated by **creatinine**
  - creatinine is freely filtered and not excreted

- **FF** = filtration fraction: normally 20%

Summary: Glomerular/Arteriole Drugs

- **ANP** = <u>Atrial</u> Natriuretic Peptide
  - greater Na+ filtration at glomerulus
  - inc GFR

- **NSAIDs** prevent dilation of afferent arterioles
  - Results in prerenal-ARF if too effective.

- **ACE-I** prevent constriction of efferent arterioles
  - Results in dec BP

Summary: ACE Inhibitors

- **ACE-I** → Less angiotensin II = dec BP (and inc serum pH)
  - less vascular constriction and more vasodilation
  - less blood volume

  - **Captopril, Lisinopril, Enalapril**
    - -april & -opril
  - 1st Line for <u>HTN</u> and <u>CHF</u>

  - If pt develops a **cough**, move them to **ARBs**
  - Not w/ bilateral renal artery stenosis → prerenal ARF

Glomerulus and Brush Border 2

Resorb, Excrete -- Concentrate

What goes up, what comes down?

Review

- **Renal Blood Flow (RBF)** estimate by **PAH**
- **GFR** estimated by **creatinine**

- **ANP** = <u>Atrial</u> Natriuretic Peptide
  - greater Na+ filtration at glomerulus
  - inc GFR, RBF same, FF increases
- **NSAIDs** prevent dilation of the afferent arterioles
  - Results in prerenal-ARF if too effective.
- **ACE-I** prevent constriction of the efferent arterioles
  - Results in dec BP

Review: ACE Inhibitors

- **ACE-I** → Less angiotensin II = dec BP
  - **Captopril, Lisinopril, Enalapril**
    - -april & -opril
  - 1st Line for <u>HTN</u> & <u>CHF</u>
  - If pt develops a **cough**, move them to **ARBs**
  - Not w/ bilateral renal artery stenosis
    - Leads to prerenal-ARF

PCT = Proximal Convoluted Tubule

- From Bowman's capsule to the loop of Henle.
  - Contains brush border cells
- **Brush Border**
  - aka. the <u>striated border</u>
  - densely packed microvilli
  - greatly increase surface area of the epithelial cells
  - each cell is packed w/ mitochondria
    - very busy and needs energy

PCT: This is a Busy Area

- Many ions and molecules are reabsorbed and excreted
- Resorbed:
  - 100% of organic solutes (amino acids and glucose)
  - Salt and water (Na+, Cl-, H20); CO2;
    - 80% of Na+ reabsorbed in PCT (the most in kidney)
  - Most potassium, urea, phosphate, citrate
- Secreted
  - Medications
  - Ammonium
    - Glutamine —> glutamate —> alpha-ketoglutarate —> bicarb

PCT: Brush Border Activity
[Tubular fluid] / [Plasma]

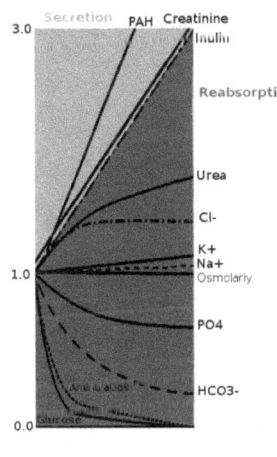

- Glucose and amino acids are immediately resorbed
  - *Don't waste your energy or your building blocks*
  - then bicarb and then phosphorous

- PAH: freely filtered + excreted
  - PAH measures **renal blood flow (RBF)**

- Creatine and inulin are freely filtered, their concentrations change as water is absorbed
  - They have no excretion component like PAH
  - Creatinine measures **GFR (glomerular filtration rate)**

- Cl- resorbed slowly in first 1/3, then equals Na+ last 2/3

- Na+ drives water resorption, so it matches Osmolarity
  - 80% of Na+ reabsorbed in PCT (the most in kidney)

PCT Pathology

- **Renal Cell Carcinoma**
  - the most common kidney cancer
  - brush border is most active with the highest turnover rate
- **ATN = Acute Tubular Necrosis**
  - induced by drugs (eg. antibiotics), myoglobin (from rhabdomyolysis), sepsis
  - also occurs along the remainder of the tubules
- **Proximal Renal Tubular Acidosis**
  - aka. RTA-Type 2
    - *Don't forget, type 2 is proximal. Type 1 is distal.*
  - Defect in bicarb reabsorption → serum acidosis
  - Often caused by **Fanconi syndrome**
    - Failure to reabsorb glucose, amino acids, bicarb, phosphate

Acute Tubular Necrosis

- ATN presents as AKI and can lead to AKF (or ARF)
  - **ATN** = acute tubular necrosis
    - something has insulted the epithelial cells of the tubules and they are unable to repair themselves
    - a drug, such as an aminoglycoside antibiotic (eg. **gentamicin**) or contrast from imaging w/ **contrast**
    - myoglobin from **rhabdomyolysis**
    - septic shock, blood transfusion, or trauma
  - **AKI** = acute kidney injury
    - when the kidney suddenly starts having problems
  - **AKF** = acute kidney failure = acute renal failure = **ARF**

ATN: Treatment

- Stop offending agent
- Maintain fluids equal to urine produced
- Restrict substances normally removed by kidneys:
  - protein, sodium, potassium
- Meds
  - to control K+ in blood
  - to remove fluid from body

Temporary dialysis may be needed, but ATN is very reversible

Summary

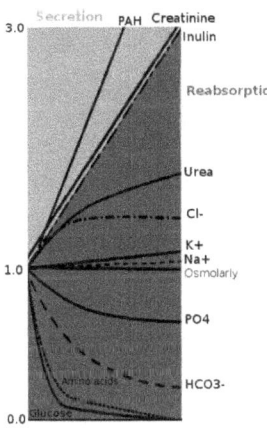

- **Brush Border** = striated border
  - Densely packed microvilli packed w/ mitochondria
- Resorbed:
  - 100% of organic solutes (amino acids and glucose)
  - Salt and water (Na+, Cl-, H20); CO2;
  - Most potassium, urea, phosphate, citrate
- Secreted
  - Medications
  - Ammonium
  - Glutamine → glutamate → α-ketoglutarate →bicarb

- Glucose and amino acids are immediately resorbed
  Don't waste your energy or your building blocks
- PAH: freely filtered + excreted
- Creatine & inulin conc changes as water is absorbed
- Cl- resorbed slowly in first 1/3, then equals Na+ last 2/3
- Na+ drives water resorption, so it matches Osmolarity
  - 80% of Na+ reabsorbed in PCT (the most in kidney)

Summary: PCT Pathology

- Renal Cell Carcinoma
- ATN = Acute Tubular Necrosis induced by
  - drugs: gentamicin, contrast
  - myoglobin (from rhabdomyolysis)
  - sepsis/shock
  - *also occurs along the remainder of the tubules*
- **Proximal** Renal Tubular Acidosis = RTA-Type 2
  - Defect in bicarb reabsorption → serum acidosis

Glomerulus and Brush Border 3

Other system's problems, causing us problems

Review

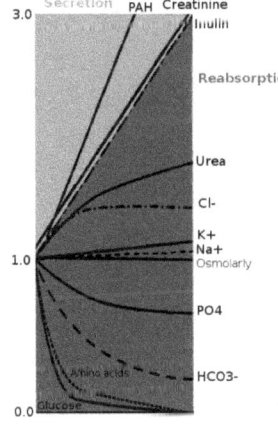

- **Brush Border** = striated border
  - Densely packed microvilli packed w/ mitochondria
- Resorbed:
  - 100% of organic solutes (amino acids and glucose)
  - Salt and water (Na+, Cl-, H20); CO2;
  - Most potassium, urea, phosphate, citrate
- Secreted
  - Medications
  - Ammonium
  - Glutamine → glutamate → α-ketoglutarate →bicarb

- Glucose and amino acids are immediately resorbed
  Don't waste your energy or your building blocks
- PAH: freely filtered + excreted
- Creatine & inulin conc changes as water is absorbed
- Cl- resorbed slowly in first 1/3, then equals Na+ last 2/3
- Na+ drives water resorption, so it matches Osmolarity
  - 80% of Na+ reabsorbed in PCT (the most in kidney)

Review: PCT Pathology

- Renal Cell Carcinoma
- ATN = Acute Tubular Necrosis induced by
  - drugs: gentamicin, contrast
  - myoglobin (from rhabdomyolysis)
  - sepsis/shock
  - *also occurs along the remainder of the tubules*
- **Proximal** Renal Tubular Acidosis = RTA-Type 2
  - Defect in bicarb reabsorption → serum acidosis

Renal Tubular Acidosis (RTA) **Type 2**

- aka. **Proximal** Renal Tubular Acidosis
- Defect in bicarb reabsorption
  - Urinary bicarb wasting → serum acidosis
  - Hypokalemia + hypophosphatemia
- Often used interchangeably w/ **Fanconi syndrome**
  - Fanconi syndrome is actually a failure to reabsorb glucose, amino acids, bicarb, phosphate

RTA-2 Causes

- Can be **Familial**
  - problem w/ <u>amino acid processing</u>
    - cystinosis or tyrosinemia
  - problem w/ <u>energy storage</u>
    - galactose, glycogen, fructose
      - ie. **Glycogen Storage Disease Type 1 (von Gierke's)**
- Can be **Acquired**
  - **Multiple myeloma**
  - HAART, ifosfamide
  - Lead, cadmium

RTA-2 Tx

- Reverse the acidosis
  - **Thiazides**: leads to contraction alkalosis
  - Generally **don't** give bicarb
    - leads to bicarb-wasting and diuresis further exacerbating
    - as well as hypokalemia

RTA-Type 2: Summary

- RTA-2 = **Proximal RTA**
  - Often used interchangeably w/ **Fanconi syndrome**
    - Fanconi syndrome is actually a failure to reabsorb glucose, amino acids, bicarb, phosphate
  - Defect in bicarb reabsorption
  - **Hypokalemia + hypophosphatemia**
  - May be caused by familial conditions such as **GSD-1** (von Gierke's) or by acquired conditions such as **MM** (Multiple Myeloma)
  - Tx: **thiazides**, NOT bicarb

GSD Type 1 = von Gierke's

- Most common Glycogen Storage Disease
- Deficiency of **glucose-6-phosphatase** (G6Pase)
  - Found in endoplasmic reticulum
  - Leads to
    - **Hypoglycemia**
    - **Lactic Acidosis**
    - **Hypertriglyceridemia**
    - **Hyperuricemia**
- Tx: frequent feedings with **cornstarch**/carbs

GSD Type 1: Effects on Liver

- Can't produce glucose from glycogen nor from gluconeogenesis
  - Liver is responsible for providing most of the glucose the body uses during fasting
    - Leads to severe hypoglycemia
- Increased glycogen storage in liver (**hepatomegaly**)
  - and kidneys

GSD Type 1: Biochemistry

- When fasting continues for more than a few hours, falling insulin levels permit catabolism of muscle and triglycerides (**TG**) from adipose tissue
  - Leads to amino acids (mostly <u>alanine</u>), FFA (free fatty acids), **LA** (lactic acid)
  - FFA breakdown → ketones and acetyl-CoA
- Gluconeogenesis:
  - amino acids + LA → **G6P** (glucose-6-phosphate)
  - G6P dephosphorylation via G6Pase → glucose + PO4
    - **final step of gluconeogenesis and glycogenolysis**
  - The build up of G6P inhibits gluconeogenesis and glycogenolysis via feedback inhibition
    - Lack of G6Pase prevents breakdown and inhibits even attempting to begin the process

GSD-1 (von Gierke's): Summary

- Deficiency of **glucose-6-phosphatase** (G6Pase)
- Biochemistry
  - Fasting → catabolism of muscle and **TG** from adipose tissue → amino acids (mostly <u>alanine</u>), FFA, **LA**
    - FFA → ketones and acetyl-CoA
  - Gluconeogenesis:
    - amino acids + LA → G6P → via G6Pase → glucose + PO4
      - final step is same in gluconeogenesis and glycogenolysis
      - no G6Pase → build up of G6P inhibiting TG breakdown → no glucose
- Symptoms
  - **Hypoglycemia, Lactic Acidosis**
  - Hypertriglyceridemia, Hyperuricemia
  - **Hepatomegaly**
- Tx: **cornstarch**

PCT Pathology Summary

- RTA-2 = **Proximal** RTA (Often caused by **Fanconi syndrome**)
  - Defect in bicarb reabsorption
  - **Hypo-K,-PO4**
  - May be caused by **GSD-1** or **MM**
  - Tx: **thiazides**, NOT bicarb
- GSD-1 (von Gierke's)
  - Deficiency of **glucose-6-phosphatase** (G6Pase)
  - Catabolism of muscle & **TG** (from adipose tissue) → alanine, FFA, **LA**
    - FFA → ketones and acetyl-CoA
    - Gluconeogenesis: amino acids + LA → G6P → via G6Pase → glucose + PO4
      - no G6Pase → build up of G6P inhibiting TG breakdown → no glucose
  - Symptoms
    - **Hypoglycemia, Lactic Acidosis,** Hypertriglyceridemia, Hyperuricemia
    - **Hepatomegaly**
  - Tx: **cornstarch**

Glomerulus and Brush Border 4

My symptoms could be caused by
other things? How do I really know?
What should I do?

PCT Pathology Review

- RTA-2 = **Proximal** RTA (Often caused by **Fanconi syndrome**)
  - Defect in bicarb reabsorption
  - **Hypo-K,-PO4**
  - May be caused by **GSD-1** or **MM**
  - Tx: **thiazides**, NOT bicarb
- GSD-1 (von Gierke's)
  - Deficiency of **glucose-6-phosphatase** (G6Pase)
  - Catabolism of muscle & **TG** (from adipose tissue) → alanine, FFA, **LA**
    - FFA → ketones and acetyl-CoA
    - Gluconeogenesis: amino acids + LA → G6P →via G6Pase → glucose + PO4
      - no G6Pase → build up of G6P inhibiting TG breakdown → no glucose
  - Symptoms
    - **Hypoglycemia, Lactic Acidosis,** Hypertriglyceridemia, Hyperuricemia
    - **Hepatomegaly**
  - Tx: **cornstarch**

Hypoglycemia

- Commonly thought of as shakiness w/ altered mood and thinking
- < 60 mg/dL is below normal, but symptoms generally don't appear till **50 mg/dL**
- Symptoms
  - Principally due to dec glucose to brain
    - so any neuroglycopenic manifestation is a symptom
  - Adrenergic
    - palpations/tachycardia, sweating, cold/clammy, dilated pupils
  - Glucagon
    - hunger, nausea, vomiting, headache

Hypoglycemia: Causes & Tx

- Principal Causes
  - Diabetes mellitus medications and insulin
  - Drugs/poisons/alcohol
  - Hyperinsulinemia, **inborn errors of metabolism**, hormone deficiencies
  - Prolonged starvation, organ failure, metabolism altered by infection
- Treatment
  - Increase the frequency of feedings
  - Drugs: octreotide, glucocorticoids
  - Partial pancreatectomy

Lactic Acidosis

- Primarily an impairment of gluconeogenesis
  - Liver and muscle generate LA
    - LA oxidized by NAD+ to pyruvic acid
    - Pyruvic acid converted via gluconeogenesis to G6P
      - accumulated G6P inhibits lactate to pyruvate conversion
- In general, LA is generated by liver and muscle or by G6Pase deficiency due to Glycogen Storage Disease Type 1 (von Gierke's)
  - Indirectly leads to hypertriglyceridemia

Hyperuricemia

- Inc production and dec excretion of uric acid
  - inc G6P metabolized via pentose phosphate pathway → inc uric acid as byproduct of purine degradation
- LA and uric acid compete w/ each other for excretion in the kidneys
- Eventually leads to renal and joint damage
- Tx: allopurinol prevents nephropathy and gout

GSD-1 Symptom Summary

- **Hypoglycemia**
  - Shakiness w/ altered mood and thinking
  - Glucose around **50 mg/dL** or less
  - Symptoms
    - Principally due to dec glucose to brain
    - Adrenergic: palpations/tachycardia, sweating, cold/clammy, dilated pupils
- **Lactic Acidosis (LA)**
  - Liver and muscle generate LA
    - LA oxidized by NAD+ to pyruvic acid → via gluconeogenesis→ G6P
      - accumulated G6P inhibits lactate to pyruvate conversion
  - Indirectly leads to **Hypertriglyceridemia**
- **Hyperuricemia**
  - G6P →via pentose phosphate pathway→ uric acid
    - byproduct of purine degradation
  - LA and uric acid compete w/ each other for excretion in the kidneys
    - Eventually leads to renal and joint damage
  - Tx: allopurinol prevents nephropathy and gout

Glomerulus and Brush Border 5

50/50 if you live 5 years.

Begin to worry around 50yo

PCT Pathology: ATN & RTA-2

- ATN = Acute Tubular Necrosis induced by
  - drugs: gentamicin, contrast
  - myoglobin (from rhabdomyolysis)
  - sepsis/shock
  - *also occurs along the remainder of the tubules*
- RTA-2 = Proximal RTA (Often caused by **Fanconi syndrome**)
  - Defect in bicarb reabsorption
  - **Hypo-K,-PO4**
  - May be caused by **GSD-1** or **Multiple Myeloma**
  - Tx: **thiazides**, NOT bicarb

PCT Pathology: GSD-1 (von Gierke's)

- Deficiency of **glucose-6-phosphatase** (G6Pase)
  - Gluconeogenesis: amino acids + LA → G6P →via G6Pase → glucose + PO4
    - **no G6Pase → build up of G6P inhibiting TG breakdown → no glucose**
- Symptoms
  - **Hypoglycemia**
    - Glucose around **50 mg/dL** or less
    - Confused. Palpations, sweaty, cold/clammy, dilated pupils
  - **Lactic Acidosis (LA)**
    - Liver and muscle generate LA
    - Indirectly leads to **Hypertriglyceridemia**
  - **Hyperuricemia**
    - G6P →via pentose phosphate pathway→ uric acid
      - byproduct of purine degradation
    - LA and uric acid compete w/ each other for excretion in the kidneys
      - Eventually leads to renal and joint damage
  - Hepatomegaly
- Tx: **cornstarch**

Multiple Myeloma (MM)

- **Multiple Myeloma Monoclonal M-protein spike**
  - (**M**ade of IgG or IgA)
- Arises in the bone marrow
  - plasma cells w/ "fried-egg" appearance and "clock-face chromatin"
- Production of cytokines (esp. IL-6) is what leads to the osteoporosis
  - ie. punched-out bone lesions in spine on CXR
- Production of paraprotein, an abnormal protein, that accumulates in the brush border of the PCT causes **RTA-2** and other kidney problems
  - ie. amyloidosis (which interferes w/ charge barrier → nephrotic)
    - Bence Jones proteins in urine

MM: Epidemiology

- Most common bone marrow tumor in > 50yo
- 2nd most common hematological malignancy in U.S.
- African-Americans to European-Americans
  - 2:1
- Median survival: 3y. With Tx advances to 7y.
- 5y-survival rate: 45%.

MM: What to Remember So Far

- Arises from bone marrow
  - plasma cells w/ "fried-egg" appearance and "clock-face chromatin"
- Punched out bone lesions on CXR
- Paraprotein build up in kidneys → RTA-2
  - ie. amyloidosis in brush border of PCT
    - which interferes w/ charge barrier → nephrotic
      - **Bence-Jones** proteins in urine
  - RTA-2 = Proximal RTA: urinary loss of bicarb
    - serum pH acidic
- Very common in middle-aged, and treatment make a difference

MM: Treatment

Incurable but treatable

- Steroids, chemo
  - *It's a cancer, so this is to be expected*
- **bortezomib** (proteasome inhibitor), **thalidomide** (teratogenic)
  - *These are the ones to know.*
- Bone specific
  - Bisphosphonates
  - Radiation therapy to reduce bone pain

MM: Associated symptoms

- **CRAB**
  - hyper**C**alcemia, **R**enal insufficiency, **A**nemia, **B**ack pain/**B**one lytic lesions
- Ie.
  - cytokine release (eg. IL-6) leads to lytic bone lesions in back → hypercalcemia
  - paraprotein buildup in brush border of PCT (ie. amyloidosis) → RTA-2 (ie. proximal RTA)
    - which interferes w/ charge barrier → nephrotic
      - Bence Jones proteins in urine
  - arises from bone marrow, disease of plasma cells → bone pain and anemia
    - plasma cells w/ "fried-egg" appearance and "clock-face chromatin"

Multiple Myeloma:
Versus Other Conditions

- MM is confused w/ MGUS and Waldenstrom's
  - MGUS = Monoclonal Gammopathy of Undetermined Significance
    - plasma cell expansion without the MM symptoms
      - no CRAB (hyperCa, Renal, Anemia, Bone/Back lesions)
    - 1% develop into MM every year
  - Waldenstrom's Macroglobinemia
    - the M-spike is Ig<u>M</u>
      - (the M-spike in MM is Ig<u>G</u> and/or Ig<u>A</u>)
    - Symptoms: nothing really stands out.
      - Fatigue/weakness, wt loss, blood oozing from nose/mouth
      - Vision changes, stroke/coma

MM: In The Real World

- Realistically, when you see a middle-aged or elderly person with kidney problems (eg. HTN, urinary changes), you're going to get a UA and CBC.
  - If the UA shows hyperCalcemia, your going to get an CXR.
    - If the CXR shows punched-out lesions in the spine, you're pretty sure you've got MM.
    - If the patient is also anemic, this is further evidence.
    - Time to do **protein ELP** and look for an M-spike of IgG and IgA.
- If you get an elderly patient with bone/back pain, you're going to get a CXR.
  - If the CXR shows punched-out lesions, you're going to suspect MM.
  - You'll then do a full workup: CBC, BMP, and UA before you order a **SPE**.

MM: In The Real World

- If you get an elderly patient with bone/back pain, you should inquire into kidney issues like HTN or changes in urination just by habit (LIQOR PAM HUGS FOSS).
  - If you get a yes to either, you'll automatically do a CXR, CBC, BMP, and UA.
    - Once you receive the results, you'll order the **SPEP**.
- If you get a middle-aged woman who has significant, lasting back pain after a minor fall, you better be in the habit of taking a good HPI (LIQOR PAM HUGS FOSS).
  - What's her past medical history? Maybe she'll tell you about her chronic anemia.
  - What meds is she on? Maybe you'll note her antihypertensives even though she never told you about having high blood pressure.
  - Urinary changes?
  - These questions will control whether you just do the CXR, see what looks like a compression fracture, and then start freaking out about why a middle-aged woman would have osteoporosis and then order a CBC, BMP, and UA.
    - When you get the results, you'll order an **IFE**.

Why Does Everything Have a Thousand Names!!!!

- Protein ELP (Protein electrophoresis) =
- SPE (serum protein electrophoresis) =
- SPEP (serum protein electrophoresis) =
- IFE (Immunofixation Electrophoresis)

PCT Pathology: ATN & RTA-2

- ATN = Acute Tubular Necrosis induced by
  - drugs: gentamicin, contrast
  - myoglobin (from rhabdomyolysis)
  - sepsis/shock
  - *also occurs along the remainder of the tubules*
- RTA-2 = Proximal RTA (Often caused by **Fanconi syndrome**)
  - Defect in bicarb reabsorption
  - **Hypo-K,-PO4**
  - May be caused by **GSD-1** or **MM**
  - Tx: **thiazides**, NOT bicarb

PCT Pathology: GSD-1 (von Gierke's)

- Deficiency of **glucose-6-phosphatase** (G6Pase)
  - Gluconeogenesis: amino acids + LA → G6P →via G6Pase → glucose + PO4
    - no G6Pase → build up of G6P inhibiting TG breakdown → no glucose
- Symptoms
  - **Hypoglycemia**
    - Glucose around **50 mg/dL** or less
    - Confused. Palpations, sweaty, cold/clammy, dilated pupils
  - **Lactic Acidosis (LA)**
    - Liver and muscle generate LA
    - Indirectly leads to **Hypertriglyceridemia**
  - **Hyperuricemia**
    - G6P →via pentose phosphate pathway→ uric acid
      - byproduct of purine degradation
    - LA and uric acid compete w/ each other for excretion in the kidneys
      - Eventually leads to renal and joint damage
  - Hepatomegaly
- Tx: **cornstarch**

PCT Pathology: MM

- **M**-protein spike. **M**ade of IgG or IgA.
- Plasma cell: "fried-egg" & "clock-face chromatin"
- Symptoms: **CRAB**
    - hyper**C**alcemia, **R**enal insufficiency, **A**nemia, **B**ack pain/ **B**one lytic lesions
        - RTA-2 + <u>Bence Jones</u> proteins in urine
- Tx
    - Steroids, chemo
    - **bortezomib, thalidomide**
    - Bone: Bisphosphonates + radiation reduce bone pain

Glomerulus and Brush Border 6

Lets review the PCT.

I got a little extra, too.

Pertinent Kidney Stats

- **Renal Blood Flow (RBF)** estimate by **PAH**
  - PAH is freely filtered, not reabsorbed, but is excreted.
- **GFR** estimated by **creatinine**
  - creatinine is freely filtered and not excreted
- **FF** = filtration fraction: normally 20%

Drugs Affecting
Glomerulus/Arterioles

- **ANP** = <u>Atrial</u> Natriuretic Peptide
  - hormone released by heart
  - greater Na+ filtration at glomerulus
  - inc GFR

- Prostaglandins dilate the afferent arterioles
  - inc RBF and GFR
  - **NSAIDS** block prostaglandin synthesis. Results in prerenal-ARF if too effective.

- **ACE-Inhibitors:** less vascular constriction and more vasodilation; less blood volume
  - dec BP (and inc serum pH)
  - **Captopril, Lisinopril, Enalapril**
    - -april & -opril
  - 1ˢᵗ Line for <u>HTN</u> and <u>CHF</u>
  - If pt devlops a **cough**, move them to **ARBs**
  - Contraindications: bilateral renal artery stenosis → prerenal ARF

Drugs/Hormones
Affecting Brush Border

- **PTH** = parathyroid hormone
  - **In PCT: dec phosphorous reabsorption & activate Vit D (1,25)**
  - In DCT: inc Ca reabsorption
  - Inc calcium and phosphorous absorption in gut

- **Acetazolamide**
  - Carbonic anhydrase inhibitor
  - Used w/ **methotrexate** to reduce kidney damage
  - **Decreases bicarb resorption in proximal convoluted tubules**
    - alkalinization of urine → increased methotrexate excretion due to higher solubility within the urine
    - ie. ion-trapping

Drugs/Hormones Affecting Brush Border

- **Mannitol**
  - Used to maintain kidney function with
    - shock
    - drug overdose
    - on cardiopulmonary bypass
  - **<u>Prevents swelling of endothelial cells</u> in the PCT and increases fluid osmolarity**
    - **increased urine flow**
  - Most testable use:
    - Treatment for **intracranial/intraocular pressure**
    1. <u>Prevents swelling of the endothelial cells</u> of the blood brain barrier
       - stretches the tight junctions of the BBB
    2. <u>Artery becomes more hyperosmotic</u>
    3. Water leaks through the tight junctions and enters the artery

Brush Border Concentration Patterns

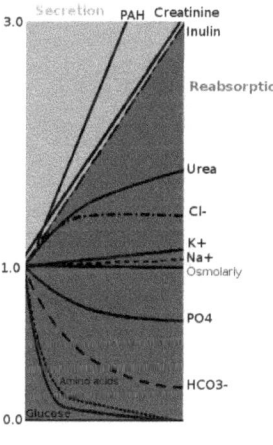

- **Brush Border** = striated border
  - Densely packed microvilli packed w/ mitochondria
- Resorbed:
  - 100% of organic solutes (amino acids and glucose)
  - Salt and water (Na+, Cl-, H2O); CO2;
  - Most potassium, urea, phosphate, citrate
- Secreted
  - Medications
  - Ammonium
  - Glutamine → glutamate → α-ketoglutarate →bicarb

- Glucose and amino acids are immediately resorbed
  Don't waste your energy or your building blocks
- PAH: freely filtered + excreted
- Creatine & inulin conc changes as water is absorbed
- Cl- resorbed slowly in first 1/3, then equals Na+ last 2/3
- Na+ drives water resorption, so it matches Osmolarity
  - 80% of Na+ reabsorbed in PCT (the most in kidney)

Important PCT Diseases

- **Renal Cell Carcinoma**
- ATN = Acute Tubular Necrosis induced by
  - drugs: **gentamicin, contrast**
  - myoglobin (from **rhabdomyolysis**)
  - sepsis/shock
  - *also occurs along the remainder of the tubules*
- **Proximal** Renal Tubular Acidosis = RTA-Type 2
  - Defect in bicarb reabsorption → serum acidosis

RTA-2 Familial Cause
GSD-1 (von Gierke's)

- Deficiency of **glucose-6-phosphatase** (G6Pase)
- Biochemistry
  - Fasting → catabolism of muscle and **TG** from adipose tissue → amino acids (mostly alanine), FFA, **LA**
    - FFA → ketones and acetyl-CoA
  - Gluconeogenesis:
    - amino acids + LA → G6P →via G6Pase → glucose + PO4
    - final step is same in gluconeogenesis and glycogenolysis
    - **no G6Pase → build up of G6P inhibiting TG breakdown → no glucose**
- Symptoms
  - **Hypoglycemia, Lactic Acidosis**
  - Hypertriglyceridemia, Hyperuricemia
  - **Hepatomegaly**
- Tx: **cornstarch**

RTA-2 Familial Cause:
GSD-1 Symptom Summary

- **Hypoglycemia**
  - Shakiness w/ altered mood and thinking
  - Glucose around **50 mg/dL** or less
  - Symptoms
    - Principally due to dec glucose to brain
    - Adrenergic: palpations/tachycardia, sweating, cold/clammy, dilated pupils
- **Lactic Acidosis (LA)**
  - Liver and muscle generate LA
    - LA oxidized by NAD+ to pyruvic acid → via gluconeogenesis→ G6P
    - Accumulated G6P inhibits lactate to pyruvate conversion
  - Indirectly leads to **Hypertriglyceridemia**
- **Hyperuricemia**
  - G6P →via pentose phosphate pathway→ uric acid
    - byproduct of purine degradation
  - LA and uric acid compete w/ each other for excretion in the kidneys
    - Eventually leads to renal and joint damage
  - Tx: allopurinol prevents nephropathy and gout

RTA-2 Acquired Cause
Multiple Myeloma

- **M**-protein spike. **M**ade of IgG or IgA.
- Plasma cell: "fried-egg" & "clock-face chromatin"
- Symptoms: **CRAB**
  - hyper**C**alcemia, **R**enal insufficiency, **A**nemia, **B**ack pain/ **B**one lytic lesions
    - RTA-2 + Bence Jones proteins in urine
- Tx
  - Steroids, chemo
  - **bortezomib, thalidomide**
  - Bone: Bisphosphonates + radiation reduce bone pain

PCT Drugs/Hormones: Summary

- **PTH** = parathyroid hormone
  - **In PCT: dec P04 & activates Vit D (1,25).** In DCT: inc Ca reabsorption
    - (Inc Ca & PO4 absorption in gut)
- **Acetazolamide** (Carbonic anhydrase inhibitor)
  - **Inc HCO3 in urine**
    - alkalinization → ion-trapping of methotrexate
- **Mannitol**
  - **Prevents swelling of endothelial cells in PCT & inc fluid osmolarity**
    - **Inc urine flow**
    - Maintain kidney function with shock, drug OD, on cardiopulmonary bypass
  - **Tx intracranial/intraocular pressure**
    1. Prevents swelling of the endothelial cells of BBB → leaky tight junctions
    2. Artery becomes more hyperosmotic
    3. Water leaks through the tight junctions and enters the artery

DCT, NDI, and Thiazides 1

Warren G's DCT needs to regulate

DCT = Distal Convoluted Tubule

- Between the loop of Henle and the collecting ducts in the cortex of the kidney
- Regulates Na+, Ca+, K+ and pH
  - **Na+**/Cl- co-transport
    - indirectly controls **K+**
  - Ca2+ channel & Ca/Na exchanger
    - **PTH** stimulates Ca2+ reabsorption in the DCT
  - **pH**
    - reabsorbs bicarb and excretes H+ OR can do reverse
- **Macula densa**

DCT: Macula Densa

- **Macula densa** is the point where the **DCT** contacts the afferent arterioles
- When the macula densa senses low NaCl
  - *Low NaCl = low renal volume, hence low BP*
  - Macula densa dilates the afferent arterioles
    - inc RBF, GFR
  - Stimulates renin release from the juxtaglomerular cells of the afferent and efferent arterioles
    - leads to increase in blood volume and pressure

Juxtaglomerular Apparatus

1. **Macula densa**
   - Cells in the DCT that signal juxtaglomerular cells to release renin when NaCl levels are low in DCT
     - indicates low renal pressure, hence low BP
     - renin is essential component of RAAS
       - **RAAS = renin-angiotensin-aldosterone system:** blood pressure and volume regulation
2. **Juxtaglomerular cells**
   - Cells of the afferent & efferent arterioles that store and release renin. Afferent >> efferent
   - Have β **1 adrenergic receptors**
     - respond to epinephrine or NE → renin release
     - this is why β 1-blockers help with BP
3. **Extraglomerular mesangial cells**
   - Cells outside the glomerulus that produce **erythropoietin (EPO)**
   - EPO: hormone that controls erythropoiesis, ie. RBC production

DCT: Arginine Vasopressin Receptor 2 ie. V2 Receptors

- **AVPR2 = <u>V2</u> Receptors**
  - Found in the DCT & collecting ducts
  - Water reabsorption
    - signal the displacement of **aquaporins** into the membrane to reabsorb water
  - LOF → **Nephrogenic Diabetes Insipidus** (NDI)
    - LOF = loss of function

Distal Convoluted Tubule: Summary

- Regulates Na+, Ca+, (indirectly) K+ and pH
  - **PTH** stimulates Ca2+ reabsorption in the DCT

- **Macula densa** are cells in the **DCT**

- Juxtaglomerular Apparatus
  1. **Macula densa** of the DCT
     - signal juxtaglomerular cells to release renin when NaCl levels
  2. **Juxtaglomerular cells** of the afferent & efferent arterioles store and release renin.
     - Have β 1 adrenergic receptors (respond to Epi, NE, β 1-blockers)
  3. **Extraglomerular mesangial cells** produce **erythropoietin**

DCT: Summary – AVPR2 = **V2**

- V2 = Arginine Vasopressin Receptor 2 (**AVPR2**)
  - Found in the **DCT** & collecting ducts
  - Water reabsorption
    - LOF → **Nephrogenic Diabetes Insipidus** (NDI)

DCT, NDI, and Thiazides 2

Can't keep fluids in, can't get rid of
them fast enough

Distal Convoluted Tubule: Review

- Regulates Na+, Ca+, (indirectly) K+ and pH
    - **PTH** stimulates Ca2+ reabsorption in the DCT

- **Macula densa** are cells in the **DCT**

- Juxtaglomerular Apparatus
    1. **Macula densa** of the DCT
        - signal juxtaglomerular cells to release renin when NaCl levels
    2. **Juxtaglomerular cells** of the afferent & efferent arterioles store and release renin
        - Have β 1 adrenergic receptors (respond to Epi, NE, β 1-blockers)
    3. **Extraglomerular mesangial cells** produce **erythropoietin**

DCT: Review – AVPR2 = V2

- V2 = Arginine Vasopressin Receptor 2 (**AVPR2**)
  - Found in the **DCT** & collecting ducts
  - Water reabsorption
    - LOF → **Nephrogenic Diabetes Insipidus** (NDI)

Nephrogenic Diabetes Insipidus

- Diabetes = excessive discharge of urine. Insipidus = without taste. ie. The urine doesn't taste sweet (hyperglycemic)
- Polydipsia, polyuria + inability to concentrate urine due to lack of response to ADH
- Cause:
  - Hereditary or Secondary to
    - hypercalcemia, lithium, demeclocyline (an ADH antagonist)
- Tests
  - Urine specific gravity < 1.006
  - Serum osmolality > 290 mOsm/L
- Tx
  - hydrochloro**thiazide**, indomethacin
    - causes mild hypovolemia → inc salt water uptake in PCT
  - amiloride
    - also blocks Li uptake

DCT: Thiazides

- Mechanism
  - Inhibit NaCl reabsorption in DCT
  - Inhibit Ca2+ excretion
- Treats
  - HTN, CHF
  - Idiopathic hypercalciuria
  - Nephrogenic Diabetes Insipidus
    - causes mild hypovolemia → inc Na/H2O uptake in PCT
      - could've also use indomethicin

DCT: Thiazides, Side Effect

- SE:
  - hyponatremia
  - hypokalemic metabolic acidosis
    - dec Na+ uptake leads to charge issue and K+ drainage
    - RAAS activation due to dec Na+ → inc aldosterone
      - aldosterone stimulates Na/K exchanger → loss of K+
    - inc flow rate in nephron → loss of K+
  - hyper**GLUC**
    - hyper: -**G**lycemia, -**L**ipidemia, -**U**ricemia, -**C**alcemia

DCT: Thiazides, Contraindications

- Contraindications
  - Inc risk of DM2, ie. may worsen diabetes
    - due to hyperglycemia SE
  - Gout
    - due to hyperuricemia SE
  - Lithium therapy (Li/Na/water balance)
    - due to hyponatremia
  - Sulfa allergy
  - Breast feeding

Distal Convoluted Tubule: Summary

- Regulates Na+, Ca+, (indirectly) K+ and pH
  - **PTH** stimulates Ca2+ reabsorption in the DCT

- **Macula densa** are cells in the **DCT**

- Juxtaglomerular Apparatus
  1. **Macula densa** of the DCT
     - signal juxtaglomerular cells to release renin when NaCl levels
  2. **Juxtaglomerular cells** of the afferent & efferent arterioles store and release renin.
     - Have β **1 adrenergic receptors** (respond to Epi, NE, β 1-blockers)
  3. **Extraglomerular mesangial cells** produce **erythropoietin**

DCT: Summary – AVPR2 (ie. V2) & NDI

- V2 = Arginine Vasopressin Receptor 2 (**AVPR2**)
  - Found in the **DCT** & collecting ducts
    Water reabsorption
    - LOF → **Nephrogenic Diabetes Insipidus** (NDI)

- **Nephrogenic Diabetes Insipidus**
  - Polydipsia, polyuria and lack of response to ADH
  - Causes
    - Hereditary or Secondary to hyperCa, Li, or demeclocyline
  - Ur SG < 1.006; Serum osmolality > 290 mOsm/L
  - Tx
    - hydrochloro**thiazide**
    - indomethacin, or amiloride

DCT: Summary Thiazides

- Inhibit NaCl reabsorption
- Inhibit Ca2+ excretion
- Treats
  - HTN, CHF
  - Idiopathic hypercalciuria
  - Nephrogenic Diabetes Insipidus
    - causes mild hypovolemia → inc Na/H2O uptake in PCT
- SE:
  - hypokalemic metabolic acidosis
  - hyponatremia
    - not w/ lithium therapy
  - hyper**GLUC**
    - hyper: -**G**lycemia, -**L**ipidemia, -**U**ricemia, -**C**alcemia
    - not w/ DM2, hyperlipidemia, gout
  - A sulfa drug that is transmitted in breast milk

Aldosterone, RTA-2, and Sjögren's 1

From cell to acidity

CT = Collecting Tubules

- From the distal convoluted tubules to the renal pyramids
- Begins in **cortex**, continues through the **medulla**, merges to form **papillary ducts** near the apex of each renal **pyramid** before releasing filtrate (urine) into a **minor-calyx**
  - 2-3 minor calyces join to form a **major-calyx** before passing urine into the renal **pelvis**
  - "Staghorn calculi" may extend into the renal calyces

CT: Two Special Cell Types

- **Principal cells**
  - Na+/K+ balance and water reabsorption
    - Na+/K+ balance regulated by **aldosterone**
    - Water resorption regulated by **ADH** (ie. **vasopressin**)
      - via **aquaporins**
- **Intercalated cells**
  - Regulate acid-base homeostasis
  - **Alpha cells**: excrete acid (H+), reabsorb bicarb
  - **Beta cells**: excrete bicarb, reabsorb acid (H+)
  - Damage to alpha cells = **Distal Renal Tubular Acidosis**
    - ie. **RTA-1** or **classical RTA**

Distal Renal Tubular Acidosis

- This was the first RTA described so you can guess how important this one is.
  - aka. **RTA-1** or **Classical RTA** or dRTA
- Alpha intercalated cells can't excrete H+
  - Can't get urine pH below **5.3** → serum **acidemia**
  - Also, can't resorb K+ → **hypokalemia**

RTA-1: Symptoms

- Calcium deposits at higher pH
  - **Bilateral** kidney stones (not w/ any other type of RTA)
  - **Nephrocalcinosis** and other stones
  - **Hypocalcemia**
    - Leads to bone demineralization: **rickets** (kids), **osteomalacia**
- **Normal anion gap metabolic acidosis**
  - only caused by diarrhea (most), RTA-1, RTA-4 (mild)
- **Hypokalemia**, hyperchloremia
- Sjögren's syndrome

CT Summary: The Cells

- **Principal cells**
  - Na+/K+ balance and water reabsorption
    - Regulated by **Aldosterone** and **ADH** (ie. **vasopressin**)
- **Intercalated cells**
  - Regulate acid-base homeostasis
  - **Alpha cells**: excrete <u>a</u>cid (H+), reabsorb bicarb
    - Damage to <u>alpha</u> cells → **distal RTA = RTA-1**
  - **Beta cells**: excrete <u>b</u>icarb, reabsorb acid (H+)

CT Summary
Distal Renal Tubule Acidosis = RTA-1

- Urine pH > **5.3**
  - Calcium deposits at higher pH
    - **Bilateral** kidney stones (not w/ any other type of RTA)
    - **Nephrocalcinosis** and other stones
    - **Hypocalcemia**
      - Leads to bone demineralization: **rickets** (kids), **osteomalacia**
- **Hypokalemia**
- **Normal anion gap metabolic acidosis**
  - only caused by diarrhea (most), RTA-1, RTA-4 (mild)
- Sjögren's syndrome

Aldosterone, RTA-2, and Sjögren's 2

Drying Up

CT Review: The Cells

- **Principal cells**
  - Na+/K+ balance and water reabsorption
    - Regulated by **Aldosterone** and **ADH** (ie. **vasopressin**)
- **Intercalated cells**
  - Regulate acid-base homeostasis
  - <u>A</u>**lpha cells**: excrete <u>a</u>cid (H+), reabsorb bicarb
    - Damage to <u>alpha</u> cells → **distal RTA = RTA-1**
  - <u>B</u>**eta cells**: excrete <u>b</u>icarb, reabsorb acid (H+)

CT Review:
Distal Renal Tubule Acidosis = RTA-1

- Urine pH > **5.3**
  - Calcium deposits at higher pH
    - **Bilateral** kidney stones (not w/ any other type of RTA)
    - **Nephrocalcinosis** and other stones
    - **Hypocalcemia**
      - Leads to bone demineralization: **rickets** (kids), **osteomalacia**
- **Hypokalemia**
- **Normal anion gap metabolic acidosis**
  - only caused by diarrhea (most), RTA-1, RTA-4 (mild)
- Sjögren's syndrome

SS = Sjögren's Syndrome

Just saying "Sjögren's" leaves one w/ dry mouth and dry eyes.

- WBCs destroy exocrine glands, eg. **salivary and lacrimal glands**
  - ie. xerostomia & keratoconjunctivitis **sicca**
  - **Sicca syndrome** = dry eyes, nose, mouth, and vagina w/ reflux esophagitis, chronic bronchitis; but **NO** arthritis
- Everything can be dry, and invasion of parotid glands can give swollen cheeks (**chipmunk cheeks**)
  - Dry: skin, nose, vagina, kidneys, vessels, lungs, liver, biliary, pancreas, nerves, brain
- This is a autoimmune disease, and like all other rheumatic diseases, they have a tendency to come in groups.
  - Sjögren's occurs w/ **rheumatoid arthritis** frequently.
  - Sjögren's triad: **xerophthalmia, xerostomia, arthritis**

SS: Autoimmune Disease (ie. Rheumatic)

- **ANA** = Anti-Nuclear Antibody
  - Signifies Abs against own cell nuclei
  - Different cell types have different nuclei, and each particular ANA is named as such
    - ie. anti-Ro, anti-La, anti-Sm, anti-nRNP, anti-Scl70, anti-dsDNA, anti-histone, anti-centromere
  - A critical point w/ ANA is when you have more than **1 in 320 cells** is an ANA cell
    - Lots of destruction going on. Maybe one type of ANA is out of control or many different types.
- SS specific ANA: **anti-Ro/SSA & anti-La/SSB**

- Tests for SS Confirmation (Need one of #1 + one of #2)

  #1: xerophthalmia or prove xerostomia

  #2: prove the level of autoimmune dz state
  1. **Schemer test** (paper in eye to soak up tears for 5 min)
  - **or Saxon test** or **sialometry** (test for salivary hypofunction)
  2. anti-Ro/SSA and/or anti-La/SSB
  - **or** a well-established rheumatic disease: eg. RA, SLE, systemic sclerosis
  - **or** anti-centromere Abs (found with scleroderma)
  - **or** ANA > 1:320 + positive RF

CT Summary: Sjögren's Syndrome

Just saying "Sjögren's" leaves one w/ dry mouth and dry eyes.

- WBCs destroy exocrine glands, eg. **salivary and lacrimal glands**
  - Invasion of the parotid glands by lymphocytes can give **chipmunk cheeks.**
  - Everything in the body can be dry:
    - skin, nose, vagina, kidneys, vessels, lungs, liver, biliary, pancreas, nerves, brain
- Autoimmune diseases generally come in groups. **SS** occurs w/ **RA** frequently.
  - **Sjögren's triad: xerophthalmia, xerostomia, arthritis**

- Tests for SS Confirmation (Need one of #1 + one of #2)

  #1: xerophthalmia or prove xerostomia

  #2: prove the level of autoimmune dz state
  1. **Schemer test** (paper in eye to soak up tears for 5 min)
  - **or Saxon test** or **sialometry** (test for salivary hypofunction)
  2. anti-Ro/SSA and/or anti-La/SSB
  - **or** a well-established rheumatic disease: eg. RA, SLE, systemic sclerosis
  - **or** anti-centromere Abs (found with scleroderma)
  - **or** ANA > 1:320 + positive RF

Aldosterone

- Synthesized in zona glomerulus (outer **adrenal cortex**)
  - Stimulated by
    - angiotensin II & III (a metabolite of II)
    - ACTH (minor role)
    - **hyperkalemia, plasma acidosis** (generally go hand and hand)
    - stretch receptors in the atria
- Reabsorbs Na+ and water while excreting K+ and H+
- Mechanism:
  - binds to aldosterone-receptor in **CT** and DCT
    - activates Na+/K+ pumps and K+ excretion
    - upregulates **ENaCs** (epithelial sodium channels)
  - stimulates Na+ and water absorption from gut, salivary & sweat glands (in exchange for K+)
- Aldosterone deficiency can cause **RTA-4**

RTA-4 = Hyperkalemic RTA

- Not actually a tubular disorder
  - Can be due to aldosterone deficiency or resistance
- Causes
  - **Aldosterone Inhibitors:**
    - **SEAT**: Spironolactone, Eplerenone, Amiloride, Trimethoprim
  - NSAIDs, ACE-I/ARBs
- Symptoms
  - Decrease in PCT ammonium excretion (2° to hypoaldosteronism)
    - Urine buffer capacity dec → **hyperkalemia**
      - other RTA's have hypokalemia, hence other name: Tubular Hyperkalemia
    - Mild normal anion gap metabolic acidosis

CT Summary:
Aldosterone & Hyperkalemic RTA-4

- Synthesized in **adrenal cortex**
  - Stimulated by
    - angiotensin II & III (a metabolite of II), stretch receptors in atria
    - **hyperkalemia, plasma acidosis** (generally go hand and hand)
- Reabsorbs Na+ and water while excreting K+ and H+
  - binds to aldosterone-receptor in **CT** and DCT
    - activates Na+/K+ pumps & upregulates **ENaCs** = epithelial sodium channels
  - stimulates Na+ & water absorption from GI (in exchange for K+)
- Aldosterone deficiency can cause **RTA-4 = Hyperkalemic RTA**

- **RTA-4 = Hyperkalemic RTA**
  - Causes
    - **Aldosterone Inhibitors:**
      - **SEAT**: Spironolactone, Eplerenone, Amiloride, Trimethoprim
    - NSAIDs, ACE-I/ARBs
  - Symptoms (2° to hypoaldosteronism)
    - Dec PCT NH4 excretion → Urine buffer capacity dec → **hyperkalemia**
    - Mild normal anion gap metabolic acidosis

CT Summary: Sjögren's Syndrome

Just saying "Sjögren's" leaves one w/ dry mouth and dry eyes.

- WBCs destroy exocrine glands, eg. **salivary and lacrimal glands**
  - Invasion of the parotid glands by lymphocytes can give **chipmunk cheeks.**
  - Everything in the body can be dry:
    - skin, nose, vagina, kidneys, vessels, lungs, liver, biliary, pancreas, nerves, brain
- Autoimmune diseases generally come in groups. **SS** occurs w/ **RA** frequently.
  - **Sjögren's triad: xerophthalmia, xerostomia, arthritis**

- Tests for SS Confirmation (Need one of #1 + one of #2)
  #1: xerophthalmia or prove xerostomia
  #2: prove the level of autoimmune dz state
  1. **Schemer test** (paper in eye to soak up tears for 5 min)
  - **or Saxon test** or **sialometry** (test for salivary hypofunction)
  2. **anti-Ro/SSA and/or anti-La/SSB**
  - **or** a well-established rheumatic disease: eg. RA, SLE, systemic sclerosis
  - **or** anti-centromere Abs (found with scleroderma)
  - **or** ANA > 1:320 + positive RF

CT Summary:
Aldosterone & Hyperkalemic RTA-4

- Synthesized in **adrenal cortex**
  - Stimulated by
    - angiotensin II & III (a metabolite of II), stretch receptors in atria
    - **hyperkalemia, plasma acidosis** (generally go hand and hand)
- Reabsorbs Na+ and water while excreting K+ and H+
  - binds to aldosterone-receptor in **CT** and DCT
    - activates Na+/K+ pumps & upregulates **ENaCs** = epithelial sodium channels
  - stimulates Na+ & water absorption from GI (in exchange for K+)
- Aldosterone deficiency can cause **RTA-4 = Hyperkalemic RTA**

- **RTA-4 = Hyperkalemic RTA**
  - Causes
    - **Aldosterone Inhibitors:**
      - **SEAT**: Spironolactone, Eplerenone, Amiloride, Trimethoprim
    - NSAIDs, ACE-1/ARBs
  - Symptoms (2° to hypoaldosteronism)
    - Dec PCT NH4 excretion → Urine buffer capacity dec → **hyperkalemia**
    - Mild normal anion gap metabolic acidosis

Aldosterone, RTA-2, and Sjögren's 3

Potassium Sparing & ADH

CT Review: Sjögren's Syndrome

Just saying "Sjögren's" leaves one w/ <u>dry mouth and dry eyes.</u>

- WBCs destroy exocrine glands, eg. **salivary and lacrimal glands**
  - Invasion of the parotid glands by lymphocytes can give **chipmunk cheeks.**
  - Everything in the body can be dry:
    - skin, nose, vagina, kidneys, vessels, lungs, liver, biliary, pancreas, nerves, brain
- Autoimmune diseases generally come in groups. **SS** occurs w/ **RA** frequently.
  - **Sjögren's triad: xerophthalmia, xerostomia, arthritis**

- Tests for SS Confirmation (Need one of #1 + one of #2)
  #1: xerophthalmia or prove xerostomia
  #2: prove the level of autoimmune dz state
  1.   **Schemer test** (paper in eye to soak up tears for 5 min)
  -   **or Saxon test** or **sialometry** (test for salivary hypofunction)
  2.   **anti-Ro/SSA and/or anti-La/SSB**
  -   **or** a well-established rheumatic disease: eg. RA, SLE, systemic sclerosis
  -   **or** anti-centromere Abs (found with scleroderma)
  -   **or** ANA > 1:320 + positive RF

CT Review:
Aldosterone & Hyperkalemic RTA-4

- Synthesized in **adrenal cortex**
  - Stimulated by
    - angiotensin II & III (a metabolite of II), stretch receptors in atria
    - **hyperkalemia, plasma acidosis** (generally go hand and hand)
- Reabsorbs Na+ and water while excreting K+ and H+
  - binds to aldosterone-receptor in **CT** and DCT
    - activates Na+/K+ pumps & upregulates **ENaCs** = epithelial sodium channels
  - stimulates Na+ & water absorption from GI (in exchange for K+)
- Aldosterone deficiency can cause **RTA-4 = Hyperkalemic RTA**

- **RTA-4 = Hyperkalemic RTA**
  - Causes
    - **Aldosterone Inhibitors:**
      - **SEAT**: Spironolactone, Eplerenone, Amiloride, Trimethoprim
    - NSAIDs, ACE-I/ARBs
  - Symptoms (2° to hypoaldosteronism)
    - Dec PCT NH4 excretion → Urine buffer capacity dec → **hyperkalemia**
    - Mild normal anion gap metabolic acidosis

K+ Sparing Diuretics

- **Potassium Sparing Diuretics: SEAT**
  - **Spironolactone**, **Eplerenone**, **Amiloride**, Triamterene
    - Competitive inhibitor of **aldosterone** in cortical collecting duct
- Uses:
  - Hyperaldosteronism, Hypokalemia, CHF
- SE:
  - can lead to **hyperkalemia** (arrhythmias)
  - Effects endocrine system:
    - **Spironolactone** causes **gynecomastia** and **antiandrogen effects**
      - *Your boobs grow, but your sex organs appear questionable*

ADH = Antidiuretic Hormone
ie. Vasopressin

- Reabsorbs water and constrict blood vessels
- Synthesized in **hypothalamus** and stored in **posterior pituitary**
  - Most is released into bloodstream to effect blood vessels and renal convoluted tubule
  - Some released into brain
    - Plays role in social behavior, sexual motivation, pair bonding, and maternal responses to stress
- **ADH** binds to **V2** receptor in **CT** (and DCT)
  - V2 = AVPR2 = Arginine Vasopressin Receptor 2
  - Signal for displacement of **aquaporins** into the luminal basement membrane allowing for **reabsorption of water**

The other actions and mechanisms of ADH don't often come up.

CT Summary:
K+ Sparing Diuretics & ADH

- **Potassium-Sparing Diuretics** = Aldosterone Inhibitors: **SEAT**
  - **S**pironolactone, **E**plerenone, **A**miloride, **T**riamterene
  - Uses:
    - Hyperaldosteronism, **Hypokalemia**, CHF
  - SE:
    - can lead to **hyperkalemia** (arrhythmias)
    - **Spironolactone: gynecomastia & antiandrogen effects**

- Antidiuretic Hormone = **ADH** = Vasopressin
  - Reabsorbs water and constrict blood vessels
  - Synthesized in **hypothalamus** and stored in **posterior pituitary**
    - Most is released into bloodstream to effect vessels and kidney
    - Some released into brain
      - Plays role in social motivation, sexual motivation, pair bonding, and maternal responses to stress
  - **ADH** binds to **V2 receptor** in **CT** (and DCT)
    - **Aquaporins** displace into the luminal basement membrane
      - allowing for **reabsorption of water**

CT Summary: The Cells

- **Principal cells**
  - Na+/K+ balance and water reabsorption
    - Regulated by **Aldosterone** and **ADH** (ie. **vasopressin**)
- **Intercalated cells**
  - Regulate acid-base homeostasis
  - <u>A</u>**lpha cells**: excrete <u>a</u>cid (H+), reabsorb bicarb
    - Damage to <u>alpha</u> cells → **distal RTA = RTA-1**
  - <u>B</u>**eta cells**: excrete <u>b</u>icarb, reabsorb acid (H+)

CT Summary
Distal Renal Tubule Acidosis = RTA-1

- Urine pH > **5.3**
  - Calcium deposits at higher pH
    - **Bilateral** kidney stones (not w/ any other type of RTA)
    - **Nephrocalcinosis** and other stones
    - **Hypocalcemia**
      - Leads to bone demineralization: **rickets** (kids), **osteomalacia**
- **Hypokalemia**
- **Normal anion gap metabolic acidosis**
  - only caused by diarrhea (most), RTA-1, RTA-4 (mild)
- Sjögren's syndrome

CT Summary: Sjögren's Syndrome

Just saying "Sjögren's" leaves one w/ dry mouth and dry eyes.

- WBCs destroy exocrine glands, eg. **salivary and lacrimal glands**
  - Invasion of the parotid glands by lymphocytes can give **chipmunk cheeks.**
  - Everything in the body can be dry:
    - skin, nose, vagina, kidneys, vessels, lungs, liver, biliary, pancreas, nerves, brain
- Autoimmune diseases generally come in groups. **SS** occurs w/ **RA** frequently.
  - **Sjögren's triad: xerophthalmia, xerostomia, arthritis**

- Tests for SS Confirmation (Need one of #1 + one of #2)
  #1: xerophthalmia or prove xerostomia
  #2: prove the level of autoimmune dz state
  1. **Schemer test** (paper in eye to soak up tears for 5 min)
  - **or Saxon test** or **sialometry** (test for salivary hypofunction)
  2. **anti-Ro/SSA and/or anti-La/SSB**
  - **or** a well-established rheumatic disease: eg. RA, SLE, systemic sclerosis
  - **or** anti-centromere Abs (found with scleroderma)
  - **or** ANA > 1:320 + positive RF

CT Summary: Aldosterone & Hyperkalemic RTA-4

- Synthesized in **adrenal cortex**
  - Stimulated by
    - angiotensin II & III (a metabolite of II), stretch receptors in atria
    - **hyperkalemia, plasma acidosis** (generally go hand and hand)
- Reabsorbs Na+ and water while excreting K+ and H+
  - binds to aldosterone-receptor in **CT** and DCT
    - activates Na+/K+ pumps & upregulates **ENaCs** = epithelial sodium channels
  - stimulates Na+ & water absorption from GI (in exchange for K+)
- Aldosterone deficiency can cause **RTA-4 = Hyperkalemic RTA**

- **RTA-4 = Hyperkalemic RTA**
  - Causes
    - **Aldosterone Inhibitors:**
      - <u>**SEAT**</u>: Spironolactone, Eplerenone, Amiloride, Trimethoprim
    - NSAIDs, ACE-1/ARBs
  - Symptoms (2° to hypoaldosteronism)
    - Dec PCT NH4 excretion → Urine buffer capacity dec → **hyperkalemia**
    - Mild normal anion gap metabolic acidosis

CT Summary:
K+ Sparing Diuretics & ADH

- **Potassium-Sparing Diuretics** = Aldosterone Inhibitors: **SEAT**
  - **S**pironolactone, **E**plerenone, **A**miloride, **T**riamterene
  - Uses:
    - Hyperaldosteronism, **Hypokalemia**, CHF
  - SE:
    - can lead to **hyperkalemia** (arrhythmias)
    - Spironolactone: gynecomastia & antiandrogen effects

- Antidiuretic Hormone = **ADH** = **Vasopressin**
  - Reabsorbs water and constrict blood vessels
  - Synthesized in **hypothalamus** and stored in **posterior pituitary**
    - Most is released into bloodstream to effect vessels and kidney
    - Some released into brain
      - Plays role in social behavior, sexual motivation, pair bonding, and maternal responses to stress
  - **ADH** binds to **V2 receptor** in **CT** (and DCT)
    - **Aquaporins** displace into the luminal basement membrane
      - allowing for reabsorption of water

Metabolic Acidosis 1

Is primarily a fall in serum bicarb

$$H^+ + HCO_3 <> H_2CO_3 <> H_2O + CO_2$$

- A fall in bicarb results from
  - addition of protons = right shift
  - loss of bicarb = left shift
  - *either is a gain of* H^+

Causes of H^+ Increase

- Enzyme dysfunction → organ dysfunction
- H^+ is accompanied by an anion to maintain electrical neutrality
  - Cl^-
  - lactate or ketone
  - phosphate or sulfate
  - an ingested anion

Normal Anion Gap = 12 ± 4

$$[Na^+] - ([Cl^-] + [HCO_3^-])$$

- The unmeasured anions
  - albumin
  - phosphates & sulfates

High Anion Gap Metabolic Acidosis

- Condition results in _____
  - Oxidative phosphorylation ➔ ATP
    - Lactic acidosis Type A
      - fail to oxidatively phosphorylate (pyruvate ➔ lactate)
    - Lactic acidosis Type B
      - lactate production overwhelms lactate metabolism
  - Diabetic ➔ ketones
  - Uremia ➔ sulphate/phosphate
  - ASA ➔ salicylate
  - Methanol ➔ formate; Ethylene glycol ➔ oxalate

Lactic Acidosis Type A:
Failure of ETC

- Due to decreased O2 delivery
  - shock
  - severe hypoxemia
  - severe anemia
- Due to inhibitors
  - CO, CN

Lactic Acidosis Type B

- Due to
  - Malignancies (post chemothcrapy)
  - Hepatic failure
  - Drugs
    - Metformin
    - AZT
    - INH

Metabolic Acidosis 2

Normal vs High-Anion Gap Acidosis

Review

- $H^+ + HCO_3 <> H_2CO_3 <> H_2O + CO_2$
- $AG = [Na^+] - ([Cl^-] + [HCO_3^-])$
- Always ask, what anion was accompanying the proton
    - Cl
    - lactate or ketone
    - phosphate or sulfate
    - ingested anion

NAGMA vs. HAGMA

- Normal Anion Gap Metabolic Acidosis results from
  - increased production of Cl- or
  - increased excretion of bicarbonate
- High Anion Gap Metabolic Acidosis results from
  - producing too much acid or
  - not producing enough bicarb

Normal Anion Gap Metabolic Acidosis (12±4)

- HARD-UPS
  - Hyperalimentation
    - nutrients are oversupplied: obesity, vitamin/iron poisoning, fad diets, low sodium diet
  - Acetazolamide (carbonic anhydrase inhibitors)
  - Renal tubular acidosis
  - Diarrhea
    - Hyperchloremic metabolic acidosis
      - loss of bicarb compensated by an increase in [Cl-]
  - Ureteroenteric fistual
    - fistula between a ureter and the GI tract
  - Pancreaticoduodenal fistula
  - Spironolactone

RTA = Renal Tubular Acidosis

- Type 1 = distal
  - defect in collecting tubule's ability to excrete H^+
  - hypokalemia, Ca kidney stones
- Type 2 = proximal
  - defect in proximal tubule HCO_3^- resorption
  - hypokalemia, hypophosphatemic rickets
- Type 4 = **hyper**kalemic
  - dec **aldosterone** affect
    - hypoaldosteronism or
    - lack of response in collecting tubules to aldosterone
  - inhibition of **ammonium** excretion in proximal tubule
    - decreased urine pH due to decreased buffering capacity

Review: The Anions ~ HAGMA

- Oxidation issues cause lactic acidosis

- Diabetics produce ketones

- Uremia accompanied by sulphates/phosphates

- Aspirin leaves salicylates

- **Methanol → formate**; ethylene glycol → oxalate

High Anion Gap Metabolic Acidosis

- MUDPIIIILES
  - Methanol
  - Uremia (CKD)
  - Diabetic ketoacidosis
  - Propylene glycol
  - Infection, Iron, Isoniazid, Inborn errors of metab
  - Lactic acidosis
  - Ethylene glycol
  - Salicylates

Nephrotic-Nephritic 1

You should separate the learning of two
similar named things by time and place to
make them less similar.

(I'm breaking a rule, but painting a picture. Anyway, lets get real.
You aren't going to finish this is one sitting)

NephrOtic = LOss of PrOtein

Relax, this is the only page I'm going to emphasize the 'O'. Everyone
emphasizes the 'O'!

- The fact that the kidney is letting proteins through often leads
  students to believe nephrOtic conditions are worse than
  nephritic. This is not the case. NephrOtic is better. Most
  nephrOtic syndromes can be managed for a long time, and
  some actually fully recover. All that has occurred is the
  negatively-charged filter (of the glomerulus's 3 filters), which
  repels prOteins, has lost its charge.

Oh, thank gOOdness I'm frOthing and lOsing prOtein.
This is nephrOtic.

Nephrotic: From Best to Worst

- Define nephrotic
  - proteinuria **> 3.5g/day**: <u>frothy urine</u>
    - inc risk of infection due to loss of immunoglobulins
    - inc risk of thrombosis due to loss of antithrombin
  - hyperlipidemia, **fatty casts**

- MCD = Minimal Change Disease
- Membranous Glomerulonephritis
- FSGS = Focal Segmental Glomerulosclerosis
- Renal Amyloidosis
- Diabetic Glomerulosclerosis

MCD = Minimal Change Disease

- A **child** recently had a cold. This triggered an immune response.
- The damage to the glomerulus can't even be seen w/ a light microscope.
- Give the kid **corticosteroids**, and she'll be fine.

Nephrotic:
Membranous Glomerulonephritis

- Most common cause of nephrotic syndrome in **adult**s.
- 1/3 spontaneously resolve. 1/3 continue but don't progress. 1/3 progress to ESRD and dialysis.
- The name
  - **Membranous** = lots of membrane = GBM thickening
  - **Glomeruli** = having to do with the glomerulus
  - **-itis** = dz characterized by inflammation
  - Lots of membrane and inflammation of the glomerulus
    - ie. **inflammation of the glomerular membrane leading to membrane thickening**
- Mechanism
  - Immune complex formation in the glomerulus activates C5b-C9 —> MAC (membrane attack complex) —> stimulates release of proteases and oxidants by mesangial and epithelial cells —> damages capillary walls which now leak
  - Epithelial cells secrete substance that reduces **nephrin** synthesis
    - **nephrin is needed for a functioning renal filtration barrier**, hence loss of negative charge filter, hence proteinuria

Nephrotic:
Membranous Glomerulonephritis

- Here you might use an electron microscope and see "**spike and dome**".
  - spikes = immune complexes on the GBM
  - domes = hyaline deposits that have overfilled the hole
- Just like minimal change disease in kids, membranous glomerulonephritis can be caused by **recent infection**.
  - Actually, anything that reacts with your immune system such as **drugs**, autoimmune diseases (esp. **SLE**), and **tumors**.
- Tx
  - Do you suppress the immune system or not? This is the art of medicine. Corticosteroids get mixed results. All the other immunosuppressives are possible. When in doubt, base on how bad the prognosis is.
  - Low risk: no medications
  - Moderate risk: **cyclophosphamide**
  - High risk: glucocorticoids + (cyclophosphamide)
    - woman of **child-bearing age**: glucocorticoids + **cyclosporine**
  - Severe and relapsing get stronger immunosuppressives.

Nephrotic: FSGS
Focal Segmental Glomerulosclerosis

- Most common glomerular disease in **HIV** pt's
  - also heroin users
- May have similar cause as minimal change disease
- **Doesn't respond to corticosteroids**
- Leads to ESRD

Really, if you have a patient w/ a nephrotic condition and HIV (or on heroin), think FSGS

Nephrotic:
Renal Amyloidosis

- What causes amyloid deposits in the kidney?
  - **Rheumatoid Arthritis,** Multiple Myeloma, TB.
    - A lot of condition do, but these are the big ones
- How well can you control the primary condition determines the outcome.
  - You may manage for a long time, or not.
- Confirm w/ light microscopy
  - **congo red stain: apple-green birefringence**

Nephrotic:
Diabetic Glomerulosclerosis

- Diabetic Glomerulosclerosis = Diabetic Nephropathy
- Primarily a nephrotic condition which progresses to nephritic.
  - Initially, the negative-filter is damaged, but as time progresses, just as w/ diabetic peripheral neuropathy, the damage gets worse until the size barrier gets involved. Big items like RBCs pass through, and you get hematuria. However, you just start off with foamy urine and advance to bloody urine over time, but you can prevent this by **managing pt's diabetes**.
- Massive mesangial growth = **Kimmelstiel Wilson** nodules

Nephrotic Summary

- MCD:
  - Child, recent cold → Px steroids
- Membranous Glomerulonephritis:
  - Immune complexes, "spike and dome",
  - Tx: none → immunosuppressants
- FSGS:
  - HIV
  - No response to steroids
- Amyloidosis:
  - Tx Cause: Rheumatoid Arthritis, Multiple Myeloma, TB
  - Congo red, apple-green birefringence

Nephrotic-Nephritic 2

MCD, GCs

Nephrotic Review

- Nephrotic means you lost the charge barrier in the glomerulus.
- The following pages progress from better to worse.

Nephrotic:
MCD = Minimal Change Disease

- A child w/ a recent cold that triggered an immune response
- Give them steroids and watch.

GCs = Glucocorticoids

- In practice, corticosteroid = glucocorticoid
  - Technically,
    - Corticosteroids = Glucocorticoids & Mineralocorticoids
    - Mineralocorticoids main function is to influence salt and water balances
    - This is all we will say about mineralocorticoids as this time.
- Glucocorticoids: **gluco**se + **cort**ex + ster**oid**
  - Regulates metabolism of glucose
  - Synthesized in the adrenal cortex
  - Has a steroidal structure

(GC) Glucocorticoid Basics

- **Cortisol**:
  - Most important human glucocorticoid
  - Regulates/supports: immunologic, metabolic, homeostatic, and cardiovascular functions.
    - Synthetic GCs are produced specifically to effect these functions.
- GCs are generally classified as immunologic or metabolic
  - The ones we deal with the most are the immunologic ones, so I will limit the scope of this topic to those
    - Mostly inhibit lymphocytes and help w/ side effects
    - They still have some effect on metabolic functions.
    - They still have some metabolic function side effects.

GCs

- Inhibits phospholipase A2 and COX2
  - Dec leukotrienes and prostaglandins
    - **Inhibit inflammation**
- Interfere w/ abnormal mechanisms of cancer
- SE:
  - **Iatrogenic Cushing's syndrome**
    - buffalo hump, moon facies, truncal obesity, easy bruising, osteoporosis, peptic ulcers, diabetes
  - When stop suddenly → **adrenal insufficiency**.

Glucocorticoid Potency (Cortisol is 1)

- Weak
  - Cortisone = Hydrocortisone: 0.8
- Strong
  - Prednisone: 3.5-5
  - Prednisolone: 4
  - Methylprednisolone: 5-7.5
- Stronger
  - Betamethasone: 25-30
  - Dexamethasone: 25-80

GCs: Some High Points

- Cortisone/Hydrocortisone
  - Cortisone is activated through hydrogenation, so it is often called hydrocortisone
- Prednisone & Prednisolone & Methylprednisolone
  - **Prednisone**: *When in doubt, think of prednisone first.*
  - **Prednisolone**: Prednisone converted to Prednisolone by the liver.
    - It has no significant biological effects until after the conversion.
  - **Methylprednisolone**: The **IV** variant of prednisolone.
    - *The IV-version of another drug is generally stronger*
- Betamethasone: 25-30
  - Deliverable as IV, IM, PO. Notable as a topical cream for eczema, psoriasis
- **Dexamethasone**
  - **When you need something stronger than prednisone.**
  - **Maturation of premie lungs**
  - High-altitude cerebral edema and high-altitude pulmonary edema
  - Stronger side effects

Prednisone

- Inhibits synthesis of nearly all cytokines
- Inactivate NF-κB
  - the TF that induces production of TNF-α and others
- May trigger apoptosis
- Used in cancer treatment **a lot**
- SE:
  - Cushing-like
    - immunosuppression, cataracts, acne, osteoporosis, HTN, peptic ulcers, hyperglycemia, psychosis

Prednisone Summary

- Uses
  - Immunosuppressant
  - Interfere w/ abnormal mechanisms of cancer
  - *When in doubt, think prednisone first*
    - If need something stronger, think dexamethasone
- **Prednisone** converted to **Prednisolone** by the liver.
  - **Methylprednisolone** is the IV variant of prednisolone
- SE
  - Cushing-like **A PIG CHOP**
    - **A**cne, **P**eptic ulcers, **I**mmunosuppression, hyper**G**lycemia, **C**ataracts, **H**TN, **O**steoporosis, **P**sychosis
      - *This drug is used a lot. You better know these SE.*

Nephrotic Summary

- MCD:
  - Child, recent cold → Px steroids
- Membranous Glomerulonephritis:
  - Immune complexes, "spike and dome",
  - Tx: none → immunosuppressants
- FSGS:
  - HIV
  - No response to steroids
- Amyloidosis:
  - Tx Cause: Rheumatoid Arthritis, Multiple Myeloma, TB
  - Congo red, apple-green birefringence

Prednisone Summary

- Uses
  - Immunosuppressant
  - Cancer
  - If need something stronger, think dexamethasone
- **Prednisone** converted to **Prednisolone** by the liver.
  - **Methylprednisolone** is the IV variant of prednisolone
- SE
  - Cushing-like **A PIG CHOP**
    - Acne, Peptic ulcers, Immunosuppression, hyperGlycemia, Cataracts, HTN, Osteoporosis, Psychosis
      - *This drug is used a lot. You better know these SE.*

Nephrotic-Nephritic 3

Thicken GBM and
Immunosuppressants

Nephrotic Review

- MCD:
  - Child, recent cold → Px steroids
- Membranous Glomerulonephritis:
  - Immune complexes, "spike and dome",
  - Tx: none → immunosuppressants
- FSGS:
  - HIV
  - No response to steroids
- Amyloidosis:
  - Tx Cause: Rheumatoid Arthritis, Multiple Myeloma, TB
  - Congo red, apple-green birefringence

Nephrotic:
Membranous Glomerulonephritis

- ie. inflammation of the glomerular membrane with membrane **thickening**
  - **Adult**
  - Immune complex formation on **GBM** (glomerular basement membrane)
  - Destruction of membrane w/ protease destruction of capillary wall: leaks
    - Epithelial cells inhibit **nephrin** secretion → filtration problems
- What causes immune response in adults?
  - recent infection, drugs, autoimmune dz (esp. SLE), tumors
- "**spike and dome**" on **EM**
  - spikes = immune complexes; domes = overfilled deposits
- Tx based on a continuum of prognosis
  - **No treatment** → **cyclophosphamide** → + steroids
    - (if could get pregn, change cyclophosphamide to **cyclosporine**)
  - Keep using stronger immunosuppressives

Cyclophosphamide

- **Alkylating agent**:
  - Activated by the liver → **crosslinks DNA** at guanine N-7
    - **teratogenic**
- Uses
  - Immunosuppression: used with autoimmune disorders
  - Cancer: NHL, breast & ovarian
- SE
  - **Hemorrhagic cystitis** (bleeding in bladder)
    - Prevent w/ **Mesna:**
      - Mesna binds toxic metabolite
  - Myelosuppression
  - If taking for autoimmune dz and have an acute crisis
    - move to methotrexate or azathioprine

Cyclosporine

- Mechanism
  - Binds to cyclophilins → inhibits calcineurin
    - Inhibits IL-2 → inhibits T-cell differentiation and activation
- Uses
  - Suppresses organ rejection
  - Autoimmune disorders
- SE
  - **Nephrotoxic**: preventable w/ **Mannitol**
  - **Gout**
    - also kidney related.

Cyclosporine has a thing for kidneys!
Weird that something used to prevent renal transplant rejection's big
SE are renal related, ie uremia, and nephrotoxicity.

Summary: Immunosuppressants

- **Cyclophosphamide**
  - **Alkylating agent**: crosslinks DNA → <u>teratogenic</u>
  - Autoimmune d/o's, Cancer (NHL, breast & ovarian)
  - SE:
    - **Hemorrhagic cystitis** (Prevent w/ **Mesna**)

- **Cyclosporine**
  - **Inhibits IL-2 → inhibits T-cell differentiation and activation**
  - Autoimmune d/o's, Suppresses organ rejection
  - SE
    - **Nephrotoxic**: preventable w/ **Mannitol**
    - **Gout**

Nephrotic Summary

- MCD:
  - Child, recent cold → Px steroids
- Membranous Glomerulonephritis:
  - Immune complexes, "spike and dome",
  - Tx: none → immunosuppressants
- FSGS:
  - HIV
  - No response to steroids
- Amyloidosis:
  - Tx Cause: Rheumatoid Arthritis, Multiple Myeloma, TB
  - Congo red, apple-green birefringence

Summary: Immunosuppressants

- **Cyclophosphamide**
  - **Alkylating agent**: crosslinks DNA → <u>teratogenic</u>
  - Autoimmune d/o's, Cancer (NHL, breast & ovarian)
  - SE:
    - **Hemorrhagic cystitis** (Prevent w/ **Mesna)**

- **Cyclosporine**
  - **Inhibits IL-2 → inhibits T-cell differentiation and activation**
  - Autoimmune d/o's, Suppresses organ rejection
  - SE
    - **Nephrotoxic**: preventable w/ **Mannitol**
    - **Gout**

Nephrotic-Nephritic 4

FSGSclerosis, Amyloidosis, RA

Nephrotic Review

- MCD:
  - Child, recent cold → Px steroids
- Membranous Glomerulonephritis:
  - Immune complexes, "spike and dome",
  - Tx: none → immunosuppressants
- FSGS:
  - HIV
  - No response to steroids
- Amyloidosis:
  - Tx Cause: Rheumatoid Arthritis, Multiple Myeloma, TB
  - Congo red, apple-green birefringence

Nephrotic: **FSGS**
Focal Segmental Glomerulosclerosis

- **HIV** (or heroin) user
- **No response to steroids**
- Leads to ESRD

Nephrotic: **Renal Amyloidosis**

- Due to **Rheumatoid Arthritis**, MM, TB
  - **RA** ~ got gnarly looking knuckles
  - MM ~ middle aged w/ lytic bone lesions in spine
  - TB ~ coughing up blood
- Control the condition
- Confirm w/ congo red stain:
  - apple-green birefringence
  - You should know this by now.
    - Always the same: **amyloid - congo red - green bifringence**

RA = Rheumatoid Arthritis

- Define
  - Rheumatic = dz affecting joints or connective tissue
  - Arthro = joint
- 50% of the risk is genetic. Smoking increases risk by 3x
- Rheumatoid Arthritis can produce inflammation in the
  - joints (primarily), nodules in skin
  - lungs, heart, and sclera
- Joints:
  - Pain is nociceptive and not neuropathic.
    - ie. body is sending signals of painful stimuli and not nerve damage
  - **Inflammation of the synovial** membrane
    - **swollen, tender, warm, stiff**
  - In the early stages, gentle movements can provide relief.
  - Later stages: **erosion —> deformity**

RA Sequela

- Joints
  - **Ulnar deviation**:
    - Swelling of metacarpophalangeal joint (the big knuckles) cause finger to displace toward digit 5
  - **Boutonniere deformity**:
    - PIP (joint nearest the knuckle) permanently bent toward the palm while DIP is bent away from the palm
  - **Swan neck**:
    - Fingertip is permanently bent toward the palm while PIP is bent away
- Other
  - Lungs: fibrosis
  - Heart:
    - fibrosis → atherosclerosis > MI, stroke
    - pericarditis, endocarditis, valvulitis
  - Eyes: episcleritis, keratoconjunctivitis sicca → blindness
  - Kidney:
    - chronic inflammation leads to **renal amyloidosis**. Some direct effect as well.

RA: Dx

- Tests
  - **ESR, CRP, RF, ANA, CCP** Abs (anti-cyclic citrullinated peptide)
  - X-rays
  - When uncertain: arthrocentesis.
- Dx:
  - Base on all the classic findings of the dz
  OR
  - **≥ 3 joints** for **> 6w** + (**RF or CP** positive) + (**inc CRP or ESR**)
  - without evidence of diseases w/ similar clinical features

RA: Tx

- Directed toward control of **synovitis** and prevention of joint injury

- **DMARD**
  - (Disease-Modifying Anti-Rheumatic drug),
    - DMARDs slow, sometimes stop, the dz
  - **Methotrexate**
    - else: **etanercept, adalimumab,** or leflunomide
- **NSAIDs**: all who can
- Prednisone: as needed

RA Summary

- 50% of the risk is genetic. Smoking increases risk by 3x
- Rheumatoid Arthritis can produce inflammation in the
  - joints (primarily), nodules in skin
  - lungs, heart, and sclera
- Joints:
  - **Inflammation of the synovial** membrane → → erosion → deformity
    - **swollen, tender, warm, stiff**
  - **Ulnar deviation**:
    - Swelling of metacarpophalangeal joint cause finger to displace toward pinkie
  - **Boutonniere deformity**:
    - PIP permanently bent toward the palm, DIP is bent away from the palm
  - **Swan neck**:
    - Fingertip is permanently bent toward the palm while PIP is bent away
- Kidney: **renal amyloidosis** (due to chronic inflammation)

RA Summary: Dx & Tx

- Tests: **ESR, CRP, RF, ANA, CCP;** X-rays
- Dx
  - Base on all the classic findings of the dz
  OR
  - **≥ 3 joints** for **> 6w** + (**RF or CP** positive) + (**inc CRP or ESR**)
  - without evidence of diseases w/ similar clinical features
- Tx
  - **Methotrexate** (DMARD)
    - else: **etanercept, adalimumab, or leflunomide**
  - **NSAIDs**: all who can
  - Prednisone: as needed

Nephrotic Summary

- MCD:
  - Child, recent cold → Px steroids
- Membranous Glomerulonephritis:
  - Immune complexes, "spike and dome",
  - Tx: none → immunosuppressants
- FSGS:
  - HIV
  - No response to steroids
- Amyloidosis:
  - Tx Cause: Rheumatoid Arthritis, Multiple Myeloma, TB
  - Congo red, apple-green birefringence

RA Summary

- Sequela:
  - **Ulnar deviation:**
    - Swelling of metacarpophalangeal joint cause finger to displace toward pinkie
  - **Boutonniere deformity:**
    - PIP permanently bent toward the palm, DIP is bent away from the palm
  - **Swan neck:**
    - Fingertip is permanently bent toward the palm while PIP is bent away
  - **Renal amyloidosis**
- Tests: **ESR, CRP, RF, ANA, CCP**; X-rays
- Dx
  - Base on all the classic findings of the dz
  - OR
  - **≥ 3 joints** for **> 6w** + (**RF or CP** positive) + (**inc CRP or ESR**)
  - without evidence of diseases w/ similar clinical features
- Tx
  - **Methotrexate** (else: **etanercept, adalimumab**, or leflunomide)
  - **NSAIDs:** all who can
  - Prednisone: as needed

Nephrotic-Nephritic 5

Review

Nephrotic Summary

- MCD = Minimal Change Disease
  - Child, recent cold, immune response → Px steroids and watch

- Membranous Glomerulonephritis
  - ie. glomerular inflammation leading to GBM thickening
  - Adult: recent infection, drugs, SLE, or tumor
  - "Spike and dome" = immune complexes and overfilled deposits
  - Px immunosuppressives equal to the dz
    - none → cyclophosphamide (baby makers get cyclosporine instead) → + steroids → stronger

- FSGS = Focal Segmental Glomerulosclerosis
  - HIV (or heroin user); no response to steroids; eventual ESRD

- Renal Amyloidosis
  - Control the primary condition: MM, TB, RA
  - Confirm w/ congo red stain revealing apple-green birefringence

- Diabetic Glomerulosclerosis
  - Progresses from nephrotic to nephritic; Control the diabetes
  - Kimmelstiel Wilson nodules: massive mesangial growth

Summary: Immunosuppressants

- **Prednisone**
  - **Prednisone** –liver→ **Prednisolone**
    - **Methylprednisolone** is the IV variant of prednisolone
    - If need something stronger, think **dexamethasone**
  - Immunosuppressant; Cancer
  - SE: Cushing-like **A PIG CHOP**
    - **A**cne, **P**eptic ulcers, **I**mmunosuppression, hyper**G**lycemia, **C**ataracts, **H**TN, **O**steoporosis, **P**sychosis

- **Cyclophosphamide**
  - **Alkylating agent**: crosslinks DNA → <u>teratogenic</u>
  - Autoimmune d/o's; Cancer (NHL, breast & ovarian)
  - SE: **Hemorrhagic cystitis** (prevent w/ **Mesna**)

- **Cyclosporine**
  - **Inhibits IL-2** → **inhibits T-cell differentiation and activation**
  - Autoimmune d/o's; Suppresses organ rejection
  - SE: **Nephrotoxic** (preventable w/ **Mannitol**); Gout

RA Summary

- Sequela:
  - **Ulnar deviation**:
    - Swelling of metacarpophalangeal joint cause finger to displace toward pinkie
  - **Boutonniere deformity**:
    - PIP permanently bent toward the palm, DIP is bent away from the palm
  - **Swan neck**:
    - Fingertip is permanently bent toward the palm while PIP is bent away
  - **Renal amyloidosis**
- Tests: **ESR, CRP, RF, ANA, CCP;** X-rays
- Dx
  - Base on all the classic findings of the dz
  OR
  - **≥ 3 joints** for **> 6w** + (**RF or CP** positive) + (**inc CRP or ESR**)
  - without evidence of diseases w/ similar clinical features
- Tx
  - **Methotrexate** (else: <u>**etanercept, adalimumab**, or leflunomide</u>)
  - **NSAIDs**: all who can
  - Prednisone: as needed

Nephrotic Re-summary

- MCD:
  - child, recent cold → Px steroids
- Membranous Glomerulonephritis:
  - immune complexes, "spike and dome"
  - Px none → immunosuppressants
- FSGS:
  - HIV, no response to steroids, eventual ESRD
- Amyloidosis:
  - Control MM, TB, RA
  - congo red, apple-green birefringence

Re-summary: Immunosuppressants

- **Prednisone/Prednisolone/Methylprednisolone →
  Dexamethasone**
  - SE: Cushing-like **A PIG CHOP**
    - **A**cne, **P**eptic ulcers, **I**mmunosuppression, hyper**G**lycemia, **C**ataracts, **H**TN, **O**steoporosis, **P**sychosis

- **Cyclophosphamide**
  - **Alkylating agent**: crosslinks DNA → teratogenic
  - Autoimmune d/o's; Cancer (NHL, breast & ovarian)
  - SE: **Hemorrhagic cystitis** (prevent w/ **Mesna**)

- **Cyclosporine**
  - **Inhibits IL-2 → inhibits T-cell**
  - Autoimmune d/o's; Suppresses organ rejection
  - SE: **Nephrotoxic** (preventable w/ **Mannitol**); **Gout**

RA Re-summary

- Sequela
  - **Ulnar deviation, Boutonniere deformity, Swan neck**
  - **Renal amyloidosis**
- Tests: **ESR, CRP, RF, ANA, CCP;** X-rays
- Dx
  - Base on all the classic findings of the dz
  OR
  - **≥ 3 joints** for **> 6w** + (**RF or CP** positive) + (**inc CRP or ESR**)
  - without evidence of diseases w/ similar clinical features
- Tx
  - **Methotrexate** (else: **etanercept, adalimumab, or leflunomide**)
  - **NSAIDs**: all who can
  - Prednisone: as needed

RPGN Sucks Usually 1

Alport and Crescent Shapes

Nephritic

- *Maybe nephritic doesn't have to be that bad, but where nephrotic is an interference w/ the charge barrier, nephritic is destruction of the size barrier. Doesn't that just sound worse?*
- *Sometimes it is, sometimes it isn't. When it's bad, it can kill your pt quick!*
  - *When it's good, they recover. Usually a kid.*
- Nephritic conditions
  - Alport Syndrome
  - **Rapidly Progressive (Crescentic) Glomerulonephritis (RPGN)**
    - Often when physicians say RPGN, they mean the worst prognosis, but RPGN is actually a range of conditions.

Alport Syndrome

- A mutation in type IV collagen → split basement membrane
- Recurrent hematuria & proteinuria before 20yo
- Pt presents w/ nerve disorder
  - vision changes
  - deafness
  - neuropathy
- Expect a family history of nephritis
  - **XR** (75%), AR (25%)

Alport = *Red, frothy urine w/ blindness +/- deafness* → *ESRD*

(**RPGN**) Rapidly Progressive (Crescentic) Glomerulonephritis

- Crescentic describes the appearance under light microscopy and w/ immunofixation (**IF**)
  - Crescents are made from **fibrin** and plasma proteins
  - Crescents seen in > 50% of cases
- Immune response at parietal cells due to C3b, monocytes, and macrophage activities
- Possible 50% loss of GFR in 3m
  - Progresses to ARF → death within months

RPGN Overview

- Symptoms
  - Hematuria, RBC casts, proteinuria
  - Possible HTN + edema (due to loss of protein)
  - When severe: oliguria or anuria (ie. kidneys not working)
- Types
  - Type I, Hypersensitivity Type II rxn:
    - antibodies against the glomerular basement membrane (**GBM**)
  - Type II, Hypersensitivity Type III rxn:
    - deposition of immune complexes into the GBM/mesangium
  - Type III = Pauci-Immune RPGN:
    - glomeruli damaged possibly due to the activation of neutrophils

RPGN Overview

- Dx
  - Type I: **GBM Abs** (GBM = glomerular basement membrane)
  - Type II: **ANA** (Anti-Nuclear Abs)
    - supports Type II RPGN, does not confirm
  - Type III: **ANCA** (Anti-Neutrophil Cytoplasmic Abs)
- Tx: corticosteroids ± immunosuppressives ± plasmapheresis
  - Immunosuppressives: **C R pregnant CAT**
  - **Cyclophosphamide** or **Rituximab**
    - If pregnant: **Cyclosporine** or **Azathioprine** or **Tacrolimus**
  - Possible plasma exchange to clear antibodies
  - Prophylaxis for opportunistic infections: **TMP/SMX**

Summary: Alport & RPGN

- **Alport Syndrome**
  - Recurrent hematuria & proteinuria < 20yo, & blind or deaf
  - Mutation type IV collagen → **split GBM**
  - FHx of nephritis: **XR** (75%), AR (25%)

- **RPGN = Rapidly Progressive (Crescentic) Glomerulonephritis**
  - Dx
    - Type I: **GBM Abs**;
      - Hypersensitivity Type II rxn
    - Type II: **ANA**;
      - Hypersensitivity Type III rxn
    - Type III, aka Pauci-Immune RPGN: **ANCA**
  - Tx: corticosteroids ± immunosuppressives ± plasmapheresis
    - Immunosuppressives: **C R pregnant CAT**
      - **C**yclophosphamide or **R**ituximab
      - If pregnant: **C**yclosporine or **A**zathioprine or **T**acrolimus
    - Plasmapheresis to clear antibodies.
    - Prophylaxis for opportunistic infections: **TMP/SMX**

RPGN Sucks Usually 2

Henoch and the
Self-Resolving RPGN Type II's

Review: Alport & RPGN

- **Alport Syndrome**
  - Recurrent hematuria & proteinuria < 20yo, & blind or deaf
  - Mutation type IV collagen → **split GBM**
  - FHx of nephritis: **XR** (75%), AR (25%)

- **RPGN = Rapidly Progressive (Crescentic) Glomerulonephritis**
  - Dx
    - Type I: **GBM Abs**;
      - Hypersensitivity Type II rxn
    - Type II: **ANA**;
      - Hypersensitivity Type III rxn
    - Type III, aka Pauci-Immune RPGN: **ANCA**
  - Tx: corticosteroids ± immunosuppressives ± plasmapheresis
    - Immunosuppressives: C R pregnant CAT
      - **C**yclophosphamide or **R**ituximab
      - If pregnant: **C**yclosporine or **A**zathioprine or **T**acrolimus
    - Plasmapheresis to clear antibodies.
    - Prophylaxis for opportunistic infections: **TMP/SMX**

RPGN Type I
Goodpasture Syndrome

- Many causes. Basically any irritant of the vessels taking blood to/from the lungs can activate the immune system abnormally resulting in Goodpasture.
  - *Therefore, don't worry about the cause for test purposes.*
- Antibodies against basement membrane **Type-IV collagen**
  - **Hypersensitivity Type II rxn**
- Lungs & kidneys
  - hemoptysis + hematuria
- Males: 25-30

RPGN Type I: Dx & Tx

- IF:
  - **linear deposits in basement membrane**
    - due to the Abs against type-IV collagen in the GBM
- Tx:
  - glucocorticoids + immunosuppressives
    - ± plasmapheresis
- *With treatment, the 5y survival rate is >80%*

RPGN Type II
Deposition of Immune Complexes

- **Hypersensitivity Type III Reaction**
  - Any disease that results in immune complex depositions in the kidney may progress to RPGN Type II
    - Henoch-Schönlein Purpura
    - Streptococcal infections
    - SLE
      - Drug-induced Lupus
- RPGN Type II Diseases
  - Self-Resolving
    - IgA Nephropathy = Berger's Disease
    - Poststreptococcal Glomerulonephritis
  - Nephrotic and/or Nephritic
    - Membranoproliferative Glomerulonephritis (MPGN)
    - Diffuse Proliferative Glomerulonephritis

MPGN Type II:
IgA Nephropathy (aka Berger's Dz)

- **IgA-based** immune complexes in the **mesangium**
  → mesangial proliferation
- Flares up as sequela of URI or acute gastroenteritis
- May be due to **Henoch-Schönlein Purpura**

Henoch-Schönlein Purpura

- Child with **previous URI** (eg. sore throat) develops
  - Arthritis, abdominal pain, and **palpable purpura in the lower body**
- Systemic vasculitis due to deposition of **immune complexes containing IgA**
- Kidney involvement consists of minor hematuria and proteinuria that usually goes unnoticed
  - can progress to **IgA Nephropathy**
    - aka. **Berger's Disease**

Henoch-Schönlein Purpura: Dx & Tx

- Dx
  - Inc **IgA**; Inc **CRP** &/or **ESR**
  - Assess kidney function: Inc serum **Cr** and **urea**;
  - **Plt count** may be raised which helps differentiate this condition from ITP and TTP
- Tx:
  - Generally treat w/ analgesics and resolves within weeks.
  - Immunosuppression may be required

RPGN II: **Poststreptococcal GN**

- Common complication of cellulitis or pharyngitis due to Streptococcus bacteria is, aka.
  - **Poststreptococcal Glomerulonephritis**
  - aka. **Postinfectious Glomerulonephritis**
  - aka. **Acute Proliferative Glomerulonephritis**
- Type III hypersensitivity rxn:
  - immune complex accumulate → inflammatory response
    - In this case, the immune complexes accumulate in the glomerulus → glomerulonephritis
- Usually children with
  - **recent cold**
  - **peripheral and periorbital edema** and dark urine

RPGN II: Post-streptococcal GN

- Dx:
  - Inc **ASO (anti-streptolysin O titer)**
  - Low **C3**
  - Renal biopsy rarely done
    - LM shows "**lumpy bumpy**"
    - IF is granular due to IgG, IgM, and C3 deposits on GBM and mesangium
- Tx:
  - Resolves spontaneously

Summary: RPGN Type II,
These Are Self-Resolving

- Overview:
  - Deposition of **immune complexes** in GBM: **Hypersensitivity Type III Rxn**
  - Causes: Henoch-Schönlein Purpura, Streptococcal infections, SLE (drugs)
  - RPGN Type II Diseases
    - Self-resolving: IgA Nephropathy (aka Berger's Dz); Poststreptococcal Glomerulonephritis
    - Nephrotic/Nephritic: Membranoproliferative GN (MPGN), Diffuse Proliferative GN

- **IgA Nephropathy,** aka. **Berger's Disease**
  - **IgA-based immune complexes in the mesangium →** mesangial proliferation
  - Flares up as sequela of **URI or acute gastroenteritis**
  - May be due to **Henoch-Schönlein Purpura**
  - May require immunosuppressants, but generally resolves spontaneously
- **Poststreptococcal Glomerulonephritis, aka Postinfectious GN**
  - Child w/ recent cold, peripheral and periorbital edema, dark urine
  - Dx:
    - Inc **ASO** + low **C3**
    - LM: "**lumpy bumpy**"
  - Tx: Resolves spontaneously

Summary: HSP

- **Henoch-Schönlein Purpura**
  - Systemic vasculitis due to deposition of **immune complexes containing IgA**
  - Child with **previous URI** (eg. sore throat) develops arthritis, abdominal pain, and **palpable purpura in the lower body**
  - **Plt count** may be raised which helps differentiate this condition from ITP and TTP

RPGN Sucks Usually 3

RPGN Type II: Nephrotic →
Nephritic

RPGN Type II Review:
Overview and The Self-Resolving

- Overview:
  - Deposition of **immune complexes** in GBM: **Hypersensitivity Type III Rxn**
  - Causes: Henoch-Schönlein Purpura, Streptococcal infections, SLE (drugs)
  - RPGN Type II Diseases
    - Self-resolving: IgA Nephropathy (aka Berger's Dz); Poststreptococcal Glomerulonephritis
    - Nephrotic/Nephritic: Membranoproliferative GN (MPGN), Diffuse Proliferative GN

- RPGN Type II: Self-Resolving
  - **IgA Nephropathy, aka. Berger's Disease**
    - **IgA-based immune complexes in the mesangium** → mesangial proliferation
    - Flares up as sequela of **URI or acute gastroenteritis**
    - May be due to **Henoch-Schönlein Purpura**
  - **Poststreptococcal Glomerulonephritis, aka Postinfectious GN**
    - Child w/ recent cold, peripheral and periorbital edema, dark urine
    - Inc **ASO** + low **C3**
    - LM: "lumpy bumpy"

RPGN Type II
(**MPGN**) Membranoproliferative GN

- **Membranoproliferative Glomerulonephritis = MPGN**
  - aka. **Mesangiocapillary Glomerulonephritis**
- Mesangium: "meso" = middle, angeion = "vessel"
  - Mesangium = Mesangial cell: These are cells that are in the middle of a bunch of capillaries. In fact, they are continuous w/ the smooth muscles of the arterioles.
    - hence "**mesangiocapillary**"
- The Glomerulus Basement Membrane (GBM) surrounds both the capillaries and the mesangium
  - ie. proliferation of mesangial cells "in the middle" of glomerular basement membranes
- Therefore the name fits the characteristic LM trait:
  - **Tram-track:** Mesangial cells grow in-between the GBM causing it to split and give a tram-track appearance
    - Compare to Alport Syndrome where a mutation in type IV collagen → split-basement membrane
      - Split-basement and tram-track do not look the same, though you don't need to know the difference on sight, for the pt HPI will tell you the rest.

RPGN Type II: MPGN Types

Can be nephrotic or nephritic.

- Once, MPGN was referred to in terms of the three types. They aren't really used anymore.
  - Type I: classical **complement** pathway
  - Type II: alternative **complement** pathway
    - 10y till ESRD
    - associated w/ deteriorating vision
  - Type III: really rare

- Instead, don't worry about the types now. Focus on some specifics
  - **Hypersensitivity Type III Rxn:**
    - immune complexes depositing in the kidney and the immune response that follows
  - Causes: HBV, **HCV**, <u>C3</u>

RPGN II: Diffuse Proliferative GN

- Diffuse Proliferative Glomerulonephritis
  - Commonly caused by MPGN or SLE
  - Epithelial **crescents** form in **Bowman's space** and capillary walls thicken and resemble **wire loops**

RPGN Type II Summary: Nephrotic → Nephritic

- **MPGN = Membranoproliferative Glomerulonephritis**
  - aka. **Mesangiocapillary Glomerulonephritis**
    - Mesangium: "meso" = middle, angeion = "vessel"
    - Mesangiocapillary = Mesangial cells are continuous w/ the smooth muscles of the arterioles.
    - The Glomerulus Basement Membrane (GBM) surrounds both the capillaries and the mesangium
  - **Tram-track**: Mesangial cells grow in-between the GBM causing it to split
  - Caused by hepatitis (HBV, **HCV**) and C3

- **Diffuse Proliferative Glomerulonephritis**
  - Commonly caused by MPGN or SLE
  - **Wire Loops**: Capillary walls thicken

RPGN Sucks Usually 4

The SLE Continuum

RPGN Type II Review:
Nephrotic → Nephritic

- **MPGN = Membranoproliferative Glomerulonephritis**
  - aka. **Mesangiocapillary Glomerulonephritis**
  - Mesangial cells grow in-between the GBM causing it to split and give a **tram-track** appearance
  - Caused by hepatitis (HBV, **HCV**) and C3
- **Diffuse Proliferative Glomerulonephritis**
  - Cause: MPGN or SLE
  - Capillary walls thicken and resemble **wire loops**

Nephrotic vs Nephritic SLE

- MGN (nephrotic) → Diffuse Proliferative GN (nephritic)
  - Nephrotic
    - SLE may cause a milder, nephrotic disease, MGN, as a result of the IC deposits in GBM w/ minimal damage caused by immune response at the GBM.
      - Membranous Glomerulonephritis (MGN)
        » *(covered in another set of concept-chunks)*
        » "Membranous": it's still a normal-ish membrane with IC deposits
        » Spike & dome: IC build up & overfilled repaired divots
  - Nephritic, aka Rapidly Progressive (Crescentic) GN
    - As a Hypersensitivity Type III rxn, SLE can result in structural damage to the GBM and the capillaries
      - **RPGN Type II: Diffuse Proliferative GN**
        » Capillary walls are so damaged that they thicken and look like **wire loops**

(**SLE**) Systemic Lupus Erythematosus

AA Female: tired, fever of unknown origin (FUO), joint & muscle pains. Butterfly rash on face with mouth ulcers.
If you don't know "FUO", you should. It's used all the time in hospitals.

- 90% female, 14-45yo
  - most common and severe in **African American females**
- It effects the whole body. Flares up then goes into remission.

- **SOAPP BRRAIN MD**
  - **S**erositis, **O**ral ulcers, **A**rthritis, **P**hotosensitivity, **P**ulmonary fibrosis
  - **B**lood cells, **R**enal, **R**aynauds, **A**NA, **I**mmunologic (anti-dsDNA, anti-Sm, anti-histone), **N**=neuropsych,
  - **M**=malar rash, **D**=discoid rash

SLE: Key Symptoms

- **Arthritis**
  - #1 reason for seeking medical attention
- Skin
  - Most famous symptom: **malar rash** (ie. **butterfly rash**) on the face.
  - **Discoid rash**: red, scaly skin patches → scarring
  - Photosensitivity
- Ulcers: **mouth**, nasal, urinary, and vaginal
- **Spontaneous abortions** and **in utero deaths**.
- Neuro/psych: various

SLE: Key Evaluations

- Heart & Lungs: CXR
  - **Libman-Sacks endocarditis**.
  - Fibrous sac, muscle, and lining.
  - **Serositis**: Pleuritis or pericarditis
- Kidney
  - MGN (nephrotic) → Diffuse Proliferative GN (nephritic)
    - Membranous Glomerulonephritis (MGN)
      - *(covered in another set of concept-chunks)*
      - spike and dome
    - RPGN Type II: Diffuse Proliferative GN
      - **Wire looping** in kidneys.
      - Renal impairment → ARF → ESRD

SLE: Various

- **Type III hypersensitivity** Rxn
  - w/ Type II involvement
- **HLA class I, II**, and III associations
- Outcome
  - Vast majority in 1st World now have normal lifespans.
  - Worse outcome for children and men.
  - Death by cardiovascular disease due to accelerated atherosclerosis
    - particularly as a sequela of **Diffuse Proliferative GN**

SLE Tests & Tx

- Tests:
  - ANA (not specific)
  - **anti-dsDNA** (very specific, poor prognosis)
  - **Anti-Smith** (ie. anti-Sm, very specific)
  - **Anti-histone** (drug-induced lupus)

- Tx.
  - Mild: Corticosteroids + **hydroxychloroquine**
  - Severe: Corticosteroids + **cyclophosphamide** (or **mycophenolate**)
    - Hydroxychloroquine concentrates in the lysosome → dec intracellular processing → dec immune cell functioning
    - Cyclophosphamide: alkylating agent, attaches to guanine7 and prevents DNA crosslinks
    - Mycophenolate: inhibits enzyme needed for T and B-cell growth

  - Drug-induced lupus goes away when drug is stopped and body given time to recover

SLE Summation

Most Common:
Tired **AA Female** with FUO, **arthritis**, myalgia, **butterfly rash** & mouth ulcers.
possible discoid rash and Hx spontaneous abortions

- CXR
  - **Libman-Sacks endocarditis. Serositis**: Pleuritis or pericarditis
- Kidney: MGN (nephrotic) → Diffuse Proliferative GN (nephritic)
  - Membranous Glomerulonephritis (MGN) *(covered in another set of concept-chunks)*
    - "Membranous": it's still a normal membrane with IC deposits on it
    - Spike & dome: IC build up & overfilled repaired divots
  - **Diffuse Proliferative GN**
    - Capillary walls so involved that they thicken and look like **wire loops**
- Dx: ANA, **anti-dsDNA, anti-Sm, anti-histone** (drug-induced lupus)
- Tx:
  - Mild: Corticosteroids + **hydroxychloroquine**
  - Severe: Corticosteroids + **cyclophosphamide** (or mycophenolate)
  - Drug-induced lupus goes away when drug is stopped and body given time to recover

Summary: SLE

Most Common:
Tired **AA Female** with FUO, **arthritis**, myalgia, **butterfly rash** & mouth ulcers.
possible discoid rash and Hx spontaneous abortions

- CXR: fibrous build up and immune response
  - **Libman-Sacks endocarditis**
- Kidney: MGN (nephrotic) → Diffuse Proliferative GN (nephritic)
  - Membranous Glomerulonephritis (MGN) *(covered in another set of concept-chunks)*
    - "Membranous": it's still a normal membrane with IC deposits on it
    - Spike & Dome: IC build up & overfilled repaired divots
  - **Diffuse Proliferative GN**
    - Capillary walls are so damaged that they thicken and look like **wire loops**
- Dx: ANA, **anti-dsDNA, anti-Sm, anti-histone** (drug-induced lupus)
- Tx:
  - Mild: Corticosteroids + **hydroxychloroquine**
  - Severe: Corticosteroids + **cyclophosphamide** (or mycophenolate)
  - Drug-induced lupus goes away when drug is stopped and body given time to recover

RPGN Sucks Usually 5

Pauci Immune, The Small of It

Review: Alport & RPGN Overview

- **Alport-X Syndrome**
  - Recurrent hematuria & proteinuria < 20yo, & blind or deaf
  - Mutation type IV collagen → **split GBM**
  - FHx of nephritis: **XR** (75%), AR (25%)

- **RPGN = Rapidly Progressive (Crescentic) Glomerulonephritis**
  - Dx
    - Type I: **GBM Abs**;
      - Hypersensitivity Type II rxn
    - Type II: **ANA**;
      - Hypersensitivity Type III rxn
    - Type III, aka Pauci-Immune RPGN: **ANCA**
  - Tx: corticosteroids ± immunosuppressives ± plasmapheresis
    - Immunosuppressives: **C R pregnant CAT**
      - **C**yclophosphamide or **R**ituximab
      - If pregnant: **C**yclosporine or **A**zathioprine or **T**acrolimus
    - Plasmapheresis to clear antibodies.
    - Prophylaxis for opportunistic infections: **TMP/SMX**

Review:
RPGN Type I & Type II Overview

- RPGN Type I: **Hypersensitivity Type II rxn**
  - **Goodpasture Syndrome**
    - Abs against GBM **Type-IV collagen**
    - Lungs & kidneys: hemoptysis + hematuria
- RPGN Type II: **Hypersensitivity Type III Rxn**
  - Overview:
    - Causes:
      - Henoch-Schönlein Purpura, Streptococcal infections, SLE (drugs)
    - RPGN Type II Diseases
      - Self-resolving:
        » **IgA Nephropathy** (aka Berger's Dz)
        » **Poststreptococcal Glomerulonephritis**
      - Nephrotic → Nephritic:
        » **Membranoproliferative Glomerulonephritis** (MPGN)
        » **Diffuse Proliferative Glomerulonephritis**
        » **Note:** MPGN may develop into Proliferative GN

RPGN Type II Review:
These Are Self-Resolving

- **IgA Nephropathy = Berger's Disease**
  - **IgA-based immune complexes in the mesangium** → mesangial proliferation
  - Flares up as sequela of **URI or acute gastroenteritis**
  - May be due to **Henoch-Schönlein Purpura**
    - **Henoch-Schönlein Purpura**
      - Child with **previous URI** (eg. sore throat) develops
        » arthritis, abdominal pain, and **palpable purpura in the lower body**
      - Get Plt count to r/o ITP and TTP
- **Poststreptococcal Glomerulonephritis, aka Postinfectious GN**
  - Child w/ **recent cold**, peripheral and **periorbital edema**, dark urine
  - Dx:
    - Inc **ASO** + low **C3**
    - LM: "**lumpy bumpy**"
  - Tx: Resolves spontaneously

RPGN Type II Review: Nephrotic → Nephritic

- **MPGN = Membranoproliferative Glomerulonephritis**
  - aka. **Mesangiocapillary Glomerulonephritis**
    - Mesangium: "meso" = middle, angeion = "vessel"
    - Mesangiocapillary
      - Mesangial cells are continuous w/ the smooth muscles of the arterioles.
  - **Tram-track**:
    - Mesangial cells grow in-between the GBM causing it to split and give a **tram-track** appearance
  - Caused by hepatitis (HBV, **HCV**) and C3
  - MPGN is not MGN!
    - MGN is the nephrotic, membrane is thicker due to IC deposits disease
    - MPGN is the nephritic, mesangium grew into the GBM disease
      - **the longer acronym has more wrong with the patient**
- **Diffuse Proliferative Glomerulonephritis**
  - Causes
    - **MPGN → Diffuse Proliferative GN**
    - **SLE**
  - **Wire Looping**:
    - Capillary walls thicken and resemble **wire loops**

MPGN Type III = Pauci-Immune RPGN

- No immune complex deposition nor anti-GBM Abs
- Glomeruli are damaged in undefined manner, perhaps by activation of neutrophils in response to **ANCA**
  - ANCA = anti-neutrophil cytoplasmic antibody
- May be isolated to glomerulus or associated with a systemic disease
  - Small-Vessel Vasculitis
    - **Microscopic Polyangiitis (MPA)**
      - aka. Microscopic Polyarteritis = Microscopic Polyarteritis Nodosa
  - Small- to Medium-Vessel Vasculitis
    - **Granulomatosis with Polyangiitis (GPA)**
      - formerly Wegener Granulomatosis
    - **Eosinophilic Granulomatosis with Polyangiitis (EGPA)**
      - aka. Churg-Strauss Syndrome (CSS) = Allergic Granulomatosis

MPGN Type III
(**MPA**) Microscopic Polyangiitis

- aka. **Microscopic Polyarteritis, Microscopic Polyarteritis Nodosa**
- This is a vague, often non symptomatic disease presenting as
  - fatigue/lethargy, loss of appetite/weight
  - hematuria + proteinuria (red and frothy)
- **Small-vessel vasculitis. RPGN → ESRD**

Microscopic Polyangiitis: Dx & Tx

- Dx
  - **p-ANCA** w/ myeloperoxidase specificity
  - Inc ESR, CRP, Cr
  - Anemia
  - UA: RBCs + protein
- Tx
  - Mild: long-term corticosteroids
  - Severe: add "**C R pregnant CAT**"
    - **Cyclophosphamide** or **Rituximab**
      - If pregnant: **Cyclosporine** or **Azathioprine** or **Tacrolimus**
  - **Plasmapheresis to remove p-ANCA**

MPGN Type III & Small Vessel Vasculitis Summary

- MPGN Type III = Pauci-Immune RPGN
  - activation of neutrophils in response to **ANCA**
  - Isolated to glomerulus or systemic disease
  - Small-Vessel Vasculitis
    - **Microscopic Polyangiitis (MPA)**
      - aka. Microscopic Polyarteritis = Microscopic Polyarteritis Nodosa
  - Small- to Medium-Vessel Vasculitis
    - **Granulomatosis with Polyangiitis (GPA)**
      - formerly Wegener Granulomatosis
    - **Eosinophilic Granulomatosis with Polyangiitis (EGPA)**
      - aka. Churg-Strauss Syndrome (CSS) = Allergic Granulomatosis
- **Microscopic Polyangiitis**
  - aka. **Microscopic Polyarteritis, Microscopic Polyarteritis Nodosa**
    - **Small-vessel vasculitis**. RPGN → ESRD
  - Often non symptomatic. Fatigue/lethargy, loss of appetite/weight. Urine: red and frothy
  - **p-ANCA w/ myeloperoxidase specificity**
  - Tx: long-term corticosteroids
    - Severe: add "**C R pregnant CAT**"
      - **C**yclophosphamide or **R**ituximab
        » If pregnant: **C**yclosporine or **A**zathioprine or **T**acrolimus
    - Plasmapheresis to remove p-ANCA

RPGN Sucks Usually 6

Pauci Immune, The Small and Medium of It

Review: MPGN
Type III & Small Vessel Vasculitis

- MPGN Type III = Pauci-Immune RPGN
  - activation of neutrophils in response to **ANCA**
  - Isolated to glomerulus or systemic disease
  - Small-Vessel Vasculitis
    - **Microscopic Polyangiitis (MPA)**
      - aka. Microscopic Polyarteritis = Microscopic Polyarteritis Nodosa
  - Small- to Medium-Vessel Vasculitis
    - **Granulomatosis with Polyangiitis (GPA)**
      - formerly Wegener Granulomatosis
    - **Eosinophilic Granulomatosis with Polyangiitis (EGPA)**
      - aka. Churg-Strauss Syndrome (CSS) = Allergic Granulomatosis
- **Microscopic Polyangiitis**
  - aka. **Microscopic Polyarteritis, Microscopic Polyarteritis Nodosa**
    - **Small-vessel vasculitis.** RPGN → ESRD
  - Often non symptomatic. Fatigue/lethargy, loss of appetite/weight. Urine: red and frothy
  - **p-ANCA w/ myeloperoxidase specificity**
  - Tx: long-term corticosteroids
    - Severe: add "**C R pregnant CAT**"
      - **C**yclophosphamide or **R**ituximab
        - » If pregnant: **C**yclosporine or **A**zathioprine or **T**acrolimus
    - Plasmapheresis to remove p-ANCA

MPGN Type III
(GPA) Granulomatosis w/ Polyangiitis

- Formerly, **Wegener's Granulomatosis**
  - [Wegener was a high-ranking Nazi physician who possibly experimented on Jews. Hence, the name change.]

- **Granulomatosis + polyangiitis**

- **Small and medium** sized vessels vasculitis.
  - primarily **lungs and kidneys**

GPA Usually Leads to ESRD

- **Granulomatosis with Polyangiitis** → ESRD
- ENT issues, notable:
  - Nose: **saddle-nose** and perforated septum
  - Oral: **strawberry gingivitis**, loose teeth, ulcers
  - Sight and hearing loss
- Lungs:
  - pulmonary nodules (**coin lesions**), cavitary lesions
  - infiltrates that appear as pneumonia pulmonary hemorrhage
- Arthritis, skin nodules

GPA Dx & Tx

- Test for <u>c</u>-**ANCA**
  - Pathophysiology suspected to be ANCA proliferation causing neutrophil activation leading to inflammation → granulomas
  - **C**-ANCA as in
    - **C**oin lesions. The **c**-shape of the horseshoe to go with saddle nose. **C** this is much worse than the other one. The one that doesn't have 'c' in the name is the one you test for **c**-**ANCA**
      - Concentrate on learning Granulomatosis with Polyangiitis is c-ANCA, and then the other one will be the one that isn't c-ANCA.
- Tx:
  - Mild disease & maintenance:
    - **corticosteroids + Methotrexate (MTX)**
  - Severe disease: replace MTX w/ "**C R pregnant CAT**"
    - <u>C</u>yclophosphamide or <u>R</u>ituximab
      - If pregnant: <u>C</u>yclosporine or <u>A</u>zathioprine or <u>T</u>acrolimus
  - Prevent relapse due to opportunistic infection with prophylactic:
    - **TMP/SMX**

With autoimmune diseases, maintenance often includes methotrexate (MTX)

RPGN Type III: **Eosinophilic Granulomatosis w/ Polyangiitis**

- **(EGPA) Eosinophilic Granulomatosis with Polyangiitis**
  - aka. **Churg-Strauss Syndrome (CSS)**
- Vasculitis of **small and medium sized vessels** in a person w/ a **Hx of atopy**
  - atopy = allergic hypersensitivity
- Three Stages
  1. **Prodromal:** airway inflammation
     - asthma ± allergic rhinitis
  2. **Hypereosinophilia:** tissue damage, esp. lungs and GI
  3. **Vasculitis:** cell death and possible systemic death

EGPA: Assess & Tx

- One pt for each
  - \> 65yo
  - Absence of ENT manifestations
  - Cardiac insufficiency
  - Renal insufficiency
  - GI involvement
- Tx
  - 1 present = Mild: glucocorticoids
  - ≥ 2 present = Severe: + **cyclophosphamide**
  - Maintenance therapy:
    - **Methotrexate (MTX)** or **Azathioprine** or Leflunomide for **18m**

RPGN Type III EGPA Summary

- (**EGPA**) **Eosinophilic Granulomatosis with Polyangiitis**
  - aka. **Churg-Strauss Syndrome (CSS)**
  - Vasculitis of **small and medium sized vessels** in a person w/ a **Hx of atopy**
  - Three Stages
    1. **Prodromal**: airway inflammation: asthma +/- allergic rhinitis
    2. **Hypereosinophilia**: tissue damage, esp. lungs and GI
    3. **Vasculitis**: eventual cell death and possible systemic death
- One pt for each:
  - \> 65yo, absence of ENT manifestations
  - Cardiac, Renal, GI
- 1 present = Mild: glucocorticoids.
- ≥ 2 present – Severe: + **cyclophosphamide**
- Maintenance therapy:
  - **Methotrexate (MTX)** or **Azathioprine** or Leflunomide for **18m**

MPGN Type III: GPA Summary

- [Formerly, **Wegener's Granulomatosis**]
  - **Small and medium** sized vessels vasculitis.
  - **Saddle-nose, strawberry gingivitis, coin lesions**
- Test for <u>**c**</u>**-ANCA**
- Tx:
  - Mild disease & maintenance:
    - **corticosteroids + Methotrexate (MTX)**
  - Severe disease: replace MTX w/ "**C R pregnant CAT**"
    - <u>**C**</u>**yclophosphamide** or <u>**R**</u>**ituximab**
      - If pregnant: <u>**C**</u>**yclosporine** or <u>**A**</u>**zathioprine** or <u>**T**</u>**acrolimus**
  - Prevent relapse due to opportunistic infection with prophylactic:
    - **TMP/SMX**

With autoimmune diseases, maintenance often includes methotrexate (MTX)

RPGN Sucks Usually 7

Round'em Up

Review
Alport & RPGN Overview

- **Alport-X Syndrome**: recurrent nephritic, blind/deaf
  - Mutation <u>type IV collagen</u> → **split GBM**
  - FHx of nephritis: **XR** (75%), AR (25%)

- **RPGN = Rapidly Progressive (Crescentic) Glomerulonephritis**
  - Types
    - I, Hypersensitivity Type II rxn: **GBM Abs**
    - II, Hypersensitivity Type III rxn: **ANA**
    - III = Pauci-Immune RPGN. **ANCA**
  - Tx: corticosteroids ± **C R pregnant CAT** ± plasmapheresis
    - **C**yclophosphamide or **R**ituximab
      - If pregnant: **C**yclosporine or **A**zathioprine or **T**acrolimus

Review
RPGN Type I & Type II Overview

- RPGN Type I, **Hypersensitivity Type II rxn: Goodpasture Syndrome**
  - Abs against GBM **Type-IV collagen.**
  - Lungs & kidneys: hemoptysis + hematuria

- RPGN Type II, **Hypersensitivity Type III Rxn**
  - Causes:
    - Henoch-Schönlein Purpura, Streptococcal infections, SLE (drugs)
  - Self-resolving:
    - **IgA Nephropathy** (aka Berger's Dz)
    - **Poststreptococcal Glomerulonephritis**
  - Nephrotic → Nephritic:
    - **Membranoproliferative Glomerulonephritis** (MPGN)
    - **Diffuse Proliferative Glomerulonephritis**
    - MPGN may develop into Proliferative GN

Review
RPGN Type II: The Self-Resolving

- **IgA Nephropathy = Berger's Disease**
  - URI or acute gastroenteritis → flare up
  - **Henoch-Schönlein Purpura**
    - Child with **previous URI** (eg. sore throat) develops
      - arthritis, abdominal pain, and **palpable purpura in the lower body**
    - **Get Plt count to r/o ITP and TTP**

- **Poststreptococcal Glomerulonephritis**
  - Child w/ **recent cold**, peripheral and **periorbital edema**, dark urine
  - Inc **ASO** + low **C3**
  - LM: "**lumpy bumpy**"

Review
RPGN Type II: Nephrotic → Nephritic

- **MPGN = Membranoproliferative Glomerulonephritis**
  - aka. **Mesangiocapillary Glomerulonephritis**
    - Mesangium: "meso" = middle, angeion = "vessel"
    - Mesangiocapillary: Mesangial cells continuous w/ smooth muscles of arterioles.
  - **Tram-track**:
    - Mesangial cells grow in-between the GBM causing it to split
  - Caused by hepatitis (HBV, **HCV**) and C3
- **Diffuse Proliferative Glomerulonephritis**
  - Causes
    - **MPGN → Diffuse Proliferative GN**
    - **SLE**
  - **Wire Looping**:
    - Capillary walls thicken and resemble **wire loops**

Review SLE

Most Common:
Tired **AA Female** with FUO, **arthritis**, myalgia, **butterfly rash** & mouth ulcers.
possible **discoid rash** and Hx **spontaneous abortions**

- CXR: fibrous build up and immune response
  - **Libman-Sacks endocarditis**
- Kidney: MGN (nephrotic) → Diffuse Proliferative GN (nephritic)
  - Membranous Glomerulonephritis (MGN) *(covered in another set of concept-chunks)*
    - "Membranous": it's still a normal membrane with IC deposits on it
    - Spike and dome: IC build up & overfilled repaired divots
  - **Diffuse Proliferative GN**
    - **Wire loops**: Capillary walls are so damaged that they thicken
- Dx: ANA, **anti-dsDNA**, **anti-Sm**, **anti-histone** (drug-induced lupus)
- Tx:
  - Mild: Corticosteroids + **hydroxychloroquine**
  - Severe: Corticosteroids + **cyclophosphamide** (or mycophenolate)
  - Drug-induced lupus goes away when drug is stopped and body given time to recover

Review MPGN
Type III & Small Vessel Vasculitis

- **MPGN Type III = Pauci-Immune RPGN**
  - activation of neutrophils in response to **ANCA**
  - Small-Vessel Vasculitis
    - **Microscopic Polyangiitis (MPA)**
      - aka. Microscopic Polyarteritis = Microscopic Polyarteritis Nodosa
  - Small- to Medium-Vessel Vasculitis
    - **Granulomatosis with Polyangiitis (GPA)**
      - formerly Wegener Granulomatosis
    - **Eosinophilic Granulomatosis with Polyangiitis (EGPA)**
      - aka. Churg-Strauss Syndrome (CSS) = Allergic Granulomatosis
- Small-Vessel Vasculitis
  - **Microscopic Polyangiitis = Microscopic Polyarteritis Nodosa**
    - Often non symptomatic. Fatigue/lethargy, loss of appetite/weight. Urine: red and frothy
    - **p-ANCA w/ myeloperoxidase specificity**
    - Long-term corticosteroids. When severe, add "**C R pregnant CAT**"
      - <u>C</u>yclophosphamide or <u>R</u>ituximab
        » If pregnant: <u>C</u>yclosporine or <u>A</u>zathioprine or <u>T</u>acrolimus

Review MPGN Type III:
Small to Medium Vessel Vasculitis

- **Granulomatosis with Polyangiitis** [Formerly, Wegener's Granulomatosis]
  - **Saddle-nose, strawberry gingivitis, coin lesions**
  - <u>c</u>-**ANCA**
  - Corticosteroids + **Methotrexate (MTX)**.
    - Severe: replace MTX w/ "C R pregnant CAT"

- **(EGPA) Eosinophilic Granulomatosis with Polyangiitis**
  - aka. **Churg-Strauss Syndrome (CSS)**
  - **Hx of atopy**
  - Three Stages
    1. **Prodromal**: airway inflammation: asthma +/- allergic rhinitis
    2. **Hypereosinophilia**: tissue damage, esp. lungs and GI
    3. **Vasculitis**: eventual cell death and possible systemic death
  - One pt for each: > 65yo, Absence of ENT, Cardiac, Renal, GI
    - 1 present = Mild: glucocorticoids.
    - ≥ 2 present = Severe: + **cyclophosphamide**
    - Maintenance therapy:
      » **Methotrexate (MTX)** or **Azathioprine** or Leflunomide for **18m**

FIRST DRUG TALK

Antibiotics 1

The Overall Groupings

This Module Is Different

- I don't know that a way exists to tie the Abx into memorable, teachable pieces.
  - This is an attempt to group them.
  - Don't try and learn them all at once. Instead, memorize them within their treatment groups.
    - The similarities of treatment become more apparent this way.
  - Separate groups by time and place.
    - Don't cover respiratory and UTI at the same time.
      - If you have to cover more material, do the respiratory + another lesson from somewhere else on Day-1, and then do UTI + another lesson from somewhere else on Day-2.
- Remember to store them in chunks.
  - No list longer than 5, preferably 3-4. If you have more items, you need deeper lists (ie. lists of lists).

Broad Types

- Interfere With
  - Cell Wall Synthesis
  - Nucleic Acid Synthesis
  - Protein Synthesis

Interferes w/ Cell Wall Synthesis

- Beta Lactams
- Vancomycin, Bacitracin
- Polymyxins
  - actually interfere with cell membrane

Beta Lactams

- Penicillins
- Cephalosporins
- Carbapenems
- Monobactams

Interferes w/ Nucleic Acid Synthesis

Be careful w/ pregnancy

- Folate Synthesis
  - Sulfonamides, Trimethoprim
- DNA Gyrase
  - Quinolones
- RNA Polymerase
  - Rifampin

Interferes w/ Protein Synthesis

- 30s Subunit
  - Tetracyclines
  - Aminoglycosides (TAGS)
    - Tobramycin, Amikacin, Gentamycin, Streptomycin
- 50s Subunit
  - Macrolides (ACE), clindamycin
    - ACE: azi-, clari-, ery-thromycin
  - Linezolid, Chloramphenicol
  - Streptogramins
    - ie. quinupristin/dalfopristin

Only Two Treatments Today

- Endocarditis:
  - Vanc (cell wall) + gent (30s)
    - Life-threatening w/ significant sequela, so we hit this infection hard.
      - Go after the cell wall to kill on contact, and we prevent further protein production limiting spread and development.
- Spontaneous bacterial peritonitis:
  - Cefotaxime (cell wall)
    - Very good, broad-spectrum 3rd-gen cephalosporin

Broad Type Summary

- Interfere With
  - Cell Wall Synthesis
    - Beta Lactams
      - Penicillins, Cephalosporins
      - Carbapenems, Monobactams
    - Vancomycin, Bacitracin
    - Polymyxins (Cell Membrane)
  - Nucleic Acid Synthesis
    - Folate Synthesis: Sulfonamides, Trimethoprim
    - DNA Gyrase: Quinolones
    - RNA Polymerase: Rifampin
  - Protein Synthesis
    - 30s Subunit: Tetracyclines, aminoglycosides (TAGS)
    - 50s Subunit
      - Macrolides (ACE), clindamycin
      - Linezolid, Chloramphenicol
      - Streptogramins (ie. quinupristin/dalfopristin)

Today's Treatment Summary

- Endocarditis: **Vanc + gent**
- Spontaneous bacterial peritonitis: **Cefotaxime**

Antibiotics 2

Respiratory

The Go to Treatments Seen in Training Hospitals Every Day

- Bacterial meningitis
  - **Ceftriaxone + vanc + steroids ± ampicillin**
  - Life and death headache, non-stroke
- Otitis Media or Sinusitis or Pharyngitis
  - **Amoxicillin**
- Lung Abscess: **Clindamycin** or **PCN**
  - aspiration ~ anaerobes
  - eg. alcoholic, very sick, horrible breath

Respiratory Infection

- CAP = Community Acquired Pneumonia
  - Outpatient: **Azithromycin** (50s) or Doxycycline (30s)
  - Inpatient, previous Abx or comorbidities:
    - **Levofloxacin** (DNA) or
    - Ceftriaxone + azithromycin
- HAP = Hospital Acquired Pneumonia
  - Ceftazidime (3rd gen) or **Cefepime** (4th gen) or
  - Carbapenems or
  - Piperacillin + tazobactam

Respiration Summary

- Bacterial meningitis
  - Ceftriaxone + vanc + steroids ± ampicillin
- Otitis Media or Sinusitis or Pharyngitis
  - Amoxicillin
- Lung Abscess: Clindamycin or PCN
  - ie. aspiration pneumonia
- CAP
  - Outpatient: **Azithromycin** (50s) or Doxycycline (30s)
  - Inpatient: **Levofloxacin** (DNA) or (Ceftriaxone + azithromycin)
- HAP: Ceftazidime (3rd gen) or **Cefepime** (4th gen) or
  - Carbapenems or (Piperacillin + tazobactam)

Treatments For Next Time

- GI: Severe infectious diarrhea:
  - **Ciprofloxacin**
- Urinary
  - UTI: Ciprofloxacin or TMP/SMX
    - If pregnant, **nitrofurantoin**
  - Cystitis: **Cephalexin**
  - Acute Prostatitis or Pyelonephritis: **amp + gent**

Antibiotics 3

GI, Urinary, GU

GI Infection

- Severe infectious diarrhea:
  - **Ciprofloxacin**

Urinary Infections

- UTI: Ciprofloxacin or TMP/SMX
  - If pregnant, **nitrofurantoin**
- Cystitis: **Cephalexin**
- Acute Prostatitis: amp + gent
- Pyelonephritis: **amp + gent**
  - If fever after 5 days of Abx, suspect abscess
  - Image: U/S or CT → Drain and treat

GU Infections

- Urethritis or PID
  - Ceftriaxone (or cefixime) + azithromycin (or doxy)
  - Get a pregnancy test
- Post-partum endometritis
  - clinda + gent

GI & GU Summary

- GI
  - Severe infectious diarrhea: Ciprofloxacin
- Urinary
  - UTI: Ciprofloxacin or TMP/SMX
    - If pregnant, **nitrofurantoin**
  - Cystitis: **Cephalexin**
  - Acute Prostatitis or Pyelonephritis: amp + gent
- GU
  - Urethritis or PID: Ceftriaxone + azithromycin
  - Post-partum endometritis: clinda + gent

For Next Time: Skin Infection

- Impetigo
  - Mild: topical, mupirocin or bacitracin
  - Severe: PO, doxy or clinda or Bactrim (TMP/SMX)
- Cellulitis
  - Mild: PO, dicloxacillin or cephalexin
    - w/ allergy: macrolide (ACE) or clinda
  - Severe: IV, nafcillin or oxacillin or cefazolin
    - w/ allergy: clinda
- MRSA
  - Vancomycin, Linezolid
  - Ceftaroline (5th gen)
- VRSA
  - Linezolid, dalfopristin/quinupristin

Antibiotics 4

Skin

Skin Infection

- Impetigo
  - Mild: topical, mupirocin or bacitracin
  - Severe: PO, doxy or clinda or Bactrim (TMP/SMX)
- Cellulitis
  - Mild: PO, dicloxacillin or cephalexin
    - w/ allergy: macrolide (ACE) or clinda
  - Severe: IV, nafcillin or oxacillin or cefazolin
    - w/ allergy: clinda

MRSA & VRSA

- MRSA
  - Vancomycin, Linezolid
  - Ceftaroline (5th gen)
- VRSA
  - Linezolid, dalfopristin/quinupristin

Skin Infection Summary

- Impetigo
  - Mild: topical, mupirocin or bacitracin
  - Severe: PO, doxy or clinda or Bactrim (TMP/SMX)
- Cellulitis
  - Mild: PO, dicloxacillin or cephalexin
    - w/ allergy: macrolide (ACE) or clinda
  - Severe: IV, nafcillin or oxacillin or cefazolin
    - w/ allergy: clinda
- MRSA
  - Vancomycin, Linezolid
  - Ceftaroline (5th gen)
- VRSA
  - Linezolid, dalfopristin/quinupristin

Think About This For Next Time

- What if your patient is losing serum protein?
- What if your patient has ARF or ESRD?
- What if you need systemic coverage including the CNS?

Antibiotics 5

Abx Considerations

Unexpected SE

- Sulfonamides compete w/ albumin
  - Thiazides & Furosemide are sulfonamides, but if you're losing albumin, your patient probably isn't hypertensive, and therefore, is not on these.
  - TMP/SMX (ie. Bactrim) interfere with the production of tetrahydrofolate, and therefore Bactrim interferes with DNA.
    - TMP/SMX is a goto drug for UTI and skin infections. It is regularly used for GI and respiratory.
      - Very easy to exacerbate hypoalbuminemia-related issues without realizing it.
- Aminoglycosides
  - Decrease ACh release into synapse
  - Acts as neuromuscular blocker
  - ie. If your patient experiences respiratory depression, check if they're on an aminoglycoside (TAGS).

Renal Clearance

- PCN's:
  - except oxacillin & nafcillin
- Cephalosporins:
  - except cefoperazone & ceftriaxone
  - inhibit exceptions w/ probenicid

- If your patient has ARF or ESRD, these are not the drugs you want.
  - Unless the pt is getting regularly hemodialysis
    - Then maybe

BBB

- Only 2nd-gen that cross:
  - cefuroxime
- All 3rd-gens cross, except:
  - cefoperazone

Disulfram-like Rxn

- Cefotetan and cefoperazone
  - Cefoperazone is exception to most 3rd-gen rules
    - All 3rd gens cross BBB except cefoperazone
    - All cephalosporins renally cleared except cefoperazone

Contraindication Summary

- Hypoalbuminemia
  - Contraindication to TMP/SMX (ie. Bactrim)
- Your patient begins to experience unexpected respiratory depression
  - Are they on a aminoglycoside (TAGS)?
- Infection w/ Kidney Failure
  - No PCNs, except oxacillin & nafcillin
  - No cephalosporins, except ceftriaxone or cefoperazone
- Do you want or not want to cross the BBB?
  - Only 2nd-gen that crosses BBB: cefuroxime
  - All 3rd-gens cross BBB, except: cefoperazone
- Your patient is experiencing a disulfram-like reaction
  - Are they receiving cefotetan and cefoperazone?

NEWBORN CENTRIC

Newborn Screenings

Newborn Screenings

- **State by state basis**
- Most
  - Measure metabolites and enzyme activity
  - Many areas are starting to screen infants for hearing loss and congenital heart defects
  - Infants who screen positive undergo further testing
  - Follow-up testing is typically coordinated between geneticists and the infant's pediatrician or PCP

PKU = Phenylketonuria

- **Deficiency of phenylalanine hydroxylase →** inc **phenylalanine** (PHE) in body fluids and CNS
- Mental and growth retardation, vomiting, athetosis, seizures
  - Athetosis = athetoid movements = slow writhing movements of body. Most likely distal
  - Generally lesions to the corpus striatum
    - caudate nucleus, putamen, globus pallidus
  - Often accompanies cerebral palsy
- **Fair hair, fair skin, blue eyes**
- Tx: **low PHE diet for life**

Cerebral Palsy

- Permanent disorders of movement and posture due to non-progressive disturbances in fetal/ infant brain development
  - ie. Don't move correctly or take postures that are normal, but condition doesn't get worse.

Classic Galactosemia

- Galactose-1-P uridylyltransferase (**G1PUDT**) deficiency
  - →accumulation of **gal-1-P**
  - → injured kidney, liver, brain
- Hepatomegaly, jaundice, hypoglycemia
- Cataract, mental retardation, seizures
- **Predisposition to E. coli sepsis**
- Tx:
  - **No lactose** in diet:
    - reverses most problems but not neurodevelopmental

Summary: PKU & Classic Galactosemia

- **PKU**
  - Deficiency of phenylalanine hydroxylase → inc PHE
  - Athetosis, lesions to corpus striatum, seizures, often accompanies cerebral palsy
    - Cerebral palsy = Permanent disorders of movement and posture due to non-progressive disturbances in fetal/infant brain development
  - **Fair hair, fair skin, blue eyes**
  - Tx: **low PHE diet for life**
- **Classic Galactosemia**
  - **G1PUDT** deficiency → inc **gal-1-P**
    - → injured kidney, liver, brain
  - **Predisposition to E. coli sepsis**
  - Tx: **No lactose** in diet

Newborn Defects 1

Baseline Assessment

APGAR Score

- This is your first evaluation of an infant. Standardization of grading helps all involved to evaluate these first critical periods and judge the progress.

- **A**ppearance/complexion
- **P**ulse rate
- **G**rimace (reflex irritability)
- **A**ctivity
- **R**espiratory effort

Really only have to memorize a couple of things past the acronym

APGAR Scoring: Max of 10

- **Appearance, Pulse, Grimace, Activity, Respiration:** Scoring
  - In general, doesn't have one of the above is a score of **0**.
  - Has a little of one of the above is a score of **1**.
  - Is normal-ish or strongly does one of the above is a score of **2**
  - Appearance:
    - blue or pale is 0
    - **blue extremities and body pink is 1**
    - no cyanosis is 2
  - Pulse:
    - absent is 0, 1pt < **100bpm** < 2

APGAR Summary

- **Appearance, Pulse, Grimace** (reflex irritability)
- **Activity, Respiratory effort**
- 0 or 1 or 2
  - blue + pink 1
  - 100bpm
- APGAR @ 1 and 5 minutes, then every 5 minutes as long as resuscitation continues
  - Not predictive of outcome, except for neurological

Gestational Age & Size Defined

Dates are measured from last day of **LMP**
- Preterm: < **37w**
- Low birth wt: < **2500g**
- Large for Gestational Age (**LGA**) = Fetal **Macrosomia**
  - Birth wt > **4500g** at term
  - Often sequela of obesity and/or diabetes
  - Increased birth injuries and congenital anomalies
- Post-term: > **42w**
  - Delivery >3w past term significantly increases mortality

VACTERAL Association

- (formerly VATER associations)
- **V**ertebral anomalies
- **A**nal atresia
- **C**ardiac defects
- **T**racheoesophageal fistula and/or **E**sophageal atresia
- **R**enal & **Radial** anomalies
- **L**imb defects
  - **If find one of these in a newborn, you must check for the rest.**
    - Not pathogenically related like a syndrome, but tend to occur together

Birth Considerations Summary

- Gestational Age and Size
  - Preterm: < **37w**. Post-term: > **42w**
  - Low birth wt: < **2500g**.
  - Macrosomia (ie. LGA): > **4500g**
- **VACTERAL** Association
  - **V**ertebral anomalies, **A**nal atresia, **C**ardiac defects
  - **T**racheoesophageal fistula and/or **E**sophageal atresia
  - **R**enal & **Radial** anomalies
  - **L**imb defects

Newborn Defects 2

Edward and Patau Make a WAGeR

Story Time

- Tina Edwards is Tony Patau's older cousin. Tina **Edwards** is a **female** adult, being **18yo**, while Tony Patau has just hit puberty at 13yo. Whenever Tina Edwards gets mad, she **clenches her hands**, sticks her **stomach out**, and **rocks back and forth on her feet**.

- <u>Both of their moms were pretty old when they had kids.</u>

18 Edwards, 13 Patau: Story

- Tina Edwards is Tony Patau's older cousin. Tina **Edwards** is a female (**80%**) adult, being **18yo** (chr18), while Tony Patau has just hit puberty at 13yo (chr13). Whenever Tina Edwards gets mad, she clenches her hands (**index over 3rd, 5th or 4th**), sticks her stomach out (**omphalocele**), and rocks back and forth on her feet (**rocker-bottom feet** and hammer toe).

13yo Patau

- **Patau**, being **13**yo never completely developed (**holoprosencephaly**). She's very quiet and doesn't talk much (**severe cleft lip and/or palate**).

Trisomy 13 = Patau

- Defect in mid face, eye, and forebrain development
- A single defect in 3w → holoprosencephaly (**failure to develop into two hemispheres**).
- Facial: severe cleft lip and/or palate

Summary: 18 Edwards, 13 Patau

- **Edwards**
  - chr18
  - female, clinched hand (2 over 3, 5 over 4), omphalocele, rocker-bottom feet
- **Patau**
  - chr13
  - holoprosencephaly, defects in mid fact (cleft lip/ palate)
    - w/ some of Edwards stuff (not the hand thing though)
      - only an 18yo clinches her hands and rocks back and forth

Newborn Defects 3

Renal Defects

& Chromosomes

Potter Sequence

- Renal agenesis or other urinary tract defect → **oligohydramnios**
  - Oligohydramnios = deficiency of amniotic fluid
    - Amniotic fluid needed for movement and spacing.
    - Lungs exchange amniotic fluid with environment to aid development
  - Lack of amniotic fluid → **fetal compression, pulmonary hypoplasia**
    - Death from respiratory insufficiency due to hypoplasia
- Potter facies
  - Wide spaced eyes, epicanthal folds
  - Flat nose and ears, micrognathia

Renal Defects Summary

- Potter Sequence
  - Renal agenesis → **oligohydramnios**
  → **facial compression, pulmonary hypoplasia**
  - Potter facies
    - Wide spaced eyes, epicanthal folds, flat nose and ears, micrognathia
- WAGR Syndrome = del 11p13
  - **W**ilms tumor, **A**niridia, **G**onad tumors, **R**etardation

WAGR Syndrome

- **W**ilms: child kidney tumor
- **A**niridia: no iris
- **G**onad tumors
- **R**etardation
- del 11p13

EDS = Ehlers-**DA**nlos Syndrome

- DA: Dominant Autosomal (or Autosomal dominant)
- Hyperextensible skin, droopy ears, easily bruised, poor healing
- Joint hyperlaxity, tendency to dislocation
- Heart dilatations, intracranial aneurysm
- Blue sclera, ectopia lentis
  - ectopia lentis = displacement of lens

Klinefelter Syndrome (XXY)

- IQ 85-90 w/ behavioral issues
- Slim w/ long limbs
- Ambiguous genitalia w/ breasts
  - Obviously Dx at puberty most of the time

Fragile X Syndrome

- Male, broken X, **CGG** repeats
  - Carrier females can be affected
- Mild to profound learning problems
- Very **Marfan-like**:
  - large ears, large jaw, long face
- **Macroorchidism** (large testes)
- Normal lifespan

Klinefelter vs Fragile X

- Slow wit, slim long limbs and boobs
  - Felter boobs
  - vs.
- Slower wit, long face, big ears, big testes

Fragile Summary

- EDS
  - Hyperextensible skin, easily bruised, poor healing
  - Joint hyperlaxity, tendency to dislocation
  - Heart dilatations, intracranial aneurysm
  - Blue sclera, ectopia lentis
- Klinefelter
  - Slow witted, slim limbs, ambiguous sex w/ breasts
  - Mnemonic: felter boobs
- Fragile X
  - Male, broken X, **CGG** repeats
  - Much slower wit, Marfan-like, macroorchidism

Newborn Defects – Heart 1

Left to Right Shunts 1

Left-to-Right Shunts

- VSD
- ASD
- Endocardial Cushion Defect
- PDA

VSD = Ventricular Septal Defect

- Most common congenital heart lesion.
  - Most are membranous
- **PVR** (pulmonary vascular resistance) to **SVR** (systemic vascular resistance) ratio determines the intensity of the shunt
  - **When PVR falls in first few weeks of life, the shunt increases**
    - SVR becomes increasingly greater than PVR making retrograde movement the direction of less pressure
    - If flow continues until PVR > SVR (**Eisenmenger's syndrome**), this causes the left-to-right shunt to become a right-to-left shunt → cyanosis. **Very bad!**

VSD = Ventricular Septal Defect

- Harsh, **holosystolic** murmur over left lower sternal border, possible thrill, and **widely split S2**
  - Can also hear across the mitral valve
- Tx
  - Small ones resolve < **2yo**
  - Surgery if
    - FTV unable to be managed medically
    - < 1yo: large defect + pulmonary HTN
    - > 2yo: pulmonary flow/systemic flow > 2/1

PDA = Patent Ductus Arteriosus

- Maternal **rubella infection or premie**
- Small ones are asymptomatic and close spontaneously
- Large: wide pulse pressure, bounding arterial pulses, dec diastolic BP
  - **Sounds like machine**
- CXR:
  - inc pulmonary artery + pulmonary markings + edema
- Tx: **premies get indomethacin** → surgery

VSD & PDA Summary

- VSD
  - As PVR/SVR decreases, left-to-right shunt increases
  - If PVR > SVR = **Eisenmenger's syndrome**
    - Becomes a right-to-left shunt → cyanosis
  - Harsh, **holosystolic** murmur over left lower sternal border, **widely split S2**
- PDA
  - Small ones close spontaneously
  - Large ones:
    - Wide pulse pressure, bounding arterial pulses, dec diastolic BP
    - **Sounds like machine**
  - CXR: inc pulmonary artery + pulmonary markings + edema
  - Tx: **premies get indomethacin** → surgery

Newborn Defects – Heart 2

Left to Right Shunts 2,
Pulmonic Stenosis

ASD = Atrial Septal Defect

- No symptoms early on but get worse as exercise demands increase.
  - Body often copes until into 20's.
- Large lesions can be heard across tricuspid valve
  - Diastolic murmur
  - Wide fixed split S2
- Cardiomegaly (enlarged right side)
  - EKG will show a right-axis deviation
- Tx: most close spontaneously → surgery

Endocardial Cushion Defect

- Structure
  - ASD contiguous w/ VSD + abnormal AV valves
  - Mild intermittent cyanosis
    - due to mix of left-to-right shunting and right-to-left shunting

- AV valve insufficiency → inc volume load on one or both sides of ventricles
  → cyanosis, FTV, hepatomegaly, and early heart failure
  - Possible sequela: Eisenmenger's Syndrome, precordial bulge

- Wide fixed split S2, pulmonary ejection murmur, rumble at left sternum and apex

- Tx: surgery in infancy or death from HF

Left to Right Shunts:
ASD & Endocardial Cushion Defects

- ASD
  - Tricuspid valve: Diastolic murmur w/ wide fixed split S2
  - Cardiomegaly. EKG: right-axis deviation
  - Tx: most close spontaneously, else surgery

- Endocardial Cushion Defect
  - ASD contiguous w/ VSD + abnormal AV valves → Mild intermittent cyanosis
    Mild intermittent cyanosis, hepatomegaly, and early heart failure
  - Left sternum and apex: Wide fixed split S2 and pulmonary ejection murmur

Pulmonic Stenosis

- Noonan Syndrome or Alagille Syndrome
- Tx: balloon valvuloplasty → surgery

Noonan Syndrome AD

- **The male version of Turner's syndrome**
  - *It's actually AD and effect both sexes, but this give you the picture*
  - Heart defects, short, learning problems, pectus excavatum, impaired blood clotting, webbed neck, flat nose bridge
- Cause: disruption of **RAS-MAPK pathway**
- Similar in frequency to Downs

Alagille Syndrome AD

- Arteriohepatic dysplasia
  - heat, liver, kidney dysplasia
  - Ranges from unnoticeable to looking like liver failure
    - Jaundice, pruritus, xanthomas
    - Heart defects
- Common:
  - broad, prominent forehead, deep-set eyes, small pointed chin

Congenital Pulmonic Stenosis Summary

- **AD: Noonan = male version of Turner's**
  - Disruption of **RAS-MAPK pathway**
  - Similar in frequency to Downs
- AD: Alagille Syndrome = Arteriohepatic Dysplasia
  - Broad, prominent forehead, deep-set eyes, small pointed chin
  - Heat, liver, kidney dysplasia.
    - Variable penetrance.

Summary Left to Right Shunt: ASD & Endocardial Cushion Defects

- ASD
  - Tricuspid valve: Diastolic murmur w/ wide fixed split S2
  - Cardiomegaly. EKG: right-axis deviation
  - Tx: most close spontaneously, else surgery

- Endocardial Cushion Defect
  - ASD contiguous w/ VSD + abnormal AV valves → Mild intermittent cyanosis
  - Mild intermittent cyanosis, hepatomegaly, and early heart failure
  - Left sternum and apex: Wide fixed split S2 and pulmonary ejection murmur

Congenital Pulmonic Stenosis Summary

- **AD: Noonan = male version of Turner's**
  - Disruption of **RAS-MAPK pathway**
- AD: Alagille Syndrome
  - ie. Arteriohepatic Dysplasia
  - Broad, prominent forehead, deep-set eyes, small pointed chin
  - Heat, liver, kidney dysplasia.
    - Variable penetrance.

Newborn Defects – Heart 3

Aortic Stenosis

Aortic Stenosis

- Most have **bicuspid aortic valve**.
  - ie. Turner Syndrome
    - Turner also has **coarctation of the aorta**
- Usually asymptomatic.
  - Williams Syndrome
- Right 2nd-intercostal space w/ radiation to neck and left midsternal border
  - Possible thrill in suprasternal notch

Williams Syndrome

- *William Shakespeare loved 7 elves*
  - *A little dim, but cheerful and can easily talk to strangers*
  - *They develop big ears, big anxieties, and slow hearts*

- del chr 7 → neurodevelopmental disorder
- **Elfin face**:
  - low nasal bridge, cheerful and ease w/ strangers
- Developmental day but **strong language skills**.
  - Develop **higher anxiety levels and phobias** along w/ hyperacusis
    - hyperacusis = high sound sensitivity at certain frequencies
- CV issues w/ transient hypercalcemia

Preductal Tubular Hypoplasia
Infantile Type

- Narrowing starting at head and/or neck vessels and extending to ductus
  - Right ventricular BF across the PDA supplies the descending aorta to perfuse the lower body
  - Upper body pink, lower body cyanotic → HF as ductus closes

- PE:
  - Cyanotic lower body, acidosis, with worsening severe HF and large heart
  - Systolic murmur along left sternal border

Preductal Tubular Hypoplasia Infantile Type

- CXR:
  - Large heart
  - Inc size of subclavian artery
  - Notching of inferior border of ribs
- EKG:
  - As neonate shows biventricular hypertrophy
    - Gets older, shows left ventricular hypertrophy
- Tx: PGE1 to maintain PDA → surgery

Preductal Tubular Hypoplasia

- Adult Type
  - Delayed femoral pulse and weaker pulses in LE in general
  - BP greater in right arm than left suggests involvement of left subclavian artery
  - Rib notching

Aortic Stenosis Summary

- Most asymptomatic **bicuspid aortic valve**.
  - Turner is bicuspid w/ **coarctation of the aorta**
- *William Shakespeare loved 7 elves*
  - *A little dim, but cheerful and can easily talk to strangers*
  - *They develop big ears, big anxieties, and slow hearts*
- *Preductal Tubular Hypoplasia*
  - Narrowing between head and ductus
  - Upper body pink, lower body cyanotic → HF as ductus closes
    - and acidosis
  - CXR: cardiomegaly, inc subclavian artery, inferior notching
  - EKG: biventricular hypertrophy → left ventricular hypertrophy
  - Tx: PGE1 to maintain PDA → surgery

Newborn Defects – Heart 4

Right to Left Shunts 1

Right-to-Left Shunts

- These are cyanotic conditions. The 5 T's
  - Tetralogy of Fallot
  - Truncus Arteriosis
  - Transposition of Great Vessels
  - Total Anomalous Pulmonary Venous Return
  - Tricuspid Atresia

Tetralogy of Fallot (**TOF**)

- Most common cyanotic heart defect
  ~ del 22, DiGeorge Syndrome, environmental
- Survival w/o surgery:
  - 75% (1yo), 60% (4yo), 30% (10yo), 5% (40yo)
  - With surgery, you can be the best in the world at snowboarding (Shaun White)
- Result of anterior malalignment of aorticopulmonary septum
  - Pulmonary infundibular stenosis
  - Right ventricular hypertrophy
  - Overriding aorta
  - Ventricular septal defect
- **Boot-shaped heart**

Pulmonary Infundibular Stenosis

- Narrowed right ventricular outflow tract
  - Generally caused by overgrowth of the heart muscle wall or overriding aorta
  - Probably secondary to pulmonic stenosis
  - The level of affect determines the severity of TOF
  - Right ventricular hypertrophy is secondary to this.
- Overriding aorta
  - Aortic valve w/ biventricular connection:
    - Above ventricular septal deflect and connected to both right and left ventricles
- Ventricular septal defect

TOF Pathophysiology

- Right-side can't pump blood into pulmonary artery correctly, so the right ventricle gets more muscular → hypertrophy → Boot-shaped heart
- Given the overriding aorta, unoxygenated blood from the right ventricle, which is having trouble going into the pulmonary artery, can flow directly out to the system, as can oxygenated blood from the left ventricle. Thus, blood flowing to the system is a mix of oxygenated and unoxygenated blood depending on the severity of the pulmonic stenosis and the degree of the overriding aorta
  - Sometimes the aorta is only 5% of the right ventricle. Sometimes it's 95%
- On top of that, the ventricular septal defect (VSD) also allows a mixing of blood. As the pulmonic stenosis gets worse, more unoxygenated blood accumulates in the left ventricle and is expelled into the system via the aortic valve or the overriding aorta.
- As you can see, the right ventricle has a lot of pressure to overcome due to this convoluted backup which gets worse as the pulmonic stenosis gets worse, and pulmonic stenosis is primarily a result of right-ventricle hypertrophy. Vicious cycle.

Blue Baby

- In neonate, you look for cyanosis.
- Older kids
  - Progressively become bluer
  - Have marked clubbing and dyspnea on exertion.
  - To overcome the dyspnea, child will squat.
    - This increases the systemic vascular resistance → dec right-to-left shunt.
- Tx:
  - Neonate get PGE1 to prevent PDA closure → surgery

TOF Summary

- Tetralogy caused by anterior malalignment of aorticopulmonary septum
  - Pulmonary infundibular stenosis → Narrowed right ventricular outflow tract
  - Right ventricular hypertrophy (results of above) → **boot-shaped heart**
  - Overriding aorta (mixing of blood)
  - Ventricular septal defect (mixing of blood)
    - As the pulmonic stenosis gets worse → inc unoxygenated blood expelled into system
      - Squatting helps inc systemic pressure to offset

Newborn Defects – Heart 5

Right to Left Shunts 2

TOF Review

- **Tetralogy** caused by anterior malalignment of aorticopulmonary septum
  - **Pulmonary infundibular stenosis** → Narrowed right ventricular outflow tract
    - Generally caused by overgrowth of the heart muscle wall secondary to pulmonic stenosis
  - → **Right ventricular hypertrophy**
    - boot-shaped heart
  - **Overriding aorta** & **Ventricular septal defect**
    - Mixing of blood
    - As the pulmonic stenosis gets worse → inc unoxygenated blood expelled into system
      - Squatting helps inc systemic pressure to offset

Truncus Arteriosus

- ~ CATCH-22 (aka. DiGeorge Syndrome)
- Single arterial trunk arise from heart and supplies all circulation
  - Truncus overlies ventral septal defect (VSD) receiving blood from both ventricles (mixing)
  - As pulmonary vascular resistance drops in first week → pulmonary BF increases → HF (Eisenmenger's Syndrome)

DiGeorge Syndrome

- aka. **22q11.2 deletion** syndrome = **Velocardiofacial** Syndrome
- Possible migration defects of neural crest-derived tissues
  - Particularly the **3rd and 4th pharyngeal pouches**
- **CATCH-22**
  - **C**ardiac anomalies (esp. Tetralogy of Fallot)
  - **A**bnormal facies
  - **T**hymic dysplasia → **T**-cell issues
  - **C**left Palate
  - **H**ypocalcemia/**H**ypoparathyroidism
  - **22**q11.2 deletion

Hypoparathyroidism

- Early:
  - Myalgia, numbness/tingling → **laryngeal and carpopedal spasms** → seizures (hypocalcemia)
    - Carpopedal spasms = spasmodic contraction of muscles of hands an feet, in particular wrists and ankles
      - kind-of like when you make a shadow-puppet of a bird
- Later:
  - Low PTH → dec Ca & inc PO4 → prolongation of QT
    - abnormal repolarization of the heart due to dec Ca
- Tx: <u>This is a neonate emergency!</u>
  - IV **calcium gluconate** → **calcitriol** (activated Vit D) → normalized Ca

Truncus Arteriosus Summary

- ~ CATCH-22
- Single arterial trunk arise from heart and supplies all circulation
  - Overlies VSD and receives blood from both ventricles
  - PVR drops in 1w → pulmonary BF increases
    - → HF due to Eisenmenger's Syndrome

DiGeorge & HypoPTH Summary

- **DiGeorge Syndrome** = Syndrome
  - **3rd and 4th pharyngeal pouches**
  - **CATCH-22**
    - **C**ardiac, **A**bnormal facies, **T**hymic dysplasia
    - **C**left Palate, **H**ypocalcemia/**H**ypoparathyroidism
    - 22q11.2 del
- Hypoparathyroidism (a neonate emergency)
  - Early:
    - Myalgia, numbness/tingling → **laryngeal and carpopedal spasms** →
      seizures
      - due to hypocalcemia
  - Later: Low PTH → dec Ca & inc PO4 → prolongation of QT
  - Tx:
    - IV **calcium gluconate** → **calcitriol** (activated Vit D) → normalized Ca

Newborn Defects – Heart 6

Right to Left Shunts 3

Truncus Arteriosus Summary

- ~ CATCH-22
- Single arterial trunk arise from heart and supplies all circulation
  - Overlies VSD and receives blood from both ventricles
  - PVR drops in 1w → pulmonary BF increases
    - → HF due to Eisenmenger's Syndrome

Ebstein Anomaly

- ~ **Maternal lithium use**
- ~ **Wolff-Parkinson-White**
- Downward displacement of abnormal tricuspid valve into right ventricle
    - → tricuspid valve regurgitates, dec right ventricle output
    - → enlarged right atrium shunts blood through foramen ovale or ASD → cyanosis
- When severe in neonate, Blue Baby, else, may not present until adulthood.
- Holosystolic murmur over anterior left chest
- Tx: PGE1 → shunt → surgery

Wolff-Parkinson-White Syndrome

- Short PR interval
- Abnormal accessory electrical conduction pathway between atria and ventricles (**bundle of Kent**) allows ventricles to depolarize prematurely
    - Can bypass the AV node which coordinates the proper depolarization of the heart
        - palpitations, dizziness, SOB, syncope
    - Can enter a depolarization loop → supra ventricular tachycardia
- Tx:
    - **Procainamide**
        - used to use amiodarone but now associated w/ vent fib
    - **Avoid AV node blockers:**
        - **adenosine, CCB (diltiazem, verapamil), or Beta-blockers**
        - makes worse and can be lethal
    - Catheter ablation

Ebstein & WPW Summary

- Ebstein Anomaly
  - Li use can cause. Ebstein Anomaly can cause WPW
  - Downward displacement of abnormal tricuspid valve into right ventricle → dec right ventricle output → enlarged right atrium shunts blood through foramen ovale or ASD
- WPW
  - Short PR interval
  - 2nd conduction pathway between atria and ventricles (**bundle of Kent**)
    - Can bypass the AV node which coordinates the proper depolarization of the heart
    - Can enter a depolarization loop → supra ventricular tachycardia
  - Tx: **Procainamide**
    - **Avoid AV node blockers:**
      - adenosine, CCB (diltiazem, verapamil), or Beta-blockers
    - Catheter ablation

Newborn Defects – Heart 7

Right to Left Shunts 4

Transposition of the Great Arteries (TGA)

- Most common **immediate** Blue Baby Syndrome
- **Increases pulmonary blood flow!**
- Aorta arises from right ventricle and pulmonary artery from the left ventricle.
  - **Require both a foramen ovale and PDA**
  - If PDA starts to close → Blue Baby
- PE: **Single loud S2, no murmurs**
- CXR: **"egg on a string"**
  - narrow heart base + no main segment of pulmonary artery
- Tx:
  - PGE1 → balloon atrial septostomy → surgery **by 2 weeks**

CXR: Snowman

- **Total Anomalous Pulmonary Venous Return (TAPVR)**
  - *Get used to seeing TAPVR, for no one wants to write out that name.*
  - Pulmonary veins drain into systemic venous system → complete mixing
    - Right atrial blood may flow normal path or go through foramen ovale or ASD to reach left atrium
  - Right-side enlarged, Left-side small
    - Big: Right atrium and ventricle, pulmonary artery
    - Small: Left atrium and possibly left ventricle
  - Obstruction of pulmonary veins → Increases pulmonary HTN → dec cardiac output → shock
  - Tx: PGE1 → surgery

Review: Right-to-Left Shunts

- These are cyanotic conditions. The 5 T's
  - Tetralogy of Fallot
  - Truncus Arteriosis
  - Transposition of Great Vessels
  - Total Anomalous Pulmonary Venous Return
  - Tricuspid Atresia

TOF Review

- **Tetralogy** caused by anterior malalignment of aorticopulmonary septum
  - **Pulmonary infundibular stenosis** → Narrowed right ventricular outflow tract
    - Generally caused by overgrowth of the heart muscle wall secondary to pulmonic stenosis
    - → **Right ventricular hypertrophy**
      - boot-shaped heart
  - **Overriding aorta** & **Ventricular septal defect**
    - Mixing of blood
    - As the pulmonic stenosis gets worse → inc unoxygenated blood expelled into system
      - Squatting helps inc systemic pressure to offset

Truncus Arteriosus & Ebstein Anomaly Summary

- **Truncus Arteriosus**
  - Single arterial trunk arise from heart and supplies all circulation
    - Overlies VSD and receives blood from both ventricles
    - PVR drops in 1w → pulmonary BF increases
      - → HF due to Eisenmenger's Syndrome

- **Ebstein Anomaly**
  - Li use can cause. Ebstein Anomaly can cause WPW
  - Downward displacement of abnormal tricuspid valve into right ventricle → dec right ventricle output → enlarged right atrium shunts blood through foramen ovale or ASD

TGA & TAPVR Summary

- **Transposition of the Great Arteries** (TGA)
  - **Increases pulmonary blood flow!**
  - Aorta arises from right ventricle and pulmonary artery from the left ventricle.
    - **Require both a foramen ovale and PDA**
      - If PDA starts to close → Blue Baby
  - CXR: **"egg on a string"**
    - narrow heart base + no main segment of pulmonary artery
  - Tx: PGE1 → balloon atrial septostomy → surgery **2w**

- Total Anomalous Pulmonary Venous Return (**TAPVR**)
  - Pulmonary veins drain into systemic venous system → complete mixing
    - Right atrial blood may flow normal path or go through foramen ovale or ASD to reach left atrium
  - Right-side enlarged, Left-side small
  - Obstruction of pulmonary veins → Inc pulmonary HTN → dec CO → shock
  - CXR: **snowman**
  - Tx: PGE1 → surgery

Newborn Defects – Liver 1

Jaundice Intro

Jaundice

- General:
  - Inc production of bilirubin from fetal RBC breakdown + immature hepatic conjugation.
  - Eliminated in first week.
- Bilirubin crosses the BBB and can lead to **Kernicterus**:
  - Unconjugated bili → basal ganglia & brain stem →
    - **Hypotonia or opisthotonos**: no tone vs. arched back
    - **Seizures, choreoathetosis**
    - **Sensorineural hearing loss**
  - Classified into type of bilirubin encephalopathies

Physiologic vs Pathologic Jaundice

- **Physiologic**
  - **ie. Physiologic Jaundice of the Neonate**
    - correct for term baby
  - Day 2 or 3: appears and soon peaks
  - Day 5: disappears
  - Peak bili < **13mg/dL**, rises at < **5mg/dL/day**
- **Pathologic**
  - Day 1 appears. Peak and resolution vary
  - Peak bili has no limit and usually rises faster than 5mg/dL/ day

  - Also, any **Direct Bili > 2mg/dL** is pathologic

Causes of
Pathologic Jaundice of Newborn

- **Direct**, due to
  - Infection
  - Hepatic issue
  - Systemic deficit
- **Indirect, Coombs (+)**
  - Immune hemolysis:
    - Rh/ABO incompatibility
    - minor blood group
- **Indirect, Coombs (-)**
  - Polycythemia
  - Anemia

Causes of
Pathologic Jaundice of Newborn

- **Direct**, due to
  - Infection
    - TORCH infections
    - Sepsis
  - Hepatic issue
    - Biliary atresia
    - Dubin-Johnson
    - Rotor Syndrome
  - Systemic deficit
    - Hypothyroidism
    - Cystic fibrosis
    - Galactosemia

Causes of
Pathologic Jaundice of Newborn

- **Indirect, Coombs (+)**
  - Immune hemolysis:
    - Rh/ABO incompatibility
    - minor blood group

Causes of
Pathologic Jaundice of Newborn

- **Indirect, Coombs (-)**
  - **Polycythcmia**
    - Just waited a bit too long to clamp the umbilical cord
    - Infant of diabetic mother
    - IUGR
      - *maybe due to being an infant of a diabetic mom*
    - Twin-twin Transfusion
    - Fetal-Maternal Hemorrhage

Causes of
Pathologic Jaundice of Newborn

- **Indirect, Coombs (-)**
  - **Anemia**
    - Caused by food Going in/Coming out
    - Trauma
    - Hepatic issue
    - Systemic deficiency

Causes of
Pathologic Jaundice of Newborn

- **Indirect, Coombs (-)**
  - **Anemia**
    - Food Going in/Coming out
      - Breast Feeding
      - Breast-feeding Jaundice vs. Breast-milk Jaundice
      - Bowel obstruction
    - Trauma
      - Cephalohematoma or Bruising; Hemorrhage
    - Hepatic issue
      - Crigler-Najjar, Gilbert Syndrome
    - Systemic deficiency
      - Spherocytosis, Elliptocytosis; G6PD deficiency

Causes of
Pathologic Jaundice of Newborn

- Lots of causes. Much better to understand the processes and deduce.
- **Direct**, due to
  - Infection: TORCH infections, Sepsis
  - Hepatic issue: Biliary atresia, Dubin-Johnson, Rotor Syndrome
  - Systemic deficit: Hypothyroidism, Cystic fibrosis, Galactosemia
- **Indirect, Coombs (+)**
  - Immune hemolysis: Rh/ABO incompatibility, minor blood group
- **Indirect, Coombs (-)**
  - **Polycythemia**
    - Just waited a bit too long to clamp the umbilical cord
    - Infant of diabetic mother, IUGR
    - Twin-twin Transfusion, Fetal-Maternal Hemorrhage
  - **Anemia**
    - Food Going in/Coming out
      - Breast Feeding: Breast-feeding Jaundice vs. Breast-milk Jaundice; Bowel obstruction
    - Trauma: Cephalohematoma or Bruising; Hemorrhage
    - Hepatic issue: Crigler-Najjar, Gilbert Syndrome
    - Systemic deficiency: Spherocytosis, Elliptocytosis; G6PD deficiency

Newborn Defects – Liver 2

Direct Pathologic Jaundice

Infections: TORCH

Causes of Direct Pathologic Jaundice Infection

- TORCH infections
- Sepsis

Causes of Direct Pathologic Jaundice Infection

- TORCH infections
  - A better mnemonic is CHEAPTORCHES, but what is a better way to think of this than that is **Vertically Transmitted Infection**
  - Any infection that a mom gets and can pass on to fetus/neonate falls into this category. Therefore, you really just need to learn the characteristics for specific ones so that you may begin treating while awaiting BCx.

  - **T**oxoplasmosis
  - **O**ther
    - Syphilis
  - **R**ubella
  - **C**MV
  - **H**erpes
    - Varicella

Causes of Direct Pathologic Jaundice Infection

- Toxoplasmosis
  - **Diffuse intracranial calcifications**, hydrocephalus, chorioretinitis
  - Unexplained mononuclear CSF pleocytosis (inc cell count) or elevated CSF protein
  - Tx: antiparasitic (**pyrimethamine + sulfadiazine**) + folinic acid (**leucovorin**)
- Other - Syphilis
  - Skeletal abnormalities: osteochondritis and periostitis
  - Pseudoparalysis
  - **Snuffles** (Persistent rhinitis)
  - Maculopapular rash on **palms and soles**
  - Tx: PCN

Causes of Direct Pathologic Jaundice Infection

- Rubella
  - Eyes: **cataracts**, glaucoma, pigmentary retinopathy
  - **Heart**: PDA (patent ductus arteriosus), peripheral pulmonary artery stenosis
  - Radiolucent bone disease
  - **Sensorineural hearing loss**
  - Tx: supportive care and surveillance
- CMV
  - Thrombocytopenia, hepatosplenomegaly
  - **Periventricular intracranial calcifications**, microcephaly
  - Sensorineural hearing loss
  - Tx: ganciclovir

Causes of Direct Pathologic Jaundice Infection

- Herpes
  - Mucocutaneous vesicles or scarring
  - CSF pleocytosis
  - Thrombocytopenia, elevated LFTs
  - Eyes: Conjunctivitis or keratoconjunctivitis
  - Tx: acyclovir
- Varicella
  - Vesicular skin lesions or scars
  - Limb hypoplasia
  - Tx: acyclovir
  - If mom is symptomatic but neonate is not, prophylaxis VariZIG (varicella-zoster Ig)

Causes of Direct Pathologic Jaundice Infection: Summary

- **T**oxoplasmosis: **Diffuse intracranial calcifications**
  - Tx: **pyrimethamine + sulfadiazine + leucovorin**
- **O**ther – Syphilis: **Snuffles,** rash on **palms and soles**
  - Tx: PCN
- **R**ubella: **cataracts**, heart issue, **sensorineural hearing loss**
  - Tx: Supportive
- **CMV: Periventricular intracranial calcifications**
  - Tx: ganciclovir
- **H**erpes: Mucocutaneous vesicles, conjunctivitis
  - Tx: acyclovir
  - Varicella: Vesicular skin lesions, limb hypoplasia
    - Tx: acyclovir ± VariZIG

Newborn Defects – Liver 3

Direct Pathologic Jaundice
Infections: TORCH Review + Sepsis

Causes of Direct Pathologic Jaundice Infection: Review

- **T**oxoplasmosis: Diffuse intracranial calcifications
  - Tx: **pyrimethamine + sulfadiazine + leucovorin**
- **O**ther – Syphilis: Snuffles, rash on palms and soles
  - Tx: **PCN**
- **R**ubella: cataracts, heart issue, sensorineural hearing loss
  - Tx: Supportive
- **C**MV: Periventricular intracranial calcifications
  - Tx: **ganciclovir**
- **H**erpes: Mucocutaneous vesicles, conjunctivitis
    - Tx: **acyclovir**
  - Varicella: Vesicular skin lesions, limb hypoplasia
    - Tx: **acyclovir ± VariZIG**

Causes of Direct Pathologic Jaundice Infection

- Sepsis
  - Most common:
    - < 3 days old: group B Strept., E. coli, Listeria monocytogenes
    - > 3 days old: Serratia marcescens, Pseudomonas aeruginosa, Citrobacter koseri
  - Dx:
    - CBC w/ differential, BCx, UA, UrCx, CXR, LP (if meningitis indicated)
    - Indications for meningitis: irritable, lethargic, hypothermia
  - Tx:
    - No meningitis: **ampicillin + gentamicin**
      - until 3d post neg Cx
    - Meningitis: + **cefotaxime**
      - 3rd-gen cephalosporin, **NOT ceftriaxone**

Causes of Direct Pathologic Jaundice Infection: Summary

- **T**oxoplasmosis: **Diffuse intracranial calcifications**
  - Tx: **pyrimethamine + sulfadiazine + leucovorin**
- **O**ther – Syphilis: **Snuffles,** rash on **palms and soles**
  - Tx: PCN
- **R**ubella: **cataracts**, heart issue, **sensorineural hearing loss**
  - Tx: Supportive
- CMV: **Periventricular intracranial calcifications**
  - Tx: ganciclovir
- **H**erpes: Mucocutaneous vesicles, conjunctivitis
  - Tx: acyclovir
  - Varicella: Vesicular skin lesions, limb hypoplasia
    - Tx: acyclovir ± VariZIG

Causes of Direct Pathologic Jaundice Infection: Summary

- Sepsis is most common
  - < 3 days old: GBS, E. coli, or Listeria
  - > 3 days old: Serratia, P. aeruginosa, Citrobacter
  - Tx: **Ampicillin + gentamicin**
    - until 3d post neg Cx
    - With meningitis: **+ cefotaxime**
      - or a 3rd-gen cephalosporin, **NOT ceftriaxone**

Newborn Defects – Liver 4

Direct Pathologic Jaundice
Hepatic and Systemic Issues

Causes of **Direct** Pathologic Jaundice
Infection: Review

- **T**oxoplasmosis: **Diffuse intracranial calcifications**
  - Tx: **pyrimethamine + sulfadiazine + leucovorin**
- **O**ther – Syphilis: **Snuffles,** rash on **palms and soles**
  - Tx: PCN
- **R**ubella: **cataracts**, heart issue, **sensorineural hearing loss**
  - Tx: Supportive
- **C**MV: **Periventricular intracranial calcifications**
  - Tx: ganciclovir
- **H**erpes: Mucocutaneous vesicles, conjunctivitis
  - Tx: acyclovir
  - Varicella: Vesicular skin lesions, limb hypoplasia
    - Tx: acyclovir +/- VariZIG

Causes of **Direct** Pathologic Jaundice
Infection: Review

- Sepsis is most common
  - < 3 days old: GBS, E. coli, or Listeria
  - > 3 days old: Serratia, P. aeruginosa, Citrobacter
  - Tx: **Ampicillin + gentamicin**
    - until 3d post neg Cx
    - With meningitis: **+ cefotaxime**
      - or a 3rd-gen cephalosporin, **NOT ceftriaxone**

Causes of **Direct** Pathologic Jaundice
Hepatic Issues

- Biliary atresia
- Dubin-Johnson
- Rotor Syndrome

Causes of Direct Pathologic Jaundice
Hepatic Issues

- Biliary atresia
- Dubin-Johnson
  - Hepatocytes can't secrete conjugated bili into bile
  - Postmortem: **black liver**
  - Dx: can't visualize gallbladder, **check isomer of coproporphyrin**
- Rotor Syndrome
  - a milder Dubin-Johnson by means of different pathophysiology
  - no black liver
  - Dx: can visualize gallbladder, check isomer of coproporphyrin

Causes of Direct Pathologic Jaundice
Systemic Issues

- Hypothyroidism
- Cystic fibrosis
- Galactosemia

Causes of Direct Pathologic Jaundice Hepatic or Systemic Issues Summary

- Hepatic
  - Biliary atresia
  - Dubin-Johnson:
    - Hepatocytes can't secrete conjugated bili into bile
    - Postmortem: **black liver**
  - Rotor Syndrome:
    - A milder Dubin-Johnson by means of different pathophysiology
    - no black liver
- Systemic
  - Hypothyroidism
  - Cystic fibrosis
  - Galactosemia

Newborn Defects – Liver 5

Indirect Pathologic Jaundice

Coombs (+) & Coombs (-)

Indirect, Coombs (+) Pathologic Jaundice via Polycythemia

- Immune hemolysis:
  - Rh/ABO incompatibility, minor blood group
    - May need transfusion, but probably just need time
    - Mom should've gotten Rhogam

Indirect, Coombs (-) Pathologic Jaundice via **Polycythemia**

- Just waited a bit too long to clamp the umbilical cord
- Infant of diabetic mother, IUGR
- Twin-twin Transfusion
  - When twins share a chorion, one may get a disproportionate amount of blood than the other
- Fetal-maternal Hemorrhage
  - Can happen in an abnormal or normal pregnancy
  - The membrane through which gas and nutrients exchange in the placenta ceases to function as a barrier

Indirect, Coombs (-) Pathologic Jaundice via **Anemia**

- Overview of causes
  - Food Going in/Coming out
  - Trauma
  - Hepatic issue
  - Systemic deficiency

Indirect, Coombs (-) Pathologic Jaundice via Anemia

- Overview of causes, more specific
- Food Going in/Coming out
  - Breast Feeding:
    - Breast-feeding Jaundice vs. Breast-milk Jaundice;
  - Bowel obstruction
- Trauma:
  - Cephalohematoma or Bruising;
  - Hemorrhage
- Hepatic issue:
  - Crigler-Najjar, Gilbert Syndrome
- Systemic deficiency:
  - Spherocytosis, Elliptocytosis; G6PD deficiency

Newborn Defects – Liver 6

Indirect Pathologic Jaundice

Coombs (-) Anemia

Indirect, Coombs (-) Pathologic Jaundice via Anemia

- Overview of causes
  - Food Going in/Coming out
  - Trauma
  - Hepatic issue
  - Systemic deficiency

Indirect, Coombs (-) Pathologic Jaundice via **Anemia**

- Overview of causes, more specific
- Food Going in/Coming out
  - Breast Feeding:
    - Breast-feeding Jaundice vs. Breast-milk Jaundice;
  - Bowel obstruction
- Trauma:
  - Cephalohematoma or Bruising;
  - Hemorrhage
- Hepatic issue:
  - Crigler-Najjar, Gilbert Syndrome
- Systemic deficiency:
  - Spherocytosis, Elliptocytosis; G6PD deficiency

Indirect, Coombs (-) Pathologic Jaundice via **Anemia**

- Going in/Coming out: Breast Feeding
  - Breast Feeding Jaundice
    - Baby isn't nursing well and so not getting many calories (1st time mom)
    - Jaundice occurs w/in few days
    - Tx: Educate
  - Breast-milk Jaundice
    - Some breast milk contains beta-glucuronidase
    - Jaundice occurs in week 2
    - Tx: phototherapy
      - Level may rise again, but it probably won't rise to the same level
      - Baby okay to safely breast feed
      - Resolves w/in 3m
- Going in/Coming out: Bowel obstruction

Indirect, Coombs (-) Pathologic Jaundice via **Anemia**

- Trauma
  - Cephalohematoma or Bruising
  - Hemorrhage
- Hepatic issue
  - Crigler-Najjar
    - Type I: **no** UDP glucuronosyltransferase 1-A1 (**UGT1A1**).
    - Type II: **reduced** UGT1A1
    - required to conjugate bili
    - Dx: treat w/ **phenobarbital** will get no response
      - phenobarbital induces CYP450 enzyme
  - Gilbert Syndrome
    - Most common hereditary cause of increased unconjugated bili
    - Dec activity of **glucuronyltransferase**
      - Similar to Crigler-Najjar Type II

Indirect, Coombs (-) Pathologic Jaundice via **Anemia** Summary

- Breast Feeding Jaundice (w/in few days)
  - Baby isn't nursing well and so not getting many calories (1st time mom)
- Breast-milk Jaundice (starts in 2w, resolves by 3mo)
  - Some breast milk contains beta-glucuronidase
  - Tx: phototherapy
- Crigler-Najjar
  - Type I: **no** UDP glucuronosyltransferase 1-A1 (**UGT1A1**).
  - Type II: **reduced** UGT1A1
  - Dx: treat w/ **phenobarbital** will get no response
    - phenobarbital induces CYP450 enzyme
- Gilbert Syndrome
  - Dec activity of **glucuronyltransferase**
    - Similar to Crigler-Najjar Type II

PEDIATRICS

Peds – Hematology 1

Look at the Thumbs

And Another

Blackfan-Diamond =
Congenital Pure Red Cell Anemia

- Dec erythroid progenitors in BM
  → normocytic or macrocytic anemia
- With Blackfan-**Diamond**, 50% **C**an't **T**ell **C**ubic-zirconia from **G**lass
- 50% have malformations: **C**raniofacial, **T**humb (or UE), **C**ardiac, **G**U
  - Short w/ **triphalangeal thumbs**
    - ie. has 3 phalanges instead of 2. It's long
- Dx
  - Inc ADA (adenosine deaminase), HbF, Fe
  - Dec RBC precursors, retic count
- Tx
  - Steroids + transfusions + deferoxamine
  - Stem cell transplant

Fanconi Anemia

- Most common congenital pancytopenia.
  - Defect in DNA repair proteins → chromosomal breaks
- Most develop AML and BM failure
- **Short**, abnormal skin and organ development.
  - **Café au lait spots**
  - **Hypoplastic thumbs**
- Dx: BM hypoplasia
- Tx: steroids + androgens → BM transplant

- Note: Don't confuse w/ Fanconi Syndrome.
  - It's a separate disease resulting in RTA-2.

Beta Thalassemia

- Thalassemia = faulty hemoglobin synthesis
  - Therefore, the name means "faulty hemoglobin synthesis due to beta-chain production"
    - ie. The pt will have **less** beta-chains.
- Types
  - Minor: del of 1 gene — microcytic anemia
  - **Intermedia**: del of 2 — normal life with occasional transfusions
  - **Major**: del of all 3 — severe microcytic anemia
    - Splenomegaly & bone deformities
      - *(maybe thumbs, I'm not sure. I hate to ruin a theme)*
    - Death before 20yo
    - Major is also called **Cooley Anemia**
    - Skeletal anomalies

Check the Thumbs Summary

- **Blackfan-Diamond** = Congenital Pure Red Cell Anemia
  - Dec erythroid progenitors in BM → normocytic or macrocytic anemia
  - Blackfan-**Diamond**, 50% **C**an't **T**ell **C**ubic-zirconia from **Gl**ass
    - 50% have malformations: **C**raniofacial, **T**humb (or UE), **C**ardiac, **GU**
      - Short w/ **triphalangeal thumbs**
  - Tx: Steroids + transfusions + deferoxamine
    - Stem cell transplant
- **Fanconi Anemia**
  - Defect in DNA repair proteins → chromosomal breaks
    - Most develop AML and BM failure
  - **Short**, abnormal skin and organ development.
    - **Café au lait spots, Hypoplastic thumbs**
  - Tx: steroids + androgens → BM transplant
  - *Note: Don't confuse w/ Fanconi Syndrome.*
    - *It's a separate disease resulting in RTA-2.*

Beta Thalassemia Summary

- **Less beta**-chains.
- Types
  - Minor: del of 1 gene — **microcytic anemia**
  - **Intermedia**: del of 2 — normal life
    - occasional transfusions
  - **Major**: del of all 3 — severe microcytic anemia
    - Bone deformities

Peds – Hematology 2

Normal Thumbs Anemia

TEC, Alpha

Quick Word on Clotting

(TEC) Transient Erythroblastopenia of Childhood

- Hypoplastic anemia between 6mo - 3yo
  - Viral infection → immune suppression of erythropoiesis
- Recovery w/in 2m

Alpha Thalassemia

- Thalassemia = faulty hemoglobin synthesis
  - Therefore, the name means "faulty hemoglobin synthesis due to alpha chain production"
  - ie. alpha is decreased, and if alpha is decreased, beta must be increased to make up for it
- Due to HBA1 and HBA2 genes which code for alpha chains 1,2,3, and 4
  - Leads to **decreased alpha**

  Can I stress this anymore – alpha-thalassemia produces less alpha
  → more beta

Alpha Thalassemia Types

- Minima = silent carriers: del of 1 gene.
  - Probably won't ever know
- **Trait**: del of 2 genes
  - Mild microcytic anemia **mistaken for iron deficiency anemia** and treated inappropriately w/ iron
  - *We could go into Asians are generally cis and Africans are generally trans, but clinically, it doesn't really matter*
- **HgB H disease**: del of 3 genes
  - Two unstable Hgb in the blood:
    - **Hgb Barts** (4 gamma chains), **Hgb H** (3 beta chains)
    - Both grab onto O2 and won't let go
  - **Target cells & Heinz bodies** & hepatosplenomegaly
    Newborns require immediate transfusion to survive.
- **Hydrops fetalis**:
  - del of 4 genes, these fetuses die. The ones who make it out die very quickly.

Alpha Thalassemia Summary

- Decreased alpha- (and increased beta-) chains
- **Trait**: del of 2 genes
  - Mild microcytic anemia **mistaken for iron deficiency anemia** and treated inappropriately w/ iron
- **HgB H disease**: del of 3 genes
  - Binds O2 tightly
  - **Target cells & Heinz bodies** & hepatosplenomegaly
  - Newborns require immediate transfusion to survive.
- del of 4 genes → **Hydrops fetalis**

Clotting (for next time)

- All clotting factors are produced exclusively in the liver
  - except factor VIII
- PTT
  - Intrinsic pathway: 8, 9, 11, 12 (VIII, IX, XI, XII)
    - *Two thrombosis factors to both sides of X, but not X*
- PT
  - Extrinsic pathway: thromboplastin + Ca, VII, VIII
- Thrombin time, the final step in clotting
  - fibrinogen → fibrin

Peds – Hematology 3

Bernard-Soulier,
Glanzmann's Alphabet, ITP

Review Clotting

- All clotting factors are produced exclusively in the liver
  - except factor VIII
- **PTT** ~ Intrinsic pathway: 8, 9, 11, 12 (VIII, IX, XI, XII)
  - *Two thrombosis factors to both sides of X, but not X*
- **PT** ~ Extrinsic pathway: thromboplastin + Ca, VII, VIII
- **Thrombin time**, the final step in clotting
  - fibrinogen → fibrin

- Low Platelet Count Disorders → Inc Bleeding Time
  - Bernard-Soulier, ITP, TTP
    - Glanzmann's Thrombasthenia has normal platelets

Defects in Platelet Plug Formation

- Bernard-Soulier
  - Dec Gp1b:
    - platelet-to-collagen adhesion impaired
- **Glanzmann's** Thrombasthenia
  - Dec **GpIIb/IIa**:
    - No platelet-to-platelet aggregation
  - **Abciximab** does the same thing

  - *Glanzmann's alphabet just can't bring 2 things together.*
    - *alphabet (abciximab), bring 2 (GpIIa/IIb)*
    - *things together (no platelet-to-platelet aggregation)*

ITP

- **ITP = Immune Thrombocytopenia Purpura = Idiopathic Thrombocytopenia Purpura**

Is anything on a pediatrics rotation more important to get down pat than ITP? It comes up all the time.

- Can be side effect of the body fighting off any insult. Can be an infection, can be a drug.
  - Foods are drugs: walnuts, cow's milk, cranberry juice, tonic water (quinine)
- The effort to fight off whatever mistakenly results in antibodies that target your own platelets. For the most part, you just have to bridge the patient until such time as that lineage of antibodies dies out.
- ITP is what it says
  - Immune (as in, anti-platelet Abs)
  - Thrombocytopenia (as in, runs out of platelets)
  - Purpura (as in, you develop a rash and petechiae from the destruction of platelets)

ITP

- Auto-antibodies against platelet surface → petechiae and purpura and possible mucosa bleeding
  - Concern for intracranial hemorrhage
- Dx: Plt < 100k
  - Plt **10-20** concern for **spontaneous bleeds**
  - Plt < 10 think autoimmune disorder
- Tx:
  - Only give transfusion if life-threatening. **Based on combination of clinical appearance and Plt count.**
    - May have Plt of 8 and look just fine
  - IVIG for 2 days → prednisone
  - Only remove spleen w/ severe disease

Summary

- Bernard-Soulier: Dec Gp1b
- **Glanzmann's** Thrombasthenia
  - Dec **GpIIb/IIa**: No platelet-to-platelet aggregation
  - **Abciximab** does the same thing
  - *Glanzmann's alphabet just can't bring 2 things together.*
- *ITP = Immune Thrombocytopenia Purpura*
  - Anti-platelet Ab → petechiae, purpura, mucosa bleeding
  - Dx: Plt < 100k
    - Plt **10-20** concern for **spontaneous bleeds.** Plt < 10 think autoimmune
  - Tx:
    - **Based on combination of clinical appearance and Plt count**
      - May have Plt of 8 and look just fine
    - IVIG for 2 days → prednisone
    - Only remove spleen w/ severe disease

Peds – Hematology 4

Protein S Defic, Trousseau, DIC HIT

Protein S Deficiency

- Associate with Vitamin K:
  - diSCo 1972 (protein S, protein C, IX, X, VII, II)
- Protein S activates Protein C
  - → degrades factor Va and VIIIa
- 60% bound to C4b, only when free is it activated
- Leads to **venous thrombosis**

- Protein C Deficiency is more common

Trousseau's Syndrome =
Migrating Thrombophlebitis

- **"white leg"**: due to thrombus in superficial vein

- **Trousseau Sign of Malignancy**
  - Tender clot felt as nodule under skin
  - ~ pancreatic, gastric and lung CA.

- Don't confuse w/
  - Trousseau Sign of Latent Tetany: hypoCa
    - So, Trousseau's Syndrome & Trousseau Sign of Malignancy are related, but this other one is a reach.

DIC = Disseminated
Intravascular Coagulation

- DIC is a consumptive coagulopathy complicating disease
  - Widespread activation of the clotting cascade
  - Blood clots damage multiple organs
  - Clotting factors and platelets are all consumed
  - Normal clotting can't occur → severe bleeding

- ie. Microvascular thrombosis → TTP
  - → Dec clotting factors
  - → Severe bleeding, end-organ damage
  - → Severe sepsis & septic shock

~ Solid tumors and large aortic aneurysms

HIT =
Heparin Induced Thrombocytopenia

- Usually occurs w/in 5-10d
- Early onset:
  - If pt was exposed to heparin w/in past 3 months, the next exposure could result in **HIT within hours**
    - *Extremely important questions to answer before giving heparin, "Have you been exposed to heparin before? When? Have you had a problem with bleeding before? When? Have you had problems with bruising, bleeding gums, wounds that won't heal, ...? When?"*
      - *Seriously, ask like 20 questions on this, for they might say yes on question number 19.*
- Delayed Onset (10-15%):
  - several days post-exposure

Summary

- **Protein S Deficiency**
  - Vitamin K: diSCo 1972 (S, C, X, IX, VII, II)
  - Protein S activates Protein C —> degrades factor Va and VIIIa
  - Leads to venous thrombosis

- Trousseau's Syndrome = **Migrating Thrombophlebitis**
  - "white leg" due to thrombus in superficial vein
- **Trousseau Sign of Malignancy**
  - Tender clot felt as nodule under skin. ~ pancreatic, gastric and lung CA.

- **DIC** = Consumptive Coagulopathy
  - Microvascular thrombosis → TCP → dec clotting factors
    → bleeding, end-organ damage → Severe sepsis & septic shock

- **HIT** = Heparin Induced Thrombocytopenia
  - Usually occurs w/in 5-10d
  - Early onset: if exposed w/in 3m, next exposure could cause HIT w/in hours
  - Delayed Onset (10-15%): several days post-exposure

Peds – Hematology 5

Leukemoid vs ?,
Hodgkin Lymphoma

Leukemoid Reaction vs
Leukemia vs Lymphoma

- Leukemoid Rxn:
  - Inc WBC count w/ left shift (80% bands) AND inc leukocyte alkaline phosphatase
    - **Left-shift = banding**:
      - inc # of immature leukocytes in peripheral blood, particularly neutrophil band cells
      - Not a malignancy. May be lymphoid or myeloid.
  - Response to infection, drugs, hemorrhage or other stress. Often mistaken for CML.
- Leukemia:
  - Tumor cells formed in peripheral blood
    → lymphoid neoplasms widespread in BM
- Lymphoma: Arise from lymph nodes

Leukemoid Reaction

- In other words, **a stressor** to the system (infection, drugs, hemorrhage, or emotional stress) results in an **overreaction by the immune system**
- Lots of **WBCs** are produced, and during this rapid ramp-up, many **immature leukocytes** get into the peripheral blood (**particularly neutrophil-band cells**)
- Leukocyte alkaline phosphatase is found within WBCs. Therefore, when the rapid overproduction of WBC is going on, some break. Maybe some of the immature ones break. Whatever, the spill leukocyte alkaline phosphatase into the serum → **inc LAP**

Hodgkin's Lymphoma = Hodgkin Disease (**HD**)

- Most often 15-19 yo. ~ EBV
- **Reed-Sternberg** cell:
  - Large cell w/ multiple or multi-lobed nuclei
- Clinically
  - **Painless, firm cervical or supraclavicular nodes**
  - **Anterior mediastinal mass**
  - B-cell symptoms
- Tx: chemo + radiation
- Very curable when caught early.
  - Depending on type

HD Types

- **Nodular Sclerosing** (most common)
  - Large tumor nodules w/ **few RS cells** and many inflammatory cells and <u>varying degrees of **sclerosis**</u>
    - ie. collagen fibrosis
- **Mixed-Cellularity**
  - <u>Lots of RS cells & inflammatory cells</u>. No sclerosis
- **Lymphocyte Predominant** (best prognosis)
  - <u>Lots of lymphocytes, few RS cells</u>.
  - Confused w/ B-cell NHL
- **Lymphocyte Depleted** (worst prognosis)
  - Few RS-cells, few lymphocytes.

HD Types

- The names of the types actually say what they are.
  - **Nodular Sclerosing** (most common)
    - few RS cells + sclerosis
  - **Mixed-Cellularity**
    - Lots of RS cells & inflammatory cells. No sclerosis
  - **Lymphocyte Predominant** (best prognosis)
    - Lots of lymphocytes, few RS cells.
  - **Lymphocyte Depleted** (worst prognosis)
    - Few RS-cells or lymphocytes.

Summary

- Leukemoid Rxn: system stressor
  → inc WBC w/ left-shift (ie. banding) + inc LAP
- Leukemia: Tumor cells formed in peripheral blood → lymphoid neoplasms widespread in BM
- Lymphoma: Arise from lymph nodes

HD Summary

- ~ EBV
- Commonality
  - **Reed-Sternberg** cells: large cell w/ multiple or multi-lobed nuclei
  - Symptoms
    - **Painless, firm cervical or supraclavicular nodes. Anterior mediastinal mass**
    - B-cell symptoms
  - Tx: chemo + radiation
  - Very curable when caught early.
- Types
  - Nodular Sclerosing (most common)
    - sclerosis + few RS cells, many inflammatory cells
  - Mixed-Cellularity
    - Lots of RS cells and inflammatory cells. No sclerosis
  - Lymphocyte Predominant (best prognosis)
    - **Lots of lymphocytes, few RS cells.**
  - Lymphocyte Depleted (worst prognosis)
    - Few RS-cells, few lymphocytes.

Peds – Hematology 6

NHL, Intro to ALL

NHL = Non-Hodgkin Lymphoma

- No RS cells
- Lymphomas arise from lymphocytes in lymph nodes
- Big test question:
  - **Burkitt's Lymphoma: t(8;14), c-myc, EBV**
    - **Starry-sky**: sheets of lymphocytes w/ interspersed macrophages
    - Picture of big jaw in Africa

NHL = Non-Hodgkin Lymphoma

- No RS cells
- Lymphomas arise from lymphocytes in lymph nodes
- Types
  - Mature B cell neoplasms
  - Mature T cell and NK cell neoplasms
  - Precursor lymphoid neoplasms
  - Immunodeficiency-associated lymphoproliferative disorders
- **Any lymphoma that isn't Hodgkin Lymphoma (presence of RS-cells) is NHL**
  - Don't learn them as NHL. Learn them as lymphomas
    - Ask yourself, if one had uncontrolled propagation of a cell line, what would the pt look like

ALL = Acute Lymphoblastic Leukemia

- Leukemia = Cancer of blood cells.
  - Most blood cells form in the bone marrow. In leukemia, cancerous blood cells form and crowd out the healthy blood cells in the bone marrow.
  - Primarily a result of damage to DNA by whatever means (eg. radiation, chemicals)
- Lymphoblastic = Overproduction of cancerous, immature WBCs (ie. lymphoblasts)
- Cause damage to normal cell lines
  - ie. RBCs, normal WBCs, platelets are all damaged or destroyed
- Peak incidence is 2-5yo (with another peak in the elderly)
  - ie. *You think a kid might have cancer – r/o ALL first*

ALL Symptoms

- Symptoms are mostly SE of damaged cell lines
- Fever, infections, SOB, CP, cough, vomit, change in bowel habits
- Bleeding, thrombocytopenia, anemia, tachycardia, fatigue, bruising
- Enlarged lymph nodes, liver, and/or spleen
- Wt loss, dec appetite

ALL Symptoms:
What's Really Important to Notice

- Unexplained fever, **recurrent infections**
- **Bleeding/bruising**, thrombocytopenia, anemia
- **Enlarged lymph nodes, liver, and/or spleen**
- **Wt loss**, dec appetite

NHL Summary

- NHL = Non-Hodgkin Lymphoma
  - Basically, any lymphoma w/o RS cells
  - Arise from lymphocytes in lymph nodes
  - Types
    - Mature B cell neoplasms
    - Mature T cell and NK cell neoplasms
    - Precursor lymphoid neoplasms
    - Immunodeficiency-associated lymphoproliferative disorders

ALL Summary

- Lymphoblastic Leukemia:
  - Damage to DNA → uncontrolled production of a lymphoblastic cell line in the BM resulting in damage to other cell lines
    - Lymphoblasts: immature WBCs
- ALL occurs in little kids (and older-elderly)
- Symptoms to Watch Out For
  - Unexplained fever, **recurrent infections**
  - **Bleeding/bruising**, thrombocytopenia, anemia
  - **Enlarged lymph nodes, liver, and/or spleen**
  - **Wt loss**, dec appetite

Next Time

- We'll cover ALL testing, classification, and treatment.

Peds – Hematology 7

ALL

ALL Review

- Acute Lymphoblastic Leukemia:
  - Acute damage to DNA → uncontrolled production of a lymphoblastic cell line in the BM resulting in damage to other cell lines
    - Lymphoblasts: immature WBCs
- ALL occurs in little kids (and older-elderly)
- Symptoms to Watch Out For
  - Unexplained fever, **recurrent infections**
  - **Bleeding/bruising**, thrombocytopenia, anemia
  - **Enlarged lymph nodes, liver, and/or spleen**
  - **Wt loss**, dec appetite

ALL: Lots of Tests
And What They Tell You

- **RNA testing**: How aggressive is the disease?
- **Cytogenetics**:
  - Is Philly chr present?
    - Philadelphia chr: t(9;22) BCR-ABL
- **Immunophenotyping**:
  - Is it myeloblastic (neutrophils, eosinophils, basophils) or lymphoblasts (B or T)?
- Check for TdT or CALLA antigens
  - CALLA found in 80% of ALL
    - but it is also found in CML-blast crisis
- Imaging to see which organs are affected

WHO International Classification

1. Acute Lymphoblastic Leukemia/Lymphoma
   i. Precursor B acute lymphoblastic leukemia/ lymphoma
      - Multiple subtypes
        - t(9;22) ABL/BCR is the one most commonly asked
        - t(8;14) C-MYC is Burkitt's Lymphoma
          » *Which is #2, so as you can see, the lines are blurry*

2. Burkitt's Leukemia/lymphoma
3. Biphenotypic acute leukemia

ALL Treatment

- The early, the better
- Aim is to induce a "lasting remission"
  - More kids live after ALL these days, so being aware of how to attend to their needs is a growing concern
  - So pay attention to what they had and what they go through, so you might know what to watch out for in 30 years.
- Treatments include chemo, steroids, radiation, BM and stem-cell transplants, growth factors,
  - and don't forget methotrexate
    - When was the last time you pooped? What did your poop look like? Did someone else witness your poop?
      - "Alex, what are the questions a physician asks a patient on methotrexate."

Treatment Phases

1. Remission Induction
2. Consolidation
3. Maintenance

Treatment Phases

- Remission **Induction**
  - Kill off as much cancer as you can, and then reassess.
  - Drugs:
    - prednisone or dexamethasone, vincristine, asparaginase, (daunorubicin in adults), cytarabine, methotrexate (MTX)
  - CNS prophylaxis is critical
    - It is started now, and it will continue through the consolidation-phase
  - Radiation may be used in combo with a drug to increase efficacy.

Treatment Phases

- **Consolidation**
  - Focused on killing off what's left with "rounds" of treatment.
    - Each round is weeks long.
  - CNS penetration and protection is very important
    - Intrathecal administration will probably be used at some point.
  - Drugs:
    - Vincristine, cyclophosphamide, cytarabine, daunorubicin, etoposide, thioguanine, mercaptopurine
  - Radiation may be used in combo with a drug to increase efficacy.

Treatment Phases

- **Maintenance**
  - Used to kill the residual cells.
  - What has been the standard treatment
    - PO Daily mercaptopurine
    - PO Weekly methotrexate
    - IV Monthly 5-day course of vincristine
      - Pt probably comes into hospital for this
    - PO Prednisone varies
  - Length of maintenance phase
    - Girls & adults: 2y
    - Boys: 3y

ALL Summary

- Acute Lymphoblastic Leukemia:
  - Acute damage to DNA → uncontrolled production of a lymphoblastic cell line in the BM resulting in damage to other cell lines
- ALL occurs in little kids (and older-elderly)
- Symptoms to Watch Out For
  - Unexplained fever, **recurrent infections**
  - **Bleeding/bruising**, thrombocytopenia, anemia
  - **Enlarged lymph nodes, liver, and/or spleen**
  - **Wt loss**, dec appetite

ALL Summary

- Testing
  - **RNA testing**: suggests aggressiveness
  - **Cytogenetics**: what's the chromosomal abnormality
  - **Immunophenotyping**:
    - Is it myeloblastic (neutrophils, eosinophils, basophils) or lymphoblasts (B or T)
  - Any special antigens to target
  - Imaging to see which organs are affected
- **WHO International Classification**
  1. Acute Lymphoblastic Leukemia/Lymphoma
     i. Precursor B acute lymphoblastic leukemia/lymphoma
  2. Burkitt's Leukemia/lymphoma
  3. Biphenotypic acute leukemia

ALL Treatment Summary

1. **Induction**: Kill off as much cancer as you can, and then reassess.
   - prednisone or dexamethasone, vincristine, asparaginase, (daunorubicin in adults), cytarabine, methotrexate (MTX)
   - CNS prophylaxis is critical. Start now, and continue through the consolidation-phase
   - Radiation may be used in combo with a drug to increase efficacy.

2. **Consolidation**: Focused on killing off what's left with "rounds" of treatment.
   - Vincristine, **cyclophosphamide**, cytarabine, daunorubicin, etoposide, thioguanine, mercaptopurine
   - CNS penetration and protection is very important
   - Radiation may be used in combo with a drug to increase efficacy.

3. **Maintenance**: Used to kill the residual cells.
   - What has been the standard treatment
     - PO Daily mercaptopurine. PO Weekly **methotrexate**, IV Monthly 5-day course of **vincristine**
     - PO Prednisone varies
   - Length of maintenance phase: Girls & adults: 2y, **Boys: 3y**

Peds – Immune System Diseases 1

Immune Deficiency Types

Complement & Phagocytic
Deficiencies

Howell-Jolly Bodies ~ asplenia

Immune Deficiencies

- Can have a deficiency in
  - Complement
  - Phagocytes
  - B-Cell (**CD19,20**) or
  - T-Cell (**CD2,3,4,8**)

Immune Deficiencies

- Complement
  - Pyogenic infections (pus)
  - Severe septicemia
  - **Neisseria** infections

Immune Deficiencies

- Phagocytes
  - NK cells: **CD16,56**
  - **Recurrent Staph and gram (-) infections**
  - Dx: respiratory burst assay w/ rhodamine dye & flow cytometry for leukocyte adhesion deficiencies

Phagocyte Deficiency

- Chronic Granulomatous Disease (CGD)
  - Neutrophils and monocytes can't produce ROS
    - → inability to kill **cat**alase-positive microorganisms
    - **No SSPAACE** for your **cat**:
      - **N**ocardia, **S**. aureus, **S**erratia, **P**seudomonas, **A**ctinomyces, **A**spergillus, **C**andida, **E**. coli
  - Dx: **DHR test**
    - Dihydrorhodamine 123 fluorescence flow cytometry test
  - Tx: BM transplant

Immune Deficiencies
Complement & Phagocyte Summary

- **Complement** Deficiencies lead to
  - Pyogenic infections (pus) or Severe septicemia
  - **Neisseria** infections

- Phagocytes (ie. NK cells: **CD16,56**) Deficiencies lead to
  - **Recurrent Staph and gram (-) infections**
  - Dx:
    - Respiratory burst assay w/ rhodamine dye
    - Flow cytometry for leukocyte adhesion deficiencies

  - Chronic Granulomatous Disease (CGD)
    - Neutrophils and monocytes can't produce ROS
      - → inability to kill **catalase**-positive microorganisms (**No SSPAACE** for your **cat**)
    - Dx: **DHR test**
    - Tx: BM transplant

Peds – Immune System Diseases 2

Immune Deficiency Types

B-Cell Deficiencies

Immune Deficiencies

- B-Cell (**CD19,20**)
    - Recurrent **encapsulated bacterial infections, enteroviral and hepatitis viruses**
    - Dx: Quantitative Ig measurements

B-Cell Deficiencies

- Bruton Agammaglobulinemia (ie. no B cells)
  - **Xq22**, boys
  - No more moms Ig after 6mo
    - So, decreased Ig → symptoms
  - Lymphoid hypoplasia
    - Lymph nodes are major site of B-cells, so if you have no B-cells, the tissue is hypoplastic
  - Tx: monthly IVIg + Abs

B-Cell Deficiencies

- Common Variable Immune Deficiency
  - Later age of onset.
  - B cells look normal, but don't provide Ig
  - Prone to normal B-Cell deficit infections + **enteroviral meningitis**
  - **Autoantibodies to IgA**
  - Inc lymphoma risk

B-Cell Deficiencies

- Selective IgA Deficiency
  - ~ Autoimmune diseases and inc malignancies
  - − Most common B-cell defect.
  - − Results in no IgA
  - − Give blood w/ IgA → anaphylactic shock

Immune Deficiencies
B-Cell Summary

- B-Cell (**CD19,20**)
  - − Recurrent **encapsulated bacterial infections, enteroviral and hepatitis viruses**
  - − Dx: Quantitative Ig measurements
- **Bruton Agammaglobulinemia** (ie. no B cells) **XR**
  - − Lymphoid hypoplasia
  - − Tx: monthly IVIg + Abs
- **Common Variable Immune Deficiency (CVID)**
  - − B cells look normal, but don't provide Ig
  - − Normal B-Cell deficit infections + **enteroviral meningitis**
  - − **Autoantibodies to IgA**
  - − Inc lymphoma risk
- **Selective IgA Deficiency** (ie. no IgA)
  - − Give blood w/ IgA → anaphylactic shock

Peds – Immune System Diseases 3

Immune Deficiency Types
T-Cell Deficiencies

Immune Deficiencies

- T-Cell (**CD2,3,4,8**)
    - Recurrent opportunistic infections, chronic diarrhea, FTV (failure to thrive)

T-Cell Deficiencies

- DiGeorge Syndrome (**CATCH-22**)
  - del 22q11.2 → dysmorphic 3rd & 4th pharyngeal pouches
    - Thymic and parathyroid hypoplasia
    - Anomalies of great vessels and heart
    - Esophageal atresia & bifid uvula
    - Dysmorphic face (eg. small jaw)
  - Neonatal hypocalcemia → seizures & tetany
    - Due to parathyroid hypoplasia
  - Opportunistic infections:
    - fungi, viruses, P. carinii
  - Tx:
    - thymic tissue transplant from sibling (preferably) or parent

Immune Deficiencies
T-Cell Summary

- T-Cell (**CD2,3,4,8**)
  - Recurrent opportunistic infections, chronic diarrhea, FTV (failure to thrive)
- DiGeorge Syndrome (**CATCH-22**)
  - **C**ardiac anomolies (esp Tetralogy of Fallot)
  - **A**bnormal facies, **T**hymic aplasia
  - **C**left palate, **H**ypocalcemia/**H**ypoparathyroidism
  - del **22**q11.2

Immune Deficiencies Summary

- Complement
  - Pyogenic infections, Severe septicemia, **Neisseria** infections
- Phagocytes (ie. NK cells: **CD16,56**)
  - **Recurrent Staph and gram (-) infections**
  - Dx:
    - Respiratory burst assay w/ rhodamine dye
    - Flow cytometry for leukocyte adhesion deficiencies
  - ie. Chronic Granulomatous Disease (CGD)
- B-Cell (**CD19,20**)
  - Recurrent **encapsulated bacterial infections, enteroviral and hepatitis viruses**
  - Dx: Quantitative Ig measurements
  - ie.
    - Bruton Agammaglobulinemia XR,
    - Common Variable Immune Deficiency,
    - Selective IgA Deficiency
- T-Cell (**CD2,3,4,8**)
  - Recurrent opportunistic infections, chronic diarrhea, FTV (failure to thrive)
  - ie. DiGeorge Syndrome (**CATCH-22**)

Peds – Immune System Diseases 4

Immune Deficiency Types
Combined Deficiencies

Combined Deficiencies

- Severe Combined Immunodeficiency (SCID) XR
- Wiskott-Aldrich Syndrome XR
- Ataxia-Telangiectasia

Combined Deficiencies Summary

- Severe Combined Immunodeficiency (SCID) XR
  - **Severe lymphopenia** from birth
    - Small thymus, absent lymphoid tissue → no Ig's
  - Tx: Bone marrow transplant or death by 1yo
  - Adenine Deaminase (ADA) Deficiency presents same way

- Wiskott-Aldrich Syndrome XR
  - WASP (Wiskott-Aldrich Syndrome Protein)
  - Symptoms
    - Atopic dermatitis, thrombocytopenia, recurrent infections
    - First symptoms is often **prolonged bleeding from circumcision**
  - Dx: Ig is highly variable. T-cells moderately decreased
  - Tx: BM transplant or death by teenager

- Ataxia-Telangiectasia (chr11 protein kinase mutation)
  - Dec response to B- and T-cell mitogens
    - ie. **Helper T-cell defect**
  - **Progressive cerebellar ataxia**, Oculocutaneous telangiectasias
  - **Mask-like facies**, tics, drooling

Severe Combined Immunodeficiency (SCID) XR

- Presents in first few months. Sick a lot from many different things
- **Severe lymphopenia** from birth
- Small thymus, absent lymphoid tissue → no Ig's
- Dx by 3mo has 95% success from treatment
- Tx: Bone marrow transplant or death by 1yo

- Note:
  - Adenine Deaminase (ADA) presents the same way (more common in Europe)

Wiskott-Aldrich Syndrome XR

- WASP (Wiskott-Aldrich Syndrome Protein)
- Symptoms
  - Atopic dermatitis, thrombocytopenia, recurrent infections
  - First symptoms is often prolonged bleeding from circumcision
- Dx
  - Ig is highly variable.
  - T-cells moderately decreased
- Tx: BM transplant or death by teenager

Ataxia-Telangiectasia

- chr11 protein kinase mutation
- Dec response to B- and T-cell mitogens
  - Mitogens induce mitosis, therefore B- and T-cells are propagating
    - ie. **Helper T-cell defect**
- Symptoms
  - **Progressive cerebellar ataxia:**
    - Walking → wheelchair by 12yo
  - Oculocutaneous telangiectasias by 6yo
  - **Mask-like facies**, tics, drooling
- High incidence of **malignancies**
  - **lymphoreticular** and other

Peds – Immunizations 1

Vaccine Types

Immunization Chart

- We all **look at the chart**.

- If you have a test coming up, try describing **the chart**. Then look at <u>the chart</u>. **Repeat**.

- Don't forget to set an alarm to remind you to **start looking at the chart**.

Look at the chart, the chart, repeat, start looking at the chart

Vaccines – Live Attenuated

Know the **Live Attenuated Ones**, in case you have questions on immunocompromised

- Viral
  - USA:
    - **MMR, varicella, nasal** influenza, **oral** rotavirus
      - *Just say these 4 all day long until you never forget them.*
  - Other countries: smallpox, yellow fever
- Bacterial
  - Other countries: BCG, oral typhoid

Vaccine Types

- All other majors vaccines are inactivated-viral, protein-based, or polysaccharide-based

- The polysaccharide based
  - **Toxoid: diptheria, tetanus**
  - Pneumococcal, meningococcal, Hib

- Important to know the live attenuated for questions on immunocompromise, and <u>toxoids are a common test question</u>.

What were the 4 vaccines you shouldn't forget?

What were the other live attenuated vaccines?

What were vaccines for toxoids?

Vaccine Types Summary

- Live Attenuated Vaccines
  - Viral
    - USA: **MMR, varicella**, **nasal** influenze, **oral** rotavirus
    - Other countries: smallpox, yellow fever
  - Bacterial
    - Other countries: BCG, oral typhoid

- The polysaccharide based
  - **Toxoid: diptheria, tetanus**
  - Pneumococcal, meningococcal, Hib

Peds – Immunizations 2

Vaccine Rules

Vaccine Rules

- Most **can be** given simultaneously
- A lapse in schedule **doesn't** require a "start over"
- When in doubt, immunize
  - Documentation on a formal immunization record is the only acceptable proof, regardless of country.
- Never reduce doses
  - **except first dose of hepB**
- If pt received Ig, delay live vaccine for 3-11m, depending.
- Immunization is based on chronological age
  - **Doesn't matter if he's a premie**

Not Contraindications to Immunization

- **Previous DTaP → <u>T < 105F,</u> redness, soreness, and swelling**

- **Mildly sick kid or concurrent antimicrobial therapy**
  - Fever: <u>only a contraindication if it suggests a moderate to severe illness</u>

- FHx of seizures or SIDS

- **MMR** made from chick embryos **not eggs**.
  - Egg allergy does **NOT apply**.
  - **Influenza and yellow fever does contain eggs**

Disease Exposures & Prophylaxis

- Measles
  - If pregnant or immunocompromised, **give Ig**
  - < 6mo (and breast-feeding), **if mom's immune**, so is kid.
    - Otherwise, give vaccine.
- Mumps & Rubella:
  - Post exposure admin of live vaccine doesn't help
- Varicella
  - **Immunocompromised, pregnant, infant < 12mo: VZIG**
  - All others: vaccine
- Hepatitis
  - hepA: 1 dose of vaccine ASAP but w/in 2w of exposure
  - hepB: hepB Ig + vaccine → repeat at 1 & 6 months

Vaccine Rules Summary

- Rules
  - Can give simultaneously & a lapse doesn't mean "start over".
  - Formal documentation is the only thing that counts (regardless of country).
  - Never reduce doses (except 1st hepB). Premie doesn't matter.
  - If pt got IVIG, wait to give live vaccine.
- **NOT** contraindications
  - Previous DTaP that resulted in a temp under 105F
  - Kid is sick (except if fever indicates <u>moderate to severe illness)</u>
  - FHx of seizures or SIDS
  - MMR w/ an egg allergy is not a contraindication.

Exposures & Prophylaxis Summary

- Measles:
  - If immunocompromised, **give Ig**
  - > 6mo or mom not breast feeding, **give vaccine**
- Mumps & Rubella:
  - Post exposure admin of live vaccine doesn't help
- Varicella
  - **Immunocompromised, pregnant, infant < 12mo: VZIG**
  - All others: vaccine
- Hepatitis
  - hepA: 1 dose of vaccine ASAP but w/in 2w of exposure
  - hepB: hepB Ig + vaccine → repeat at 1 & 6 months

Childhood Growth 1

What to Expect

Facts to Remember

- Newborn loses **10%** of BW (birth wt) in 1w
  - Back to BW by **2w**
- Gain **30g/day for 1st month**
  - 20g/day by 4th month
- **BW x 2 by 6mo**
  - **BW x 3 by 1yo**
- Height and wt inc at steady rate
  - Head-circumference rate dec between 2-5yo

Facts to Remember

- 6-12yo: Avg. 5 growth spurts /yr in 8w periods
- **7yo: Myelination of brain complete**
- 12yo: Growth acceleration begins
- Girls
  - Peak growth: **10.5yo**
  - Stop growing: **15yo**
- Boys
  - Peak growth: **13.5yo**
  - Stop growing: **18yo**

Growth Summary

- Loses **10%** of BW in 1w → back to BW by **2w**
  - **30g/day for 1st month**, 20g/day by 4th month
  - **BW x <u>2 by 6mo</u>. BW x <u>3 by 1yo</u>**
- Head-circumference rate dec between 2-5yo
  - **7yo: Myelination of brain complete**
- 12yo: Growth acceleration begins
  - Girls: Peak rate: **10.5yo.** Stop growing: **15yo**
  - Boys: Peak rate: **13.5yo.** Stop growing: **18yo**

Evaluate Growth

Note: when you're doing Peds, you always look at and chart the growth curve

- After 2yo, you stay on 1-2 growth curves
- Height percentile at 2yo ≅ adult percentile
- Low-BW infants can catch up through early school age

Childhood Growth 2

Evaluation

Growth Review

- Loses **10%** of BW in 1w → back to BW by **2w**
  - **30g/day for 1st month**, 20g/day by 4th month
  - **BW x 2 by 6mo. BW x 3 by 1yo**
- Head-circumference rate dec between 2-5yo
  - **7yo: Myelination of brain complete**
- 12yo: Growth acceleration begins
  - Girls: Peak rate: **10.5yo.** Stop growing: **15yo**
  - Boys: Peak rate: **13.5yo.** Stop growing: **18yo**

Keep in Mind

Note: when you're doing Peds, you always look at and chart the growth curve

- After 2yo, you stay on 1-2 growth curves
- Height percentile at 2yo ≅ adult percentile
- Low-BW infants can catch up through early school age

Evaluate Growth

- Chronological Age (**CA**) (obvious)
- Bone Age (**BA**): x-ray non-dominant hand
  - **bone maturity is linked more to sexual maturity** than chronologic age
- Growth Velocity (**GV**) is the slope of the change in height/change in age graph

- Compare CA and BA to access importance of pt being short or tall.

Evaluation of Growth Summary

- Height percentile at 2yo $\cong$ adult percentile
- Low-BW infants catch up through 7yo or so
- Compare CA and BA to access importance of pt being short or tall.
  - Short
    - CA > BA w/ normal GV: constitutional delay
    - CA > BA w/ **abnormal GV**: due to deficiency
    - CA = BA w/ normal GV: pt meant to be short
    - CA = BA w/ **abnormal GV**: genetic syndrome
  - Tall
    - CA $\leq$ BA w/ normal GV: pt meant to be big
    - CA $\leq$ BA w/ **abnormal GV:** genetic, endocrine, or CNS lesion

Short

- Short
  - CA > BA w/ normal GV
    - constitutional delay:
      - growth just hasn't kicked in yet
  - CA > BA w/ **abnormal GV**
    - illness, deficiency, or endocrine issue
  - CA = BA w/ normal GV
    - familial short stature
      - your family is just naturally short
  - CA = BA w/ **abnormal GV**
    - genetic syndrome

Tall

- Tall
  - CA $\leq$ BA w/ normal GV
    - familial tall or obesity
      - your just meant to be tall
  - CA $\leq$ BA w/ **abnormal GV**
    - genetic, endocrine, or CNS lesion
      - gigantisim

Evaluation of Growth Summary

- Height percentile at 2yo $\cong$ adult percentile
- Low-BW infants catch up through 7yo or so
- Compare CA and BA to access importance of pt being short or tall.
  - Short
    - CA > BA w/ normal GV: constitutional delay
    - CA > BA w/ **abnormal GV**: due to deficiency
    - CA = BA w/ normal GV: pt meant to be short
    - CA = BA w/ **abnormal GV**: genetic syndrome
  - Tall
    - CA $\leq$ BA w/ normal GV: pt meant to be big
    - CA $\leq$ BA w/ **abnormal GV:** genetic, endocrine, or CNS lesion

Childhood Growth 3

Why Are We Here

Growth Summary

- Loses **10%** of BW in 1w → back to BW by **2w**
  - **30g/day for 1st month**, 20g/day by 4th month
  - **BW x 2 by 6mo. BW x 3 by 1yo**
- Head-circumference rate dec between 2-5yo
  - **7yo: Myelination of brain complete**
- 12yo: Growth acceleration begins
  - Girls: Peak rate: **10.5yo.** Stop growing: **15yo**
  - Boys: Peak rate: **13.5yo.** Stop growing: **18yo**

Evaluation of Growth Summary

- Height percentile at 2yo $\cong$ adult percentile
- Low-BW infants catch up through 7yo or so
- Compare CA and BA to access importance of pt being short or tall.
  - Short
    - CA > BA w/ normal GV: constitutional delay
    - CA > BA w/ **abnormal GV**: due to deficiency
    - CA = BA w/ normal GV: pt meant to be short
    - CA = BA w/ **abnormal GV**: genetic syndrome
  - Tall
    - CA $\leq$ BA w/ normal GV: pt meant to be big
    - CA $\leq$ BA w/ **abnormal GV**: genetic, endocrine, or CNS lesion

Speaking of Nutrition

- Few conditions prevent a mother from breast feeding
  - **Significant** viral infections: HIV, HSV, HBV, CMV
  - **Significant** maternal dz: TB, sepsis, breast cancer
- Drugs: substance abuse, specific pharm

- **Mastitis does NOT prevent breast feeding. Continue to breast feed**

When to Introduce Solid Foods

- 4mo: Iron-Fortified cereal
- 6mo:
    1. Introduce strained veggies and fruits
    2. **Then** introduce dairy/meats
    - follow a **step-wise pattern**
        - body needs time to adapt, and this gives opportunity to identify allergies/deficiencies
- 9mo: table foods

Solid Food Specific Warnings

- **No honey before 1yo**
    - Infant botulism
- Wait till after 2yo for
    - **egg whites**, fish
    - nuts, **wheat**
    - **citrus, chocolate**

Nutrition Summary

- Don't Breast Feed
  - With significant viral infection
    - HIV, HSV, HBV, CMV
  - With maternal dz:
    - TB, sepsis, breast cancer
  - If substance abuser
  - On certain meds
- **Mastitis does NOT prevent breast feeding. Continue to breast feed**

Introduce Solid Foods Summary

- 4mo: Iron-Fortified cereal
- **6mo**: strained vegis/fruits → dairy/meats
- **9mo**: table foods
  - **no honey till 1yo**
- After 2yo
  - **egg whites**, fish
  - nuts, **wheat**
  - **citrus, chocolate**

Developmental Milestones 1

Warnings & Motor Year 1

Birth to 5yo

- The most important milestones occur before kids start school. At that point, professionals are witnessing them every day. Up till then, the physician is the most important assessor of development, outside of the parents.

Know These Like Your Own Name

- **<u>Prone</u> =** face down
  - 'P', remember you pee down

- The important milestone ages
  - 2,4,6,10,13 months old (mo)
  - 2,3,4,5 years old (yo)

- That months-old doesn't go from 10 to 12 tells you that walking occurs by 13mo. It's just too important.

Keep Saying It Till You Got It

- 2,4,6 mo
- 10,13 mo
- 2,3,4,5 yo

- 2,4,6 mo
- 10,13 mo
- 2,3,4,5 yo

How would you like to be the person playing with a kid who is showing signs of developmental delay, and you didn't even notice?

Motor: Year 1

- 2mo
  - Lifts head
- 4mo
  - Rolls over
  - Sits with support
- 6mo
  - **Sits well unsupported**
  - Switches objects between hands
- 10mo
  - **Pincer grasp**
  - **Stands with help → Crawls → Cruises**
    - Fear of falling
- 13mo
  - **Walks, Ascends stairs**
  - Kick and throw ball

Motor: Year 1 Edited

- 4mo
  - If rolling over at 4mo, then you know she was lifting her head at 2mo
  - Rolls over
  - Sits with support
    - If sits w/ support at 4mo, then you know she sits well unsupported at 6mo
- 10mo
  - If had pincer grasp at 10mo, then you know she was switching hands at 6mo
  - **Pincer grasp**
  - **Stands with help → Crawls → Cruises**
    - Fear of falling
- 13mo
  - **Walks, Ascends stairs**
  - Kick and throw ball

Too much locomotion happening at 10mo not to memorize this one. Also, people feel smart saying "pincer grasp"

Summary

- **Prone** = face down ('P', remember you pee down)

- **4mo**
    - If rolling over at 4mo, then you know she was lifting her head at 2mo
  - **Rolls over**
  - **Sits with support**
    - If sits w/ support at 4mo, then you know she sits-well unsupported at 6mo
- **10mo**
    - If had pincer grasp at 10mo, then you know she was switching hands at 6mo
  - **Pincer grasp**
  - **Stands with help → Crawls → Cruises** (Fear of falling)
    - If cruising at 10mo, then you know she was walking at 13yo

Developmental Milestones 2

Motor: Getting Ready For School

Review

- **4mo**
  - If rolling over at 4mo, then you know she was lifting her head at 2mo
  - **Rolls over**
  - **Sits with support**
    - If sits w/ support at 4mo, then you know she sits-well unsupported at 6mo
- **10mo**
  - If had pincer grasp at 10mo, then you know she was switching hands at 6mo
  - **Pincer grasp**
  - **Stands with help → Crawls → Cruises** (Fear of falling)
    - If cruising at 10mo, then you know she was walking at 13yo

Motor: Not Ready For Polite Society

- 18mo
  - **Stacks 3 cubes**
  - Hand preference emerges
- 2yo
  - **Stacks 6 cubes**
  - **Copies a line, scribbles w/ crayons**
  - Turns doorknob, unscrews lid
  - **Runs,** Walks backward, Descends stairs
  - **Aim thrown ball**
- 3yo
  - **Stacks 9 cubes**
  - **Copies a circle**
  - Unbuttons buttons, Cuts paper w/ scissors
  - Rides tricycle, Ascends stairs like adult
  - Catches ball w/ arms
  - **Toilet training**

Motor: Threes

- **3yo:**
  - Stacks (**3 cubes** * **3** yo) = 9 cubes; Rides **TRI**cycle
  - Copies a circle, Ascends stairs like adult
  - Unbuttons buttons, Cuts paper w/ scissors, Catches ball w/ arms
  - **<u>Toilet training</u>**

- <u>3yo is HUGE. One could boldface every one of these</u>
  - At 3yo, you are going out and playing with your friends. Circles and 9 cube stacks are great for inside, but outside you're going up stairs like a pro, riding around the carport on your tricycle, catching a ball with the help of your arms, and taking your clothes off and running around naked!
  - And scissors — do you have any idea of how much trouble a kid can get into with a pair of scissors? Neither does he, but he plans to find out.

Motor: Getting Ready For School

- 4yo
  - **Copies a cross**
  - Brushes teeth
  - **Hops on one foot**, Descends stairs like adult
  - Throws overhand
- 5yo
  - **Copies a square**
  - Partially dresses self
  - Catches ball with 2 hands
  - **No potty accidents**

Motor: 5yo is Common Sense

- Don't have to memorize 5yo. Just ask yourself,
  - **What does a kid need to do to go to school and not have other kids make fun of him?**
- Forget the square. He better not be pooping his pants occasionally!!!
- He has to dress himself.
- He has to be able to catch a ball w/ 2 hands.
  - or get hit in the face

Motor: Cubes and Shapes

- Stacks Cubes: **Cubes ≈ 3 * age in years**
  - 3 (18mo) → 6 (2yo) → 9 (3yo)
    - *Test makers love cubes*

- Copies Shapes
  - **line** (2yo) → **circle** (3yo) → **cross** (4yo) → **square** (5yo)
    - 1 line at 2yo, 2 lines at 4yo = a cross
    - *Test makers love copying shapes*

Motor: Do the Locomotion

- [Stands w/ help → crawls → cruises] (10mo) → Walks (13mo) → runs (2yo) → tricycle (3yo) → hops on one foot (4yo) → **skips (6yo)**
  - *Everyone loves this, not just test makers*

Motor Summary: Trends

- Stacks Cubes:
  - **Cubes ≈ 3 * age in years**
  - 3 (18mo) → 6 (2yo) → 9 (3yo)

- Copies Shapes:
  - **line** (2yo) → **circle** (3yo) → **cross** (4yo) → **square** (5yo)
    - 1 line at 2yo, 2 lines at 4yo = a cross

- Locomotion:
  - 10mo; 1,2,3,4,6yo
  - [Stands w/ help → crawls → cruises] (10mo) → Walks (13mo) → runs (2yo) → tricycle (3yo) → hops on one foot (4yo) → **skips (6yo)**

Motor Summary: Each Year

- 2yo: Terrible Two's
  - Aggressive, running around, aiming what he throws
  - Yelling "NO", opening doors, getting into things
- 3yo: Getting Cute Again
  - Unbuttoning pants and using toilet
  - Scissors
  - Riding tricycle and going up stairs like a pro
- 4yo, almost ready for school
  - Brushes teeth while hopping on one foot and throwing things overhand into the bathtub
  - Copies a cross
- 5yo, ready for school
  - Dresses self, catches with 2 hands, and doesn't have potty accidents
    - You can't go to school if you can't get ready in the morning, protect yourself from thrown objects, and are still pooping in your pants.

Developmental Milestones 3

Lets Get Social

Review

- **4mo**
  - If rolling over at 4mo, then you know she was lifting her head at 2mo
  - **Rolls over**
  - **Sits with support**
    - If sits w/ support at 4mo, then you know she sits-well unsupported at 6mo
- **10mo**
  - If had pincer grasp at 10mo, then you know she was switching hands at 6mo
  - **Pincer grasp**
  - **Stands with help → Crawls → Cruises** (Fear of falling)
    - If cruising at 10mo, then you know she was walking at 13yo

Motor Reviews: Trends

- Stacks Cubes:
  - **Cubes ≈ 3 * age in years**
    3 (18mo) → 6 (2yo) → 9 (3yo)

- Copies Shapes:
  - **line** (2yo) → **circle** (3yo) → **cross** (4yo) → **square** (5yo)
    - 1 line at 2yo, 2 lines at 4yo = a cross

- Locomotion:
  - **10mo**; 1,2,3,4,6yo
  - [Stands w/ help → crawls → cruises] (10mo) → Walks (13mo) → runs (2yo) → tricycle (3yo) → hops on one foot (4yo) → **skips (6yo)**

Motor Review: Each Year

- 2yo: Terrible Two's
  - Aggressive, running around, aiming what he throws
  - Yelling "NO", opening doors, getting into things
- 3yo: Getting Cute Again
  - Unbuttoning pants and using toilet
  - Scissors
  - Riding tricycle and going up stairs like a pro
- 4yo, almost ready for school
  - Brushes teeth while hopping on one foot and throwing things overhand into the bathtub
  - Copies a cross
- 5yo, ready for school
  - Dresses self, catches with 2 hands, and doesn't have potty accidents
    - You can't go to school if you can't get ready in the morning, protect yourself from thrown objects, and are still pooping in your pants.

Social

- 2mo: Social smile
- 6mo: Stranger anxiety
- 9mo: Pat-a-cake, Peek-a-boo
- 1yo:
  - Separation anxiety
  - Parallel play
    - Doesn't play with others but prefers their company
- 2yo:
  - Self-centered
  - May be aggressive, "NO"
  - Imitates

Social

- 3yo
  - Group play, understands taking turns
  - Fixed gender identity, knows own gender, sex-specific play
- 4yo
  - Curious about sex, imitates adult roles
  - Nightmares/monsters, imaginary friends
- 5yo
  - Conforming to peers
  - Oedipal phase, romantic feelings for others
- 6-12yo
  - "Rules of the game" important, organized sports possible, being team member important
  - Separation of sexes, sexual feeling not apparent
  - Demonstrating competence is important
- >12yo
  - Identity important but conformity most important

Social

- Development of place in society
  - Stranger anxiety (6mo) → Separation anxiety (1yo), Parallel play → Egocentric, aggressive, "NO", imitates (2yo) → **sex establishment (3yo)** → imitates adult roles (4yo) → peer pressure (5yo) → competence important (6-12yo) → Conformity over identity (teenager)
    - Don't need to memorize "Peek-a-boo" at 9mo, because you'll learn later that object permanence occurs by 1yo, therefore, peek-a-boo isn't as much fun.
      - You learn pat-a-cake when you learn peek-a-boo.
    - Don't need to memorize imaginary friends, nightmares, and monsters at 4yo, because you'll learn later that this is when you begin to tell stories. Age 4yo is like the golden age of imagination.
- Development of sex
  - **Fixed gender, knows own gender, sex-specific play (3yo)** → curious about sex (4yo) → Oedipal & romantic (5yo) → separation of sexes (6-12yo) → teenager
    - have your first love after school starts at 5yo
- Development of gameplay
  - Peek-a-boo/pat-a-cake (9mo) → Parallel play (1yo) → Group play (3yo) → Sex-specific play (4yo) → Rules of game important/organized sports (6yo

Social Summary

- 2mo: Social smile
- 6mo: **Stranger anxiety**
- 1yo:
  - Likes having someone around (**Separation anxiety**, Parallel play)
- **2yo:**
  - **Self-centered, aggressive, "NO";**
  - **Imitating**
- **3yo**
  - **Group play, Understands taking turns**
  - **Fixed gender identity, Knows own gender, Sex-specific play**
- 4yo
  - **Imagination**: Curious about sex, Imitates adult roles, Imaginary friends, Nightmares/monsters
- 5yo
  - **Conforming to peers**
  - **Oedipal** phase, **Romantic** feelings for others
- 6-12yo
  - "**Rules** of the game" important, Organized sports possible, Being team member important
  - Separation of sexes, Sexual feeling not apparent
  - Demonstrating competence is important
- >12yo
  - Identity important but conformity most important

Social Need To Know

- **Stranger anxiety** (6mo) → **Separation anxiety**, Parallel play (12mo)
- 2yo: Terrible twos → Group play, Gender Identity (3yo) → Imagination, curiousity (4yo)
- **Conform and fall in love (Oedipal)** (5yo)

- Don't worry about 6-12yo
    - We all know when we were most active in organized sports. You didn't spend much time with the other sex. You just wanted to be trusted to do it yourself.
- Don't worry about teenagers. We all remember those years
    - and what we don't remember, teenagers will remind us.

Developmental Milestones 4

He Gets IT.
He really really gets it

Cognitive

- 5mo to 1yo
  - Everything goes in mouth
  - Bang and rattle
  - No object permanence. (Would peek-a-boo be any fun with it?)
  - Solitary play and exploration
  - **Issues of trust are key.**
- **1yo : Object permanence (no more peek-a-boo?)**
- 2yo
  - Understands "objects", can use symbols, concrete
    - no abstraction
  - Very egocentric but using **transition item** to advance into world
    - transition item: woobie, teddy bear
- 3yo
  - Repeats 3 digits, points and names 3 things
  - Knows colors

Cognitive

- 4yo
  - Repeat 4 digits
  - Knows body parts.
- 5yo
  - Counts 10 objects.
- 6-12yo
  - Abstract thought develops
  - Adheres to logic. No hypotheticals. **Personal** sense of right & wrong.
  - Law of conservation.
- >12yo
  - Expand abstractions. Can handle hypotheticals
  - Past, present, and future
  - Problems-solving algorithms.

Cognitive Summary

- 5mo to 1yo: **Issues of trust are key**.
- **1yo : Object permanence (no more peek-a-boo?)**
- 2yo
  - Understands "objects", can use symbols, concrete
    - no abstraction
  - Very egocentric but using **transition item** to advance into world
    - transition item: woobie, teddy bear
- **3**yo:
  - Repeats **3** digits, points and names **3** things, Knows colors
- 4yo
  - Repeat **4** digits, Knows body parts.
- 5yo: Counts 10 objects
- 6-12yo
  - Abstract thought develops. No hypotheticals, yet.
  - Adheres to logic. **Personal** sense of right & wrong.
    - remember, "rules" are a big deal now
  - Law of conservation.

Cognitive Summary

- The first two periods are kind of obvious. We've all learned that the more frequently a child looks over their shoulder when beginning to crawl and sees a caregiver watching them, the more confidence they're expected to develop in later life. Not sure if this is true or not, but it does emphasize that **trust** is a key issue before 1yo.
- Object permanence at 1yo is just common sense. Kid better get it before getting too old
- 2yo: She is the most important thing in the world. Expects your attention when demanded. A toy is **exactly** what a toy is. Don't screw with them on this. They're already aggressive and this makes it worse. And everyone knows of a 2yo that carries something around with them everywhere they go.
- 3yo: Repeats 3 digits, points and names 3 things, Knows colors
  - 3yo 3 3 3 colors – how easy is that
- 4yo: Repeat 4 digits, 4 body parts.
  - 4yo 4 4. Body parts may actually be more than 4, but this helps to remember
- 5yo: Counts 10 objects
  - Starts school and can count all her fingers, or the number of jelly beans.
- 6-12yo
  - Abstract thought develops. No hypotheticals, yet.
    - no abstractions, so no hypotheticals
  - Adheres to logic. **Personal** sense of right & wrong.
    - remember, "**rules**" are a big deal now
  - Law of conservation.
    - Organized sports will teach one that energy needs to be conserved, therefore other things have a limit as well

Developmental Milestones 5

What you talking about...
errrr... How did you come to talk?

Language

- 6mo: Babbles
- 9mo: Repeats sounds, Mama, dada, bye-bye
- 1yo: 10 words
- **2yo**
    - **2** word sentences, **>200** words
    - Pronouns
    - Parents understand better
- 3yo
    - Complete sentences, 900 words, understands 3600 words
    - Stranger understand 3/4
    - Recognize objects in pictures
- 4yo
    - Tells stories
    - Uses prepositions, plurals, and compound sentences
- 5yo
    - Asks meaning of words and abstract words are difficult
- 6-12yo
    - Speech more socially centered

Language Makes Sense

- Babbles (6mo) → Repeats sounds, Mama, dada, bye-bye (9mo)

- 10 words (**1**yo) → **2** word sentences, > **2**00 words, strangers understand 1/**2** (2yo)
  - pronouns at 2yo – when does a kid start saying "mine"? Terrible twos.

- **3**yo: complete sentences, and multiples of **3**
  - 900 (**3***300) words, 3600 (**3***1200) words understood, **3**/4 understood
    - bigger vocabulary is more likely to identify objects in pictures by name

- 4yo: **Imagination**
  - **Tells stories** and develops more complicated sentences
    - eg. prepositions, plurals, and compound sentences
  - This is also the time of imaginary friends, monsters, nightmares, and sexual curiosity. **4yo is the Age of Imagination**

- 5yo: Asks meaning of words and abstract words are difficult
  - Naturally this follows telling stories, and abstraction doesn't develop until 6-12yo.
    - Don't need to memorize. This one is common sense

- 6-12yo: Speech more socially centered
  - In school, playing organized sports. Of course this is when kids become more socially centered.
    - Don't really need to memorize. This one is common sense.

Language Summary

- Babbles (6mo) → Repeats sounds, Mama, dada, bye-bye (9mo)

- 10 words (**1**yo) → **2** word sentences, > **2**00 words, strangers understand 1/**2** (2yo)
  - pronouns at 2yo – when does a kid start saying "mine"? Terrible twos.

- **3**yo: complete sentences, and multiples of **3**
  - 900 (**3***300) words, 3600 (**3***1200) words understood, **3**/4 understood
    - bigger vocabulary is more likely to identify objects in pictures by name

- 4yo: **Imagination**
  - **Tells stories** and develops more complicated sentences
    - eg. prepositions, plurals, and compound sentences
  - This is also the time of imaginary friends, monsters, nightmares, and sexual curiosity. **4yo is the Age of Imagination**

- 5yo: Asks meaning of words and abstract words are difficult

313

Milestone Age Summaries: 6mo

- **S**ix mo
  - 6abbles (aka. babbles)
  - **S**witches hands, **S**trangers, **S**itting

Milestone Age Summaries: 1yo

- 1yo
  - **Walk**ing away from mom causes **anxiety**
  - Stacks **3 cubes**
    - Cubes ≈ 3 * age in years
  - **Parallel play, object permanence**
  - **10 words**

Milestone Age Summaries: 2yo

- **2**yo: Terrible Twos
  - Do a **line**, stack **6 cubes**
    - Cubes ≈ 3 * age in years
  - Run, open doors, aim what you throw
  - "NO", aggressive, imitate
  - Concrete objects, using transition object
  - **2**-word sentences, > **2**00 words, 1/**2** understood by strangers

Milestone Age Summaries: 3yo

- **3**yo
  - **Tri**cycle, **3** numbers, **3** <u>colors</u>, **3** kids make a **group, 3/4** of speech understood by strangers
  - 900 (**3*300**) words, 3600 (**3***1200) understood, complete sentences
  - **Circle, scissors**
  - Can unbutton pants and **toilet train**
  - **Gender identity**

Milestone Age Summaries: 4yo

- 4yo: **The Age of Imagination**
  - Imagination: tells stories, imaginary friends, monsters, nightmares, & sexual curiosity
  - **4** body parts (head, shoulders, knees, and toes), **4/4** speech understood by strangers, things that happened be**FOUR**
  - Cross
    - At 2yo drew a line, at 4yo draw 2 lines = a cross
  - **Brushes teeth, hops on one foot**, throws overhand

Milestone Age Summaries: 6yo

- 6yo
  - skips, ties shoes, draws person with 6 parts
    - The DAP (Draw A Person) Test has somewhat been disproven, so drawing questions are less likely. However, parents still know about it and ask questions.

Pediatric Neurology 1

Immediate Post-birth Trauma Findings

Newborn Nerve Damage

- Brachial palsy
  - Full recovery in months unless nerve was lacerated
  - Tx: Partial immobilization, massage, ROM exercise for 6mo → neuroplasty (if needed)
  - Erb-Duchenne: C5/C6
    - Can't abduct shoulder
    - Externally rotate and supinate forearm
  - Klumpke: C7/C8 ± T1
    - Paralyzed hand ± Horner syndrome
- Facial Nerve palsy
  - Improves in weeks unless fibers were torn → neuroplasty

Newborn Nerve Damage

- Brachial palsy
  - C5/6: **Erb** can't **abd**-uct
    - Externally rotate and supinate forearm
  - C7/C8: **Klumpke hand** and face
    - Klumpke sounds like clumsy
- Facial Nerve palsy

Cranial Swelling

- **Cephalohematoma**
  - cephalo = relating to head or skull
  - hematoma = solid swelling of clotted blood
  - ie. a solid swelling of clotted blood in the head that **Doesn't cross suture lines**
  - Possible underlying linear fracture, resolves in 3w
- **Caput succedaneum**
  - caput = scalp; succedaneum = coming after
    - Notice blood isn't involved. This is edematous.
  - ie. edematous swelling under the scalp of a newborn from trauma sustained during birth.
  - Swelling **crosses suture** lines
  - Disappears in days → molding (as needed)

Cranial Swelling

- **Cephalohematoma**
  - Head hematoma that **doesn't cross suture lines**
    - Possible underlying linear fracture, resolves in 3w
- **Caput succedaneum**
  - Edematous swelling under the scalp post-birth.
  - Swelling **crosses** suture lines
    - Disappears in days → molding (as needed)

Newborn Nerve Damage Summary

- Brachial palsy
  - C5/6: **Erb** can't **abd**-uct
    - Externally rotate and supinate forearm
  - C7/C8: **Klumpke hand** and face
    - Klumpke sounds like clumsy
- Facial Nerve palsy

Cranial Swelling Summary

- **Cephalohematoma**
  - Head hematoma that **doesn't cross** suture lines
    - Possible underlying linear fracture, resolves in 3w
- **Caput succedaneum**
  - Edematous swelling under the scalp post-birth.
  - Swelling **crosses** suture lines
    - Disappears in days → molding (as needed)

Pediatric Neurology 2

Fluctuant Spinal Masses That Arise a
Bit Later Than Post-birth

Neural Tube Defects
Meningocele

- **Meningocele**
  - Meninges herniate through defect in posterior vertebrae → fluctuant mass covered w/ skin
  - CT scan head for hydrocephalus

Neural Tube Defects
Myelomeningocele

- Myelomeningocele = meningocele w/ muscle involved
  - Anywhere along axis but generally in the lumbosacral region
  - 80% ~ Chiari type II malformation
    + hydrocephalus and hindbrain dysfunction (trouble swallowing, breathing, talking)
  - Low sacral lesions
    - Bowel/bladder incontinence and perineal anesthesia
    - No motor impairment
  - Mid-lumbar lesions
    - Urinary dribbling and relaxed anal sphincter
    - Flaccid paralysis below lesions. No DTRs
    - Tx: shunt + surgery

Neural Tube Defects
Meningocele vs. Myelomeningocele

- Meningocele
  - Meninges herniate through defect in posterior vertebrae → fluctuant mass covered w/ skin
- Myelomeningocele
  - Anywhere along axis but generally in the lumbosacral region
  - 80% ~ Chiari type II malformation: (hydrocephalus + hindbrain)
  - In the low sacrum, can cause incontinence & perineal anesthesia but motor was higher up.
  - In mid-lumbar, just the reverse. Motor highly effected but bowl/bladder mildly dysfunctional.

Dandy-Walker

- **4th ventricle missing roof** → expands to cyst
- **Agenesis** of posterior **cerebellar vermis** & corpus callosum
  - **Ataxia**

Neural Tube Defects
Summary

- **Meningocele**: meninges herniate
  - **Meninges** herniate through defect in posterior vertebrae → fluctuant mass covered w/ skin
- **Myelomeningocele**: meninges herniate and affect muscle
  - Anywhere along axis but generally lumbosacral
  - 80% ~ Chiari type II malformation: (hydrocephalus + hindbrain)
  - Sacral: incontinence, no motor
  - Lumbar: minor incontinence, lots of motor

- **Dandy Walker**: fluid herniates
  - 4th ventricle missing roof → expands to cyst
  - **Agenesis** of posterior **cerebellar vermis** & corpus callosum
    - **Ataxia**

Pediatric Neurology 3

Seizures: Febrile & Partial

Seizures

- Febrile
- Partial:
  - ie. **Affect only one hemisphere of the brain**
  - Simple
  - Complex
- Generalized
  - Absence = petit mal
  - Tonic-clonic

Seizures

- Febrile
- Partial:
  - Affect only one hemisphere of the brain
    - **May arise from any lobe of the brain**.
  - Simple = partial seizures **w/o** dyscognitive features
    - aka. **remain conscious**
  - Complex = partial seizures <u>**w** dyscognitive features</u>
- Generalized
  - Absence = petit mal
  - Tonic-clonic

- NOTE: aura indicates focal onset

Febrile Seizures

- 6mo to 6yo, most between 12-18mo
- Generally a FHx
- Rapid temp rise to > 39C (102F) → generalized tonic-clonic
  - lasts < 15min w/ brief postictal period
    - Can last longer than 15 min and have multiple in one day w/ focal findings, but this is atypical.
      - This would actually be a Dx by exclusion
- No inc risk of epilepsy
- Tx what caused the fever and observe

Partial Seizures: Simple

- Simple, ie. **no loss of consciousness (LOC)**
  - May have an aura, may talk during it.
  - Usually lasts < 20s w/ **no postictal period**
  - May start as Simple and advance to more generalized
    - **Jacksonian March**: spreads from distal lib toward ipsilateral face
  - EEG: **spike and sharp waves or multifocal spikes**
  - Tx: **phenytoin**

Partial Seizures: Complex

- Complex (ie. **LOC**)
  - Possible aura. Impaired consciousness.
  - Automatisms:
    - lip-smacking, chewing, increased saliva
  - EEG: often reveal **temporal lobe abnormalities**
  - Tx: **carbamazepine**

Seizures Summary

- **Febrile**
  - Before school age, generally runs in family
  - Rapid temp rise → generalized tonic-clonic
    - lasts < 15min w/ brief postictal period
  - No inc risk of epilepsy

- **Partial Seizures**
  - Simple (ie. **no LOC**)
    - Lasts < 20s w/ **no postictal period**
    - May start as Simple and advance to more generalized
    - EEG: spike and sharp waves or multifocal spikes
    - Tx: **phenytoin**
  - Complex (ie. Impaired consciousness)
    - Automatisms: lip-smacking, chewing, increased saliva
    - EEG: often reveal temporal lobe abnormalities
    - Tx: **carbamazepine**

Pediatric Neurology 4

Seizures: Generalized

Seizures Review

- **Febrile**
  - Before school age, generally runs in family
  - Rapid temp rise → generalized tonic-clonic
    - lasts < 15min w/ brief postictal period
  - No inc risk of epilepsy

- **Partial Seizures**
  - Simple (ie. no **LOC**)
    - Lasts < 20s w/ **no postictal period**
    - May start as Simple and advance to more generalized
    - EEG: spike and sharp waves or multifocal spikes
    - Tx: **phenytoin**
  - Complex (ie. Impaired consciousness)
    - Automatisms: lip-smacking, chewing, increased saliva
    - EEG: often reveal temporal lobe abnormalities
    - Tx: **carbamazepine**

Generalized Seizures

- Absence = petit mal
  - EEG: **3/second spike and generalized wave** distribution
  - Tx: **ethosuximide**

Generalized Seizures

- Tonic-clonic
  - Aura → LOC → eyes roll back
    → tonic contraction → apnea
    → clonic rhythmic contractions
  - Postictal period up to 2h
  - Tx: valproic acid, phenobarbital, phenytoin, or carbamazepine
    - basically, any of the anti-seizure medications might apply

Generalized Seizures Summary

- Absence = petit mal
  - EEG: 3/second spike and generalized wave
  - Tx: **ethosuximide**
- Tonic-clonic
  - Aura → LOC → eyes roll back → tonic contraction → apnea → clonic rhythmic contractions
  - Postictal period up to 2h

Seizures Summary

- **Febrile**: young, rapid rise in temp, no inc risk of epilepsy
- **Partial**: one hemisphere
  - Simple: **no LOC**, no postictal period
    - EEG: **spike and sharp** waves **or multifocal** spikes
    - Tx: **phenytoin**
  - Complex: **Automatisms, temporal lobe**
    - Tx: **carbamazepine**
- **Generalized**
  - Absence = petit mal. Tx: **ethosuximide**
  - Tonic-clonic: Postictal period up to 2h

Pediatric Neurology 5

Seizures: Not The Traditional Seizure

Neonatal Seizures

- Immature neurology causes subtle seizures
- Causes
  - **Hypoxic ischemic encephalopathy**
    - < 24 hours post-birth
    - Most common
  - CNS infection, hemorrhage, abnormalities
  - Inborn errors of metabolism. Drug withdrawal

Infantile Spasms

- **Inc CRH** → neuronal hyperexcitability
  → symmetric contractions.
- Attack types
  - **Lightning attacks**:
    - Sudden and severe. Involves much of body in split second
      - legs in particular
  - **Nodding attacks**: Just like it sounds
  - **Salaam or jackknife attacks**: Just like it sounds
- May be a consequence of a disorder.
- EEG: **hypsarrhythmia**
  - asynchronous, chaotic bilateral spike-and-wave pattern
- Tx: **ACTH** ± prednisone
  - ACTH provides neg feedback on CRH

Myoclonic Seizure = Myoclonus

- Repetitive. Brief, symmetric muscle contraction and loss of tone
- Most common is the **myoclonic jerk** one does when falling asleep.
  - **Hiccups** are a myoclonic jerk of the diaphragm

Not Quite Traditional Seizure Summary

- **Neonatal Seizures**
  - Immature neurology causes subtle seizures due to
    - Hypoxic ischemic encephalopathy, CNS infection, hemorrhage
    - Abnormalities, Inborn errors of metabolism. Drug w/d

- **Infantile Spasms**
  - **Inc CRH** → neuronal hyperexcitability → symmetric contractions.
  - <u>Lightning attacks</u>, Nodding attacks, Salaam or jackknife attacks
  - EEG: hypsarrhythmia
  - Tx: **ACTH** ± prednisone

- **Myoclonus** = myoclonic seizure
  - Myoclonic jerk falling asleep. Hiccups

Pediatric Neurology 6

Neurocutaneous Syndromes
Are Often AD

Neurofibromatosis 1 (NF-1)

- AD, chr17
- Dx: 2 or more of the following
  - 5 cafe-au-alit spots, axillary/inguinal freckling
  - > 2 neural growths or 1 plexiform
  - bone issues, eye issues
- Gets worse as gets older
  - optic glioma, harmartoma
  - malignant neoplasms

NF-1 Shorter

- AD, chr17
- Dx: 2 or more of the following
  - spots, freckles, growths
  - bone, or eye
- Gets worse as gets older
  - Can become malignant

NF-2 AD

- Just learn NF-1 and then remember '2' for NF-2
  - NF2, chr22, **bilateral acoustic schwannomas**
    - NF2, chr 22, 2 ears

Tuberous Sclerosis AD

- **Tubers** in convolutions of cerebral hemispheres becoming calcified projecting into ventricle → hydrocephalus
- Presentation
  - Infant:
    - infantile spasms, **ash-leaf macule** (hypopigmented)
    - CT: calcified tubers
  - Child: generalized seizures + skin lesions
    - **Sebaceous adenoma** on face and **Shagreen patch** (orange-eel in lumbosacral area)
- 50% have **rhabdomyoma of the heart** as fetus which regresses after 2yo
- Renal lesion and pulmonary affected

Neurocutaneous Syndromes Are Often Autosomal Dominant Summary

- Neurofibromatosis (**NF-1**) , chr17
  - Dx: 2 or more of the following
    - 5 cafe-au-alit spots, axillary/inguinal freckling
    - > 2 neural growths or 1 plexiform
    - bone issues, eye issues
  - Gets worse as gets older. Can become malignant.
- NF2, chr22, **bilateral acoustic schwannomas**

- Tuberous Sclerosis AD
  - **Tubers** in cerebral hemispheres, calcified, projecting into ventricle → hydrocephalus
  - Infant:
    - infantile spasms, **ash-leaf macule** (hypopigmented) → CT: calcified tubers
  - Child: generalized seizures + skin lesions
    - **Sebaceous adenoma** on face and **Shagreen patch** (orange-eel in lumbosacral area)
  - **Rhabdomyoma of the heart**, renal lesion and pulmonary

Neurocutaneous Syndromes Are Often Autosomal Dominant Summary 2

- Neurofibromatosis (**NF-1**) , chr**17**
  - Dx: 2 or more of the following
    - 5 cafe-au-alit spots, axillary/inguinal freckling
    - neural growths, bone, eye
- NF**2**, chr**22**, **bilateral acoustic schwannomas**

- Tuberous Sclerosis AD
  - **Calcified tubers** into ventricle → hydrocephalus
  - Infant: spasms, **ash-leaf macule**
  - Child: generalized seizures + skin lesions
  - Can have tubers anywhere

Pediatric Neurology 7

Neurodegenerative Disorders -
Friedrich & Sphingolipidoses

Neurodegenerative Disorders

Develop a neuro ability and then progressively lose it

- Friedrich Ataxia
- Sphingolipidoses
  - Gaucher's Disease (most common)
  - Tay-Sachs.
    - It is > 10x more likely than Niemann-Pick, therefore you always r/o Tay-Sachs first.
- Purine Metabolism Disorders
  - Lesch-Nyhan.
    - Popular for it represents purine disorders and it's X-linked.
      - Test makers love X-linked
  - Adenosine Deaminase Deficiency.

Friedrich Ataxia

- Mut of gene **frataxin** (as in **fr**iedrich **ataxi**a)
- Slowly develop ataxia and explosive dysarthria before 15yo
  - some in 20's
  - May develop **hypertrophic cardiomyopathy**
    - → CHF → death

Sphingolipase Disorders (type of LSD) Gaucher's Disease

- Most common sphingolipase disorders (a LSD)
  - 1% of Americans are carriers, 9% of Ashkenazi Jews
- chr1
- Deficiency of **glucocerebrosidase** → build up of **glucocerebroside**
- Macrophages that look like crumpled tissue paper
- Symptoms
  - **Painless hepatosplenomegaly**, pancytopenia, **osteoporosis** w/ possible aseptic necrosis of femur and bone crises
  - Type I: impaired olfaction/cognitive
  - Type 2: convulsions, hypertonia, mental retardation, apnea
  - Type 3: myoclonus, convulsions, dementia, ocular muscle apraxia
- Tx:
  - Enzyme replacement therapy costs $200,000/yr for life, so doesn't get used much (and not asked about)
  - Recombinant glucocerebrosidases: a**glucerase** or other -glucerase

Sphingolipase Disorders
Gaucher's Disease

- chr1, Deficiency of **glucocerebrosidase**
- Macrophages: crumpled tissue paper
- Painless hepatosplenomegaly, osteoporosis
  - possible aseptic necrosis of femur and bone crises
- Tx: a**glucerase**

Sphingolipase Disorders
Tay Sachs

- chr15
- Deficiency of hexosaminidase A
  → GM2 ganglioside accumulation in cells
- Cherry-red spot on macula, lysosome w/ onion skin, no hepatosplenomegaly.
- Types
  - Infantile: Presents after 6mo.
    - Deterioration. Death by 4yo
  - Juvenile: Presents 2-10yo.
    - Deterioration. Death by 15yo.
  - Adult: Presents in 30's or 40's.
    - Normally not fatal.

Sphingolipase Disorders

- Gaucher's Disease
  - chr1, Deficiency of **glucocerebrosidase**
  - Macrophages: crumpled tissue paper
  - Painless hepatosplenomegaly, osteoporosis
    - possible aseptic necrosis of femur and bone crises
  - Tx: a**glucerase**
- Tay Sachs
  - chr15, Deficiency of hexosaminidase A → GM2 ganglioside accumulation
  - Cherry-red spot on macula, lysosome w/ onion skin, no hepatosplenomegaly.
  - The later it presents, the better

Summary

- **Friedrich Ataxia**
  - Mut of gene **frataxin**
  - Slowly develop ataxia and explosive dysarthria before 15yo
    - May develop **hypertrophic cardiomyopathy**

Sphingolipase Disorders
- **Gaucher's Disease**
  - chr1, Deficiency of **glucocerebrosidase**
  - Macrophages: **crumpled tissue paper**
  - Painless hepatosplenomegaly, osteoporosis
    - possible aseptic necrosis of femur and bone crises
  - Tx: a**glucerase**
- **Tay Sachs**
  - chr15, Deficiency of hexosaminidase A → **GM2 ganglioside** accumulation
  - **Cherry-red** spot on macula, lysosome w/ **onion skin**, no hepatosplenomegaly.

Pediatric Neurology 8

Neurodegenerative Disorders -
Purine Metabolism Disorders

Purine Metabolism Disorders

- Lesch-Nyhan **XR**
- Adenosine Deaminase Deficiency

Lesch-Nyhan **XR**

- Defect in purine salvage
  - due to absence of **HGPRT**
    - → excess uric acid (<u>gout</u>)
  - **He G**ot **P**urine **R**ecovery **T**rouble
- Mental retardation
- **Aggression w/ self-mutilation**
- Choreoathetosis

Adenosine Deaminase Deficiency

- 15% of all SCID cases are caused by ADA.
  - More common in Europe.
  - 3% of kids born w/ this gene in USA
- Lack of enzyme → buildup of dATP → dec DNA synthesis
  - T cells and B cells are very mitotically active, so they noticeably diminish
  - Also lack of enzyme → buildup of S-adenosylhomocysteine (don't need to know) → toxic to immature lymphocytes
- Small thymus. Bubble Boy.

Purine Metabolism Disorders Summary

- **Lesch-Nyhan**
  - **XR**
  - Defect in purine salvage: Absence of **HGPRT** → excess uric acid (<u>gout</u>)
    - **H**e **G**ot **P**urine **R**ecovery **T**rouble
  - Mental retardation, **Aggression w/ self-mutilation, Choreoathetosis**

- **Adenosine Deaminase Deficiency** (ie. ADA Deficiency)
  - 15% of all SCID cases are caused by ADA deficiency
  - Lack of enzyme → buildup of dATP → dec DNA synthesis
    - T cells and B cells noticeably diminish
      - Small thymus

Pediatric Neurology 9

Neuromuscular Diseases –
SMA, MG, ELS, MS

Neuromuscular Diseases

- Spinal Muscle Atrophy (SMA)
- Myasthenia Gravis vs. Eaton Lambert vs. MS
- Hereditary Motor Sensory Neuropathies (HMSNs)
  - ie. Marie-Charcot-Tooth Disease
- Guillain-Barre Syndrome

Spinal Muscle Atrophy (SMA)

- Denervation of muscle beginning in fetus and progressing through infancy → atrophy
- The later it presents the better.
  - SMA 1 presents in early infancy
  - SMA 2 presents in late infancy and progresses slowly
  - SMA 3 presents in even later and is a chronic condition
  - 26 overall types falling into these groups with mixed genetics (AR, AD, X-linked)
- SMA1
  - The infant progressively looks to have botulism: hypotonic and flaccid w/ little movement
    - Begins to have trouble feeding and breathing
    - Tongue and finger fasciculate and has no DTRs

Myasthenia Gravis vs. Eaton Lambert vs. Multiple Sclerosis

- Eyes, eyes, eyes. Presenting symptom is generally vision changes.
- MG:
  - Abs attach to ACh receptors in motor end plate → immune-mediated neuronal blockade
  - **Gets <u>worse</u> the more you use the muscle**
  - Neonates can get a **transient** version that lasts as long as it takes them to get mom's Abs out of their system (days to weeks)
  - EMG better than muscle biopsy (can't count on anti-Ach Abs)
- Eaton Lambert:
  - Abs attach to presynaptic voltage-gated Ca-channels preventing release of neurotransmitters
  - **Gets <u>better</u> the more you use the muscle.**
  - Usually begins in 40's
- MS:
  - **Plaques** form in CNS, CNS inflammation, and destruction of **myelin sheaths** of neurons
  - May be some combo of genetic, environment, and infection.
  - More common the farther from the equator and in northern Europeans

SMA Summary

- Denervation of muscle beginning in fetus and progressing through infancy → atrophy
- The later it presents the better.
- SMA1
  - The infant progressively looks to have botulism
    - Begins to have trouble feeding and breathing
    - Tongue and finger fasciculate and has no DTRs

MG vs Eaton Lambert vs MS Summary

- Eyes, eyes, eyes.
- MG:
  - Abs attach to ACh receptors in motor end plate → immune-mediated neuronal blockade
  - Gets **worse the more you use the muscle**
- Eaton Lambert:
  - Abs attach to presynaptic voltage-gated Ca-channels preventing release of neurotransmitters
  - **Gets better** the more you use the muscle.
- MS:
  - **plaques** form in CNS, CNS inflammation, and destruction of **myelin sheaths** of neurons
  - More common in: Northern Europeans and cold climates

Pediatric Neurology 10

Neuromuscular Diseases –
CMT, GBS

Hereditary Motor Sensory Neuropathies (HMSNs)

- ie. **Charcot–Marie–Tooth Disease (CMT)**
- Non-typical neural development and degradation of neural tissue
  → **hypertrophic demyelinated nerves or complete atrophy of neural tissue**
  - Progressive loss of muscle tissue and touch sensation across various areas of body
  - Can begin at any age. Usually the first symptom is **foot drop.**
    – Hammer toe, stork leg, pes cavus, pes planus
    – Progresses to hearing, seeing, chewing/swallowing/speaking and breathing issues
- **Vitamin C** might help.

HMSN Again

People don't remember this one because of its <u>horrible name</u>, so lets review once more.

- Hereditary Motor Sensory Neuropathies (HMSNs)
  - *descriptive, but still not a memorable name*
  - **Inherited. Motor & Sensory. Neuropathy**
    - ie. <u>Inherited</u> neuronal deficits, <u>both motor and sensory</u>
  - Commonly called Charcot–Marie–Tooth Disease (CMT)
    - *What a terrible name!!! "Tooth" throws everyone off. "CMT" has 10 different meanings.*
  - Neural development is faulty and then it **also** degrades.
    - *Yikes!*
    - The nerves get bigger as they demyelinate.
      - *Lets say this is due to clean-up damage, but does anyone really know?*
    - Neural tissue atrophies as they are no longer being used.
    - Progressive loss of muscle tissue and touch sensation across various areas of body
  - **Foot drop. Vitamin C** might help.
    - These two tidbits might just save you on a test

HMSN Again 2

- Hereditary Motor Sensory Neuropathies (HMSNs)
  - **Inherited. Motor & Sensory. Neuropathy**
  - ie. Charcot–Marie–Tooth Disease (CMT)
  - Progression
    - The nerves get bigger as they demyelinate.
    - Neural tissue atrophies as they are no longer being used.
    - **Progressive loss of muscle tissue and touch sensation across various areas of body**
    - **Foot drop.**
  - **Vitamin C** might help.

Postinfectious Polyneuropathy

- ie. **Guillain-Barre Syndrome (GBS)**
- 10 days post infection w/ Campylobacter jejuni, Mycoplasma pneumoniae, or virus → **ascending paralysis**
  - Immune system is abnormally activated and **Abs begins to attack the myelin sheath in the spinal cord.**
- Dx:
  - Inc CSF protein, normal glucose and **no** cells
  - Dec motor and sensory conduction
- Tx: admit, **IVIG** w/ **possible plasmapheresis**

CMT, GBS Summary

- Hereditary Motor Sensory Neuropathies (**HMSNs**)
  - ie. **Charcot–Marie–Tooth Disease (CMT)**
  - Non-typical neural development and degradation of neural tissue
    → **hypertrophic demyelinated nerves or complete atrophy of neural tissue**
  - Progressive loss of muscle tissue and touch sensation across various areas of body
  - **Foot drop.**
  - **Vitamin C** might help.

- **Guillain-Barre Syndrome (GBS)**
  - 10 days post infection **ascending paralysis**
    - Campylobacter jejuni, Mycoplasma pneumoniae, or virus
  - **Abs attack the myelin sheath in the spinal cord.**
  - Dx:
    - Inc CSF protein, normal glucose and **no** cells
    - Dec motor and sensory conduction
  - Tx: **IVIG** w/ **possible plasmapheresis**

Peds – Eye 1

Neonate Conjunctiva

1. Could be chemical conjunctivitis from the erythromycin drops if within first 24h
2. Ophthalmia neonatorum
   - N. Gonorrhea: 2-5 day incubation
   - C. trachomatis: 5-14 day incubation
3. Red Eye
   - Bacterial
   - Viral

Ophthalmia Neonatorum

- C. trachomatis: 5-14 day incubation
  - Most common
  - Swelling and purulent discharge
  - Cornea not usually effected, **mostly eyelids**
  - Tx: **erythromycin** PO for 14d + saline irrigation
- N. Gonorrhea: 2-5 day incubation
  - May be delayed to after 5 days due to suppression from erythromycin drops
  - Serosanguineous discharge: **thick purulent**
  - May cause **corneal ulcerations or uveitis**
  - Tx: **ceftriaxone** IM

Red Eye

- Bacterial
  - Mucopurulent exudate → crusting of lids together
    - one or both eyes
  - Cause: normal URI bacteria, S. aureus
  - Tx: warm compresses and topical Abs
- Viral
  - URI → watery discharge, bilaterally
  - Cause:
    - Adenovirus, enterovirus
    - Don't forget H. simplex

Retinopathy

- **Retinopathy of Prematurity**
  - Vasoproliferative scarring and blinding retinal detachment
  - Tx: cryosurgery or laser photocoagulation
- **Retinoblastoma**
  - Most common primary malignant intraocular tumor
  - AR, 13q14
  - Generally Dx in first 2y due to **leucokoria** (white mass in eye) and possible strabismus
    - How far it extends, like all cancers, controls the prognosis
  - Tx:
    - Enucleation by radiation, chemotherapy, or cryotherapy

Neonate Conjunctiva Summary

- **Chemical conjunctivitis**: erythromycin drops post-natal
- **Ophthalmia Neonatorum**
  - C. trachomatis: 5-14 day incubation
    - Cornea not effected, **mostly eyelids**
    - Tx: **erythromycin** PO for 14d + saline irrigation
  - N. Gonorrhea: 2-5 day incubation
    - possible 5d delay due to post-natal drops
    - **Thick purulent d/c**, May cause **corneal ulcerations or uveitis**
    - Tx: **ceftriaxone** IM
- **Red Eye**
  - Bacterial: Mucopurulent exudate → crusting of lids together
    - Cause: normal URI bacteria, S. aureus, Tx: warm compresses and topical Abs
  - Viral: URI → watery discharge, bilaterally

Retinopathy Summary

- **Retinopathy of Prematurity**
  - Vasoproliferative scarring and blinding retinal detachment
  - Tx: cryosurgery or laser photocoagulation
- **Retinoblastoma**: 13q14
  - Dx in first 2y due to **leucokoria**
  - Tx: Enucleation by rad, chemo, or cryo

Peds – ENT 1

Ear

Otitis Externa

- Most common: P. aeruginosa = Swimmer's Ear
  - 2nd most common: S. aureus
- Manipulation of outer ear causes significant pain.
- Tx: corticosteroids $\pm$ ciprofloxacin

- **Malignant External Otitis**
  + facial paralysis, vertigo, or other cranial nerve abnormalities
  - Tx: immediate BCx, IV Abs, and CT $\rightarrow$ surgery

Otitis Media

- Acute and suppurative, hearing loss
- Usually the normal URI bacteria
  - ie. S. pneumo, H. influenzae, Moraxella catarrhalis
- **The shorter, more horizontal eustachian tube in infants and toddlers allows for reflux from pharynx**
- Dx:
  - **Must have** acute onset + tympanic inflammation + effusion
- Tx:
  - Prefer to start w/ PO ibuprofen or acetaminophen
  - **Amoxicillin** (w/ PCN allergy: **azithromycin**)
  - If still in pain after 3 days
    - **amoxicillin/clavulinate** (or IM **ceftriaxone**)
  - If still not resolving
    - myringotomy or tympanoscentesis

OME (Otitis Media w/ Effusion)

- Repeated infections w/o time for effusion to resolve
- No developmental risk, but routine Abs recommended and possible **typanostomy tubes**
- Increases risk of
  - **Acute mastoiditis** due to displacement of **pinna**
    - Dx: clinical picture may suggest need for CT
    - Tx: myringotomy + IV Abs → w/ bone destruction: mastoidectomy
  - **Acquired cholesteatoma**
    - Cyst-like growth in middle ear or temporal bone
    - Progressively expands → bone resorption → intracranial → life-threatening
    - Dx: white opacity of eardrum or malodorous smell → CT
    - Tx: tympanomastoid surgery

It Has Nothing to Do With Your Colon

- Cholesteatoma
  - Non-cancerous skin cyst that develops in the middle ear.
  - May be congenital
  - May be acquired due to repeated ear infections
  - Cholesteatoma expansion can be life-threatening

Ear Summary:
Otitis Externa vs Media

- **Otitis Externa**: move the ear → pain
  - P. aeruginosa, S. aureus
  - Tx: corticosteroids ± ciprofloxacin
  - Malignant External Otitis
    + facial paralysis, vertigo, CN problem
    - Tx: immediate BCx, IV Abs, and CT → surgery

- **Otitis Media**: acute, suppurative, hearing loss
  - URI bacteria
  - Short horizontal tube in infants/toddlers → reflux from pharynx
  - Dx: **must have** acute onset + tympanic inflammation + effusion
  - Tx: Prefer to start w/ PO ibuprofen or acetaminophen
    - **amoxicillin** (or azithromycin) → **amoxicillin/clavulinate** (or IM ceftriaxone)
      → myringotomy or tympanoscentesis

Ear Summary: OME

- **OME** (Otitis Media w/ Effusion)
  - Repeated infections and effusions can't resolve
  - Tx: Abs ± typanostomy tubes
  - Increases risk of
    - **Acute mastoiditis**
      - Tx: myringotomy + IV Abs
        - → w/ bone destruction: mastoidectomy
    - **Acquired cholesteatoma**
      - Progressively expands → bone resorption → intracranial → life-threatening
      - Dx: white opacity of eardrum or malodorous smell → CT
      - Tx: tympanomastoid surgery

Ear Summary

- **Otitis Externa**: move the ear → pain
  - Tx: corticosteroids ± ciprofloxacin
  - Malignant External Otitis:
    - Tx: immediate BCx, IV Abs, and CT → surgery
- **Otitis Media**: acute, suppurative, hearing loss
  - **Must have** acute onset + tympanic inflammation + effusion
  - Tx: Prefer to start w/ PO ibuprofen or acetaminophen
    - **amoxicillin** (or azithromycin) → **amoxicillin/clavulinate** (or IM ceftriaxone)
      → myringotomy or tympanoscentesis
- **OME** (Otitis Media w/ Effusion): Repeated infections and no resolution
  - Tx: Abs ± typanostomy tubes
  - → **Acute mastoiditis**: Tx: myringotomy + IV Abs → mastoidectomy
  - → **Acquired cholesteatoma**: Tx: tympanomastoid surgery

Peds – ENT 2

ENT

Ear Review

- **Otitis Externa**: move the ear → pain
  - Tx: corticosteroids ± **ciprofloxacin**
  - Malignant External Otitis:
    - Tx: immediate BCx, IV Abs, and CT → surgery
- **Otitis Media**: acute, suppurative, hearing loss
  - <u>**Must have**</u> acute onset + tympanic inflammation + effusion
  - Tx: Prefer to start w/ PO ibuprofen or acetaminophen
    - **amoxicillin** (or azithromycin) → **amoxicillin/clavulinate** (or IM ceftriaxone)
      → myringotomy or tympanoscentesis
- **OME** (Otitis Media w/ Effusion): Repeated infections and no resolution
  - Tx: Abs ± typanostomy tubes
  → **Acute mastoiditis**: Tx: myringotomy + IV Abs → mastoidectomy
  → **Acquired cholesteatoma**: Tx: tympanomastoid surgery

Nose

- Epistaxis
  - Tx:
    1. Apply pressure, if that doesn't work
    2. Topical **oxymetazolone** or **phenylephrine** (vasoconstrictors) + Packing, if that doesn't work
    3. Cautery
- Nasal Polyps
  - Cystic Fibrosis is the most common cause

Sinuses

- Ethmoid and maxillary present at birth but only **ethmoid is pneumatized** (air filled)
- Sphenoid present at 5yo
- Frontal begins to develop at 7yo and completes in adolescence
- **Sinusitis**
  - Symptoms: nonspecific
  - Dx:
    - Persistent URI w/o improvement for > 10d
    - Severe respiratory symptoms w/ purulent d/c and temp ≥ 102F (38.9C) for ≥ 3d
  - Tx: amoxicillin/clavulinate→ cefuroxime (or azithromycin)

Indications for a Tonsillectomy

- Strept Pharyngitis
  - \> 6 documented w/in past year OR
  - 5/yr for 2y OR 3/yr for 3y OR
  - Unilateral enlarged tonsil

ENT Summary

- Epistaxis:
  - Tx: pressure → **oxymetazolone** or **phenylephrine** + packing → cautery
- Sinuses
  - Ethmoid pneumatized from birth, maxillary a bit later
  - Sphenoid by 5yo. Frontal develops from 7yo to teens
- Sinusitis
  - Persistent URI > 10d
    - Severe respiratory, purulent, temp ≥ 102F (38.9C) for ≥ 3d
  - Tx: amoxicillin/clavulinate → cefuroxime (or azithromycin)
- Indications for a Tonsillectomy
  - Strept Pharyngitis
    - \> 6 in 1y **OR** 5/yr for 2y **OR** 3/yr for 3y **OR** Unilateral enlarged tonsil

Med Summary

- Otitis Externa: go with a fluoroquinolone
  - Ciprofloxacin:
    - Good against aerobic g- bacilli (esp Enterobacter., Haemophilus), g- cocci (ie. Neisseria, Moraxella), non enteric g- bacilli (ie. P. aeruginosa, Staph).
    - Good w/ atypical pneumonias (ie. Legionella, Mycoplasma, Chlamydia).
    - Good w/ genital pathogens (ie. Chlamydia, Ureaplasma, Mycoplasma).
    - **Have to be careful of overuse, because it works so well in so many environments. Ear is a critical organ, so we usually protect it vigorously.**
- Otitis Media & Sinusitis: generally a URI pathogen
  - Otitis Media:
    - Prefer to start w/ PO ibuprofen or acetaminophen
    - **amoxicillin** → amoxicillin/clavulinate
      - If PCN sensitive: macrolide (ie. azithromycin) or clindamycin
  - Sinusitis:
    - amoxicillin/**clavulinate** → cefuroxime (or azithromycin)
      - 40% of H. influenzae and 100% of M. catarrhalis respiratory tract isolates are beta-lactamase producing

Med Summary

- Otitis externa: corticosteroids ± ciprofloxacin
- Otitis media:
  1. Prefer to start w/ PO ibuprofen or acetaminophen
  2. Amoxicillin → amoxicillin/clavulinate
     - If PCN sensitive: macrolide (ie. azithromycin) or clindamycin
- Sinusitis:
  - Amoxicillin/**clavulinate** → cefuroxime (or azithromycin)

Peds – Respiration 1

Respiratory Disorders
of the Newborn

Respiratory Disorders of the Newborn

- Some are actually respiratory-based
- Others are do to something else, and the respiratory effect is secondary

Respiratory Disorders of the Newborn

- Respiratory
  - Immature lungs
    - RDS = Respiratory Distress Syndrome
    - TTN = Transient Tachypnea of the Newborn
  - MAS = Meconium Aspiration Syndrome
  - Pneumonia
  - Non-lung developmental issue
    - Diaphragmatic hernia
    - Choanal atresia

Respiratory Disorders of the Newborn

- Nonrespiratory
  - Cardiac: cyanotic CHD
  - Blood: Anemia, polycythemia
  - Infection
  - Metabolic
  - Neurologic

Respiratory Distress Syndrome (**RDS**)

- Surfactant helps air sacs fill w/ air. It reduces the surface tension of fluid in the lungs, making alveoli more stable. This keeps them from collapsing when an individual exhales.
- Production of surfactant begins by 28w, but not until 35w is the baby producing enough to coat the entire lungs.
  - Prior to < 36w delivery, corticosteroids (**betamethasone**, dexamethasone) are given prior to delivery to increase production.
  - Preterm-newborns younger than 36w gestational age are likely to receive surfactant to overcome or prevent respiratory issues.

Respiratory Distress Syndrome (**RDS**)

- RDS: inability to maintain alveolar volume at end expiration → dec FRC & atelectasis
  - Hypoxemia, hypercarbia, respiratory acidosis
- In addition to CXR, the L/S ratio (**lecithin-to-sphingomyelin ratio**) should be obtained. This is the most accurate Dx test.
  - L/S ratio is performed on amniotic fluid prior to birth
  - L/S ratio ≥ 2: lung maturity
  - L/S ratio < 1.5: high risk of RDS
- Tx: O2, intubation → exogenous surfactant

Transient Tachypnea of the Newborn (TTN)

- Slow absorption of fetal lung fluid → dec pulmonary compliance and tidal volume w/ dec dead space
- Common w/ C-section or a rapid second stage of labor
- CXR: air-trapping, fluid, perihilar streaking
- Resolves w/in hours to days

Meconium Aspiration Syndrome (MAS)

- Meconium is the first stool of an neonate.
- Normally stored in intestines until after birth
- Expelled in response to fetal distress and hypoxia
- Amniotic fluid is greenish/yellowish

Respiratory Disorders of the Newborn Causes

- Respiratory
  - RDS, Transient Tachypnea of the Newborn
  - Meconium Aspiration Syndrome
  - Pneumonia
  - Diaphragmatic hernia, Choanal atresia
- Nonrespiratory
  - Cardiac: cyanotic CHD
  - Blood: Anemia, polycythemia
  - Infection
  - Metabolic
  - Neurologic

RDS & TTN Summary

- **RDS**
  - Insufficient surfactant to coat lungs results in respiratory distress
  - Surfactant
    - Production begins: 28w
    - Enough to coat lungs: 35w
    - Give betamethasone prior to delivery: < 36w
  - L/S ratio is performed on amniotic fluid prior to birth
    - L/S ratio – ≥ 2: lung maturity, < 1.5: high risk of RDS
- **Transient Tachypnea of the Newborn**
  - Slow absorption of fetal lung fluid → dec pulmonary compliance and tidal volume w/ dec dead space
  - Resolves w/in hours to days

Peds – Respiration 2

Stridor And What

Allergic Rhinitis,
The Less Obvious Symptoms

These are on a test.

Sometimes adding to the arsenal of diagnostic knowledge is fun in itself. Don't you love knowing what's wrong with someone when you first meet them?

- Nasal crease
  - line between upper two-thirds and lower third of nose
- Allergic shiners w/ Dennie-Morgan fold
  - Chronic dark under-eye circles which may be accompanied by a fold or line

Stridor

- High-pitched breath sound due to **turbulent air flow** in **larynx or lower bronchial tree**.
  - When stridor is heard, may help to listen to chest and then pharynx to differentiate.
- Caused by narrowed or obstructed airway.
- Inspiratory stridor in child. Most common
  1. Laryngomalacia
  2. Congenital Subglottic Stenosis
  3. Vocal Cord Paralysis
  - Also Croup (parainfluenza 1,2,3), epiglottis, foreign body, laryngeal tumor

Laryngomalacia

- Collapse of supraglottic structures during inspiration → stridor
  - Less stridor when prone
- Starts < 2 week old, progresses until 6mo
- Dx:
  - Laryngoscopy and bronchoscopy
- Tx:
  - Mild: supportive → Severe: supraglottoplasty

Congenital Subglottic Stenosis

- Recurrent croup w/ stridor unimproved by prone position
- Tx: surgery — cricoid split or reconstruction

Summary

- Stridor
  - High-pitched breath sound due to **turbulent air flow** caused by narrowing/obstruction in larynx **OR** lower bronchial tree
  - Most common causes inspiratory stridor in child
    1. Laryngomalacia
    2. Congenital Subglottic Stenosis
    3. Vocal Cord Paralysis
    - Also Croup (parainfluenza 1,2,3), epiglottis, foreign body, laryngeal tumor
- Laryngomalacia
  - Collapse of supraglottic structures during inspiration
  - Starts < 2 week old, progresses until 6mo
  - Dx: Laryngoscopy and bronchoscopy
  - Tx: supportive → supraglottoplasty

Vocal Cord Paralysis

- Causes
  - Commonly w/ meningomyelocele, Chiari malformation, hydrocephalus
  - Postsurgical repair of congenital heart defect or tracheoesophageal fistula (TEF)
- Dx:
  - **Flexible bronchoscopy**
- Tx:
  - Resolves by 1yo but may require temp tracheostomy

Peds – Respiration 3

CF, Bronchiolitis & Pneumonia

Cystic Fibrosis (CF) Tx

1. Clear airway
   - Albuterol nebulizer (inhibit bronchial muscle expansion)
   - Mucolytic: DNAse (break up mucous)
   - Physical therapy up to 4x/day (mechanically free up)
2. Abs
   - Most common infection is P. aeruginosa: aerosolized **tobramycin** (or **aztreonam**)
3. Hospitalization for 14d
   - Tx: tobramycin + **piperacillin**
- Daily:
   - Stay hydrated + pancreatic enzymes + Vitamins ADEK

Bronchiolitis

- Ages: Most severe < 2mo in winter.
  - Usually before 2yo
- Inflammation of the bronchioles, the smallest air passages of the lungs
  - By, RSV 50%, viruses, Mycoplasma
    - May lead to secondary infection.
- Air-trapping and over-inflation
  - Listen for **fine crackles** and prolonged expiratory phase
- Steroids don't help. This is not an expansion of smooth muscle but a blockage of small airways.
  - High risk pts may benefit from **palivizumab** (monoclonal Ab to RSV F protein)

Pneumonia: Bacterial vs. Viral

- Bacterial has higher inc in temp than viral
- Bacterial appears more toxic
- Bacterial is localized while viral is scattered
- With viral, Dx requires nasopharyngeal wash

Pneumonia Causes & Clinical Dx

- Bacterial:
  - **Acute onset of shaking, chills, high fever w/ dullness to percussion** (localized)
- Mycoplasma & Chlamydia pneumoniae:
  - Long lasting, clinically not too bad, and CXR looks worse than pt
  - Rales
- Chlamydia trachomatis:
  - **Staccato cough** + peripheral **eosinophilia**
    - staccato = each sound separated from the other

Pneumonia Tx

- Bacterial:
  - IV **cefuroxime**
  - If S. aureus suspected + **Vanc or Clinda**
- Chlamydia or Mycoplasma:
  - **Erythromycin** (macrolide)
- Viral:
  - Supportive, but monitor for secondary bacterial infection to begin and then see previous

Pneumonia Tx Summary

- If temp not too high, doesn't appear toxic, and no dullness to percussion
  - Viral: supportive care and monitor for secondary bacterial
- If pt appears a bit worse than just a viral or has lasted for a while, get a CXR
  - If CXR appears worse than pt, assume walking pneumonia.
    - Mycoplasma – Tx: **erythromycin**
  - If pt has staccato cough w/ peripheral eosinophilia,
    - Chlamydia – Tx: **erythromycin**
  - Else
    - Bacterial – Tx: **cefuroxime** IV

CF Tx Summary

1. Clear airway: albuterol + mucolytic + PT
2. Abs: aerosolized **tobramycin** (or **aztreonam**)
3. If hospitalization is required
   - 14d: tobramycin + **piperacillin**
- Daily: hydration + pancreatic enzymes + Vitamins ADEK

Bronchiolitis Summary

- Most severe in winter < 2mo.
  - Usually before 2yo.
- Inflammation of the bronchioles
  - → air-trapping, over-inflation
    - **Fine crackles**, prolonged expiratory phase
- Steroids don't help.
- High risk pts may benefit from **palivizumab**

Pneumonia Tx Summary

- If temp not too high, doesn't appear toxic, and no dullness to percussion
  - Viral: supportive care and monitor for secondary bacterial
- If pt appears a bit worse than just a viral or has lasted for a while, get a CXR
  - If CXR appears worse than pt, assume walking pneumonia.
    - Mycoplasma – Tx: **erythromycin**
  - If pt has staccato cough w/ peripheral eosinophilia,
    - Chlamydia – Tx: **erythromycin**
  - Else
    - Bacterial – Tx: **cefuroxime** IV

Peds – Respiration 4

Asthma

Asthma: Quick Points

- Treatment of asthma, as with HTN, is an art.
  - Be plastic in your expectations of what meds a physician might choose to use. Grab the concept of what's going on and develop your own approach as you practice.

- CXR:
  - Don't just look at lungs. Look for hyperinflation, aka flattening of the diaphragms

Asthma Dx & Episode Classification

- Gold Standard: **Spirometry during forced expiration**
  - **FEV1/FVC < 0.8 in children > 5yo**
- **Albuterol challenge**:
  - give albuterol treatment, and FEV1 improves **> 12%**

- At home PEF (peak expiratory flow) monitor
  - Take a.m. and p.m. readings for several weeks
  - Episode classification: current PEF/personal best PEF
    - Green: > 80%
    - **Yellow: 50-80%**
    - Red: < 50%

Asthma Drugs

- **Albuterol:**
  - Most popular short-acting beta-agonist
  - Could say SABA, but albuterol is so ubiquitous
- LABA: long-acting beta-agonist
  - Often **salmeterol**
- **Montelukast**
  - Most popular leukotriene receptor antagonist

Asthma Drugs, Steroids

- ICS, OCS: inhaled corticosteroid, oral corticosteroid
  - Where ICS stay in lungs, OCS spreads to entire system due to gut absorption
    - OCS is often referred to as "systemic steroids"
- ICS
  - Child < 4yo: **budesonide** (the only one that doesn't end in "**-asone**")
  - Child > 4yo: fluticasone
  - Child > 5yo: **beclomethasone**
  - Adults might get any of these plus others
- OCS
  - **Prednisone** at home, **prednisolone** in hospital, **methylprednisolone** in emergency
    - Prednisone needs to be activate by liver
    - Prednisolone is prednisone that has been activated
    - Methylprednisolone is the IV version of prednisolone

Med Use Overview

- Albuterol
  - For acute, breakthrough and pre-exercise
- ICS is used to calm the immune rxn in the lungs when persistent
  - Montelukast is sort-of the same thing
    - Long-term montelukast is preferred, so if you can get by with just it, you do.
      - Most end up w/ ICS instead or ICS + montelukast
- LABA is used to relax the bronchial smooth muscles when persistent
- OCS is when the condition just won't stop

Severity Classification

- Intermittent:
  - Daytime Symptoms: $\leq$ 2/w, Nighttime Symptoms: $\leq$ 2/m
  - Tx: albuterol
- Mild Persistent
  - Daytime and/or Nighttime more than intermittent
  - Tx: ICS + albuterol
- Moderate Persistent
  - Daily, Nighttime > 1/w
  - Tx: ICS + LABA + SABA (breakthrough) $\pm$ montelukast
- Severe Persistent
  - Worse than moderate.
  - Tx: OCS + high-dose ICS, LABA + SABA (breakthrough) + montelukast

Classification Treatment Principles

- Intermittent: **Day & Night: $\leq$ 2/w.**
  - Tx: albuterol
- Mild Persistent: **More than intermittent.**
  - Tx: + ICS

- Moderate Persistent:
  - **Daily attacks & at least 1 night/wk**
  - Give a baseline LABA + ICS. Use SABA for breakthrough.
  - If you can get away with using montelukast instead of ICS, or to diminish the use of ICS, then do it

- Severe Persistent
  - Worse than moderate.
  - Suppress the whole immune system: OCS.
  - Suppress the airway long-term:
    - Muscles: LABA. Leukotrienes: montelukast.
  - Suppress the airway short-term:
    - high-dose ICS + albuterol (breakthrough)

ED Management
of Asthma Exacerbation

1. O2
2. Albuterol q 20m for 1st hour
   - Add **ipratropium** if no response after 1st dose
     - Ipratropium is an anticholinergic
3. Depending on severity: PO prednisolone or IV methylprednisolone
4. Pt sent home when **physically normal** and O2 > **92% after 4h** on room air w/ PEF > **70%** of personal best
5. Send home on OCS for 5d

Asthma Summary

- Dx:
  - Spirometry during forced expiration. FEV1/FVC < 0.8
  - Albuterol challenge: FEV1 should improve > 12%
- At home PEF (peak expiratory flow) monitor
  - Green, Yellow, Red
  - **Yellow: 50-80%**
    - **(current-PEF/personal-best-PEF)*100%**
- Standard Asthma Treatments
  - Intermittent: Day ≤ 2/**w**, Night: ≤ 2/**m**: Albuterol
  - Mild Persistent: Add ICS
  - **Moderate Persistent: Daily + Night > 1/w**
    - **Tx: LABA + ICS + SABA (breakthrough) + montelukast**
  - Severe Persistent: Worse than moderate
    - Tx: OCS + high-dose ICS, LABA + SABA (breakthrough) + montelukast

Peds – Cardiac 1

Heart Murmur Gradation: 1-6

1. Difficult to hear
2. Easily heard
3. Louder but no thrill
4. Associated w/ thrill
5. Thrill and audible w/ edge of stethoscope
6. Thrill and audible w/ stethoscope off chest

- Note: 2/6 musical murmur at left lower midsternum in a child is normal

Regurgitant Heart Problems

- Mitral Insufficiency vs Prolapse
  - Mitral Insufficiency:
    - Mitral valve doesn't close properly when the heart pumps out blood.
      - Leaking blood backwards from the left ventricle, through the mitral valve, into the left atrium.
      - When the left ventricle contracts, blood immediately regurgitates back into the left atrium
    - **High-pitched, holosystolic murmur at apex**
  - Mitral Valve Prolapse:
    - Displacement of an abnormally thickened mitral valve leaflet into the left atrium during systole.
    - When the left ventricle contracts, the pressure exerted forces the displaced valve open (with a "click"), and blood regurgitates back into the left atrium
    - **"Click" → apical late systolic murmur**
    - ~ Marfan, EDS

Pericarditis

- Inflammation of pericardia → accumulation of fluid in pericardial space → cardiac tamponade
  - Echo: Flattening of septal motion
  - EKG: **low-voltage QRS** and **generalized ST-elevation** or T-wave inversion
  - **Drop in BP > 20 during inspiration**
- Causes
  - Infection: Most commonly viral.
    - If bacterial, will need open pericardial drainage, removal of adhesions and Abs
  - Autoimmune: RF, juvenile RA, SLE
  - Uremia, Neoplasm
- Symptoms
  - Much like heart attack but more **stabbing** than pressure
  - Made **better by siting and leaning forward. Worse by laying down**
  - Possible friction rub
- CXR: **water bottle appearance**

Infective Endocarditis

- Associations
  - No preexisting heart condition ~ S. aureus
  - Existing heart disease ~ Strept viridans
    - eg. dental procedures, give **amoxicillin prophylactically**
  - IV drug users ~ **P. aeruginosa or Serratia**
  - Indwelling catheter ~ S. epidermidis, S. saprophyticus
    - the **coagulase-neg Staphs**, part of normal flora
  - Heart surgery ~ **fungus**

Infective Endocarditis

- **S. aureus is ubiquitous and pervasive**, so when in doubt and no other risk factors, it's generally the answer in these types of things.
- Strept viridans ~ rheumatic HD ~ dental procedures
  - You probably already know this. Rx: amoxicillin
- IV ~ wet. **P. aeruginosa & Serratia like wet**.
- Catheter: this is a way for normal flora to invade.
  - **S. epidermidis & saprophyticus are normal flora.**
- Heart surgery ~ fungus.
  - How, else would fungus get to the heart?

Infective Endocarditis

- If found later, vasculitis from circulating Ag-Ab complexes cause skin issues
  - **Osler nodes**: pea-sized intradermal nodules on pads of fingers and toes
  - **Janeway lesions**: small erythematous/hemorrhagic lesions on palms/soles
  - **Splinter hemorrhage** on nail beds
  - **Roth spots** on retina

Cardiac Summary

- **Mitral Insufficiency vs Prolapse**
  - Mitral Insufficiency:
    - **High-pitched, holosystolic murmur at apex**
  - Mitral Valve Prolapse:
    - **"Click" → apical late systolic murmur**
- **Pericarditis**
  - Inflammation of pericardia → accumulation of fluid in pericardial space → cardiac tamponade
    - Echo: Flattening of septal motion
    - EKG: **low-voltage QRS** and **generalized ST-elevation** or T-wave inversion
    - **Drop in BP > 20 during inspiration**
  - Symptoms
    - Stabbing pain made **better by siting and leaning forward. Worse by laying down**
    - Possible friction rub
  - CXR: **water bottle appearance**

Infective Endocarditis Summary

- Associations
  - No-preexisting heart problems ~ S. aureus
  - Existing heart problems ~ Strept viridans
  - IV drug users ~ P. aeruginosa or Serratia
  - Indwelling catheter ~ S. epidermidis, S. saprophyticus
  - Heart surgery ~ fungus
- If found later,
  - Osler nodes
  - Janeway lesions
  - Splinter hemorrhage
  - Roth spots

Peds – GI 1

Acute Diarrhea

Acute Diarrhea, Common Causes

- Viral
  - **Norovirus**
  - Rotavirus
  - Enteric adenovirus

Acute Diarrhea, Common Causes

- Bacterial
  - **Campylobacter**, Yersinia, E. coli
  - E. coli 0157:H7, Salmonella, Shigella
  - Clostridium difficile

Acute Diarrhea, Common Causes

- Parasitic
  - **Giardia lamblia** (most common)
  - E. histolytica, Cryptosporidium parvum
  - Strongyloides (threadworm)
  - Trichuris trichiura (whipworm)
    - a type of roundworm

Diarrhea Treatment

- Generally, supportive w/ plenty of fluids
  - E. coli and associates Abs
    - Nursery, daycare
      - Enteropathogenic E. coli (EPEC): **neomycin**
    - Traveler's diarrhea or food
      - Enterotoxigenic E. Coli (ETEC), Shigella: **TMP/SMX**
    - **NEVER use antibiotics with Enterhemorrhagic E. coli**
      - aka. EHEC = E. coli 0157:H7
      - Due to increase risk of HUS

Diarrhea Treatment

- Generally, supportive w/ plenty of fluids
  - Recent Abs or travel
    - C. difficile, E. histolytica, and Giardia: **metronidazole**
  - Campylobacter recover faster w/ **erythromycin**
  - From pets
    - Y. enterocolitica: **aminoglycoside + 3rd-gen cephalosporin**
      - aminoglycoside (eg. genta-, tobra-, strepto-mycin)
      - 3rd-gen cephalosporin (cefixime, ceftriaxone, ceftazidime)
      - ie. gentamicin + ceftriaxone
  - Cryptosporidium ~ AIDS or immunocompromised:
    - raise CD4 count

Summary
Acute Diarrhea, Common Causes

- Viral
  - **Norovirus**, rotavirus, enteric adenovirus
- Bacterial
  - **Campylobacter**, Yersinia, E. coli
  - E. coli 0157:H7, Salmonella, Shigella
  - Clostridium difficile
- Parasitic
  - **Giardia lambda** (most common)
  - E. histolytica, Cryptosporidium parvum
  - Strongyloides (threadworm), Trichuris trichiura (whipworm, roundworm)

Summary
Diarrhea Treatment

- Generally, supportive w/ plenty of fluids
  - E. coli and associates Abs
    - Daycare: EPEC: **Neomycin**
    - Traveler's/food: ETEC, Shigella: **TMP/SMX**
    - **NEVER use antibiotics with EHEC**
  - Recent Abs or travel
    - C. difficile, E. histolytica, and Giardia: **metronidazole**
  - From pets
    - Y. enterocolitica: **gentamicin + ceftriaxone**
  - Cryptosporidium ~ AIDS or immunocompromised:
    - raise CD4 count

Peds – GI 2

Chronic Diarrhea

Review
Acute Diarrhea Treatment

- Generally, supportive w/ plenty of fluids
  - E. coli and associates Abs
    - Daycare: EPEC: **Neomycin**
    - Traveler's/food: ETEC, Shigella: **TMP/SMX**
    - **NEVER use antibiotics with EHEC**
  - Recent Abs or travel
    - C. difficile, E. histolytica, and Giardia: **metronidazole**
  - From pets
    - Y. enterocolitica: **gentamicin + ceftriaxone**

Chronic Diarrhea Causes

- Pancreatic Insufficiency
- Malabsorption, Brush border enzyme deficiencies
- Lymphangiectasia (Intestinal)
  - ie. Waldmann Disease

Chronic Diarrhea Causes

- **Pancreatic Insufficiency**
  1. Cystic Fibrosis
  2. **Schwachman**-Diamond
     - short w/ skeletal abnormalities, NEUTROPENIA, & **pancreatic insufficiency**

_____-Diamond

- With Blackfan- or Schwachman-**Diamond**,
  50% **C**an't **T**ell **C**ubic-zirconia from **G**lass
  - ie. Half have malformations of **C**raniofacial, **T**humb (or UE), **C**ardiac, **G**U

- **S**chwachman–Diamond: neutropenia (& diarrhea)
  vs
- **B**lackfan-Diamond: congenital erythroid aplasia
  - anemia w/o affecting the other blood components
    - ie. platelets and WBC

- **S** is for diarrhea, **B** is for RBC

Chronic Diarrhea Causes

- Malabsorption, Brush border enzyme deficiencies
  - **Giardiasis**
    - Protozoans decrease the expression of brush border enzymes, change the morphology of microvillus, and kill epithelial cells
  - Carbs:
    - CHO Malabsorption, Disaccaridase Deficiency, Celiac Disease,
  - Fat: **Abetalipoproteinemia**
    - Mutation in TG transfer protein ⟩ deficiency in apolipoproteins B-48 & B-100
      - needed for **chylomicrons** and **VLDL** synthesis and exportation

Chronic Diarrhea Causes

- Lymphangiectasia (Intestinal) = Waldmann Disease:
  - Pathologic dilation of lymph vessels → chronic diarrhea and loss of protein

Summary
Chronic Diarrhea Causes

- Pancreatic Insufficiency
  1. Cystic Fibrosis
  2. Schwachman-Diamond
     - Short w/ skeletal abnormalities, bone marrow dysfunction, & pancreatic insufficiency
- Malabsorption, Brush border enzyme deficiencies
  - Giardiasis
  - Carbs:
    - CHO Malabsorption, Disaccaridase Deficiency, Celiac Disease,
  - Fat: Abetalipoproteinemia
- Lymphangiectasia (Intestinal)

Peds – GI 3

Chronic Diarrhea Tests

& Constipation

Review
Chronic Diarrhea Causes

- Pancreatic Insufficiency
  1. Cystic Fibrosis
  2. Schwachman-Diamond
     - Short w/ skeletal abnormalities, bone marrow dysfunction, & pancreatic insufficiency
- Malabsorption, Brush border enzyme deficiencies
  - Giardiasis
  - Carbs:
    - CHO Malabsorption, Disaccaridase Deficiency, Celiac Disease,
  - Fat: Abetalipoproteinemia
- Lymphangiectasia (Intestinal)

Chronic Diarrhea Tests

- The Usual:
  - CBC, BMP w/ BUN & Cr & glucose, ESR
- The Specific
  - Sweat test
  - 72 hour Fecal Fat Test
    - Fat malabsorption = steatorrhea ~ pancreatic insufficiency
    - Sudan red stain
      - *Funnier if you say "your pants", as in "Sudan stained your pants red"*
  - Hydrogen Breath Test
    - reveals specify CHO (carbohydrate) malabsorption
- If normal in a child, consider excess fruit juice, carbonated beverages, or low fat intake

Meckel Diverticulum, The Disease of Five **2's**

- Most common congenital GI anomaly
  - Remnant of embryonic yolk sac
  - 2yo, 2% population, 2 types of tissue,
  - 2 inches long, 2ft from ileocecal valve
- Hematochezia:
  - acid-secreting mucosa
    - → intermittent painless rectal bleeding
- Dx:
  - Tc-99m pertechnetate (Meckel radionuclide scan)
- Tx: surgical excision

Constipation

- Relieve impaction:
  - enema → stool softeners
  - No prolonged use of stimulants
- May require behavioral modification, bowel training, or resolution of psych issues
  - ie. functional constipation:
    - painful BM w/ voluntary withholding to avoid pain
      - *a vicious circle*

Summary

- Chronic Diarrhea Tests
  - Sweat test
  - 72 hour Fecal Fat Test
    - Sudan red stain "your pants"
  - Hydrogen Breath Test: specific CHO malabsorption
- Meckel Diverticulum
  - 2yo, 2% population, 2 types of tissue, 2", 2'
  - Hematochezia:
    - acid-secreting mucosa → intermittent painless rectal bleeding
  - Dx: Tc-99m pertechnetate (Meckel radionuclide scan)
- Constipation
  - Relieve impaction:
    - enema → stool softeners (No prolonged use of stimulants)
  - Functional constipation:
    - painful BM w/ voluntary withholding to avoid pain

Peds – GU 1

Testicles

- Testes should be descended by 4mo
    - Or they won't descend on their own.
    - Bilateral: 50/50 if fertile. Unilateral: 85%.
    - Delay in surgery increases risk of malignancy (seminoma)
- With pain
    - Under 12yo, most common is **Torsion of Appendix Testes**
        - Gradual onset, inflamed mass at **upper pole of testis → BLUE DOT**
    - Over 12yo, most common is **Testicular Torsion**
        - Acute pain, swelling, tenderness to palpation
        - No cremasteric reflex

Epididymitis & Varicocele

- Epididymitis (ie. the Clap)
  - Gonorrhea or Chlamydia:
    - Ascend retrograde through urethra
    - Acute scrotal pain/swelling
    - Possible pyuria
- Varicocele (ie. **Bag of Worms**)
  - Abnormal dilatation of **pampiniform plexus** →
    surgery

Tumors don't transilluminate

Summary

- Testes
  - Descend by 4mo, or not on their own
  - Delay surgery, increase risk of malignancy
  - With pain
    - < 12yo, **Torsion of Appendix Testes**
      - Gradual, inflamed mass at **upper pole of testis** → **BLUE DOT**
    - > 12yo, **Testicular Torsion**
      - No cremasteric reflex
- Epididymitis, ie. the Clap: Gonorrhea or Chlamydia infection
  - Ascend retrograde through urethra
  - Acute scrotal pain/swelling. Possible pyuria
- Varicocele, ie. **Bag of Worms**:
  - Abnormal dilatation of **pampiniform plexus** → surgery

Peds – Derm 1

Newborn Derm

Mongolian Spot vs. Salmon Patch vs Hemangioma

- Mongolian Spot:
  - Blue-gray macule that usually fade after a few years.
  - Usually found on pre sacral, back, and posterior thighs
- Salmon Patch = "angel's kiss":
  - Vascular birthmark found on glabellar region or upper-eyelid
  - Normally resolves
- Hemangioma:
  - Superficial, bright red, protuberant, sharply demarcated benign tumor that often appears by 2mo on head, back, or anterior chest.
  - Rapidly expands and then stops and remains until early school age.
    - ic. self-involuting
  - Deeper ones appear blue and are less likely to regress.
  - Tx: corticosteroids, pulsed laser

Newborn Derm

- Cutis Marmorata:
  - Lacy pattern over neonate's body when cooled. Should go away by 1m.
- Milia:
  - Tiny white bumps that appear across a baby's nose, chin or cheeks
  - Can actually appear at any age, but much more common in babies
- Erythema Toxic Neonatorum:
  - Firm, yellow papules w/ an erythematous base which peak on day 2.
  - Contain eosinophils and are benign
- Neontal acne:
  - Erythematous papules on neonate face due to mother's androgens.
  - Will resolve

Newborn Derm Summary

- Mongolian Spot:
  - Blue-gray macule on backside that usually fade after a few years
- Salmon Patch = "angel's kiss":
  - Vascular birthmark on glabellar region or upper-eyelid. Resolves
- Hemangioma:
  - Superficial, bright red, protuberant, sharply demarcated benign tumor that appears head or torso.
  - Rapidly expands by 2mo and self-involutes by 9yo

- Cutis Marmorata:
  - Lacy pattern over neonate's body when cooled. Should go away by 1m.
- Milia:
  - Tiny white bumps that appear across a baby's nose, chin or cheeks
- Erythema Toxic Neonatorum:
  - Firm, yellow papules w/ an erythematous base which peak on day 2.

Peds – Derm 2

Skin Infection, Acne

Acne

- **Open comedone** = blackhead. **Closed comedone** = whitehead
- Topical therapies (use for 8w and evaluate)
  - Benzoyl peroxide
  - **Tretinoin** is most effective agent
  - Adapalene
  - Abs: **erythromycin** or **clindamycin**
- Systemic
  - Abs: **tetracycline** (or tetracycline or erythromycin or clindamycin)
  - Isoretinoin
    - Very teratogenic. Women need pregnancy test + two forms of birth control
    - Rule out liver disease

Purpura Fulminans

- Coagulation of small vessels w/in skin
  - → bloodspots/bruising
  - → skin necrosis → DIC
- Associated w/ Protein C deficiency & **meningococcal septicemia**
  - *When you picture in your head the skin of someone with meningococcal septicemia, that's purpura fulminans*

Skin Infection

- **Impetigo**:
  - Bullous and non-bullous S. aureus (or S. pyogenes) infection of top layer of skin
  - **Ecthyma** = deeper form of impetigo
- **Cellulitis**:
  - inflammation of skin and deep tissues
- **Erysipelas**: Inflammation of upper layers of skin
  - Distinct from surrounding skin. Raised, firm and sharply marked off
  - Usually face, sometimes arms & legs
  - Sometimes peau d'orange

Summary

- Acne Meds
  - Topical therapies (use for 8w and evaluate)
    - Benzoyl peroxide, Adapalene, **Tretinoin** is most effective agent
    - Abs: **erythromycin** or **clindamycin**
  - Systemic
    - Abs: **tetracycline**
    - **Isoretinoin**: req 2 forms of birth control & a liver scan

- Purpura Fulminans (~ meningococcal septicemia)
  - Coagulation of small vessels w/in skin → bloodspots → skin necrosis → DIC

- Skin Infections
  - **Impetigo**: Bullous and non-bullous S. aureus (or S. pyogenes) infection of top layer of skin
    - **Ecthyma** = deeper form of impetigo
  - **Cellulitis**: inflammation of skin and deep tissues
  - **Erysipelas**: Inflammation of upper layers of skin
    - Distinct from surrounding skin. Raised, firm and sharply marked off

Peds – Rheumatic

Arthritis

Juvenile Idiopathic Arthritis (JIA), ie. **Juvenile RA (JRA)**

- Many call it JIA, but just think of it as "juvenile RA".
- It presents the same as RA but **not red**
  - Morning stiff, later day warm and painful, but **NOT red**
  - Getting a **salmon-cored evanescent rash** is normal, but
    - if pt develops rheumatoid nodules, that's bad
- You r/o the same things as RA
  - Psoriatic arthritis, connective tissue diseases, vasculitides, Lyme, IBD
  - Because of the age, you also **r/o lymphoproliferative disorders (LPDs)**
    - lymphomas, leukemias, MM, Waldenstrom's macroglobulinemia, Wiskott-Aldrich, …
- Dx the same as RA
  - Pt may be HLA B27 (+)
  - However, if pt is RF (+) that is a worse prognosis
- Tx the same as RA — **NSAIDs + methotrexate**

HLA B27 ~ **PAIR**

- **P**soriasis, **A**nkylosing spondylitis, **I**nflammatory Bowel Disease, **R**eactive Arthritis

- **Reactive Arthritis** (formerly Reiters Syndrome)
  - Autoimmune condition where an infection in one part of the body result in arthritis somewhere else (knee)
    - Often initially a GI issue
  - Pt may also have psoriatic-like skin lesions
  - The preference is to call this Reactive Arthritis for Reiter was a Nazi who experimented on concentration camp prisoners and wrote a book called "Racial Hygiene".

Vasculitis

Henoch-Schönlein Purpura (HSP)

- URI → **Small-vessel** vasculitis
  - **IgA and C3**
- **RASH BELOW WAIST**:
  red → purple → rust-colored
- Beware of **intussusception**
- Self-resolving, but may use corticosteroids
- **Monitor the kidneys:**
  - IgA & C3 deposits → **glomerulonephritis**

Kawasaki Disease

- **Strawberry tongue**, strawberry tongue, the tongue looks like a fricken strawberry
- Cause of this **medium-vessel** vasculitis is unknown, but Asians get it the most.
  - Vast majority under 5yo
  - Most common cause of acquired heart disease in the US
  - *To this point, I've seen nearly all my cases in AA kids, so don't rely on your pt being Asian*
- **Check the heart**, check the heart, check the heart
- Just think that the whole body can be **pruritic** w/ **rash** w/ sequela skin peeling (**desquamation**).
  - Also, think of the affect on your organs when desquamation is taking place: diarrhea, hepatitis, hydrops of GB, urethritis, arthritis, even aseptic meningitis.
- Hands and feet swell

Kawasaki Disease

- Dx:
  - **CHECK THE HEART**: echo early and often. This varies in practice. At least echo at Dx then in 2w then in 6w if all is normal.
  - ECG every time.
  - Platelets + ESR
    - Platelets and ESR shoot up early on. That's what the aspirin is for. Track the platelets to aid in tracking the disease.
- Tx: **IVIG + high-dose aspirin** → low-dose aspirin
  - This is one of the very few cases where you give a kid aspirin. The concern is obviously for **Reyes Syndrome**, but aspirin knocks the temp down quick and shows rapid improvement, so we use it. However, you don't want **influenza or varicella** to set off Reye's Syndrome, so **vaccinations** for these two is of upmost importance.

Arthritis Summary

- Juvenile RA
  - It presents the same as RA but **not red**
    - **Salmon-cored evanescent rash** normal, rheumatoid nodules bad
  - You r/o the same things as RA + **lymphoproliferative disorders (LPDs**
  - Dx the same as RA, but RF (+) is worse prognosis
  - Tx the same as RA — **NSAIDs + methotrexate**

Vasculitis Summary

- **Henoch-Schönlein Purpura (HSP)**
  - Preceded by URI, **IgA and C3**
  - **RASH BELOW WAIST**
  - Beware of **intussusception**
  - Self-resolving, but may use corticosteroids
  - **Monitor kidneys**: IgA & C3 deposits → **glomerulonephritis**

- **Kawasaki Disease**
  - **Strawberry tongue**. Whole body can be **pruritic w/ desquamation**
    → diarrhea, hepatitis, hydrops of GB, urethritis, arthritis, even aseptic meningitis.
    - Hands and feet swell
  - Dx:
    - **CHECK THE HEART**: echo early and often. ECG every time.
    - Platelets + ESR: Platelets and ESR shoot up early on.
  - Tx: **IVIG + high-dose aspirin** → low-dose aspirin
    - Immunize against influenza and varicella

Pediatric – MSK 1

Hip

Hip - Mechanical

- **Slipped Capital Femoral Epiphysis** (SCFE)
  - Most common adolescent hip disorder
  - **Thin w/ recent growth spurt** or **obese**
  - **Mild limp w/ external rotation** then suddenly extreme pain & can't stand
    - *Before it was weak, then it slipped*
    - Many complain of knee pain.
  - Needs pinning (ie. open or closed reduction)
    - Else osteonecrosis and chondrolysis
      - **chondrolysis** = complete loss of cartilage

Hip - Infection

- **Transient Synovitis**
  - Kid **had a URI** → **2 weeks later** he's limping & complaining of groin and leg pain.
  - No real fever, ESR only up slightly. Doesn't look too bad.
  - Imaging normal, maybe a slight profusion.
  - Tx:
    - Bed-rest, no weight-bearing for 1wk then limited for 2wk.
  - **THIS IS NOT**
    - **Septic arthritis** is painful, red, warm, swollen. Maybe a temperature. You need to tap it and admit to hospital for IV Abs.
      - This isn't that
    - **Osteomyelitis**, ie. septic bone

Hip - Vascular

- Legg–Calvé–Perthes Disease
  - **Painless limp**
  - **Avascular necrosis** of the **capital femoral epiphysis**
    - Blood supply to the leg is being cut off. The prognosis starts at "hope for limited sequela" and goes from there.
    - Try and stop it and be supportive.
  - Tx: PT, surgery, or worse.

Hip - Summary

Mechanical:

- **Slipped Capital Femoral Epiphysis** (SCFE)
  - Thin w/ recent growth spurt or **obese**
  - **Mild limp w/ external rotation** then suddenly extreme pain & can't stand
  - Tx: Pinning (ie. open or closed reduction)

Infection:

- **Transient Synovitis**
  - Kid **had a URI → 2 weeks later** he's limping & complaining of groin and leg pain.
    - Looks okay. Minimal fever, slight inc ESR, imaging okay
  - Tx: Bed-rest 1wk → limited 2wk
  - **THIS IS <u>NOT</u> septic arthritis or osteomyelitis**

Vascular:

- Legg–Calvé–Perthes Disease
  - **Painless limp**
  - **Avascular necrosis** of the **capital femoral epiphysis** (not good)

Pediatric – MSK 2

Knee & ahhh-everywhere?

Osgood-Schlatter Disease

- Overuse → traction apophysitis of tibial tubercle
    - ie. tubercle is more prominent, swollen and tender
- Tx:
    - <u>REST</u>: dec activities, immobilize knee
    - Build back up over 1-2y

Was feeling so-good, running/exercising all the time then SH**, I won't be up till much later.

Rhabdomyosarcoma

- Cancer of connective tissue arising from skeletal muscle progenitor cells
  - Therefore, it can raise from almost anywhere
    - Head & neck (40%)
    - GU (20%), ie. **botryoid** = grapes growing out of vagina (most famous)
    - Extremities, trunk, retroperitoneal
- ~ Inc risk of neurofibromatosis

Knee & Everywhere Summary

- Knee
  - Osgood-Schlatter Disease
    - *Was feeling so-good, running/exercising all the time then SH**, I won't be up till much later.*
    - Overuse → traction apophysitis of **tibial tubercle**
    - Tx: REST. Build back up over 1-2y
- Everywhere
  - Rhabdomyosarcoma (~NF)
    - Cancer of connective tissue arising from skeletal muscle progenitor cells
      - Head & neck (40%), GU (20%)
        - » ie. **botryoid** = grapes growing out of vagina (most famous)

Pediatric – MSK 3

Bone Tumors

Bone Tumors

- Osteosarcoma ~ **sunburst**
- Ewing Sarcoma ~ **onion skin**
  - Patrick Ewing eating an onion.

- Osteoid Osteoma: **sclerosis around a clearing**

Bone Tumors

- Osteosarcoma ~ **sunburst**
  - ~ retinoblastoma (Rb) & radiation
  - Sclerotic but will spread (malignant)
  - Tx: Chemo + surgery
    - *Radiation might cause it, but you don't use radiation to eradicate it*
- Ewing Sarcoma ~ **onion skin**
  - **Lytic** activity in the lamina of the bone is what causes the onion skin appearance. It will spread (malignant)
  - Tx: Radiation + surgery
    - *Its lytic (ie. it very active). Kill it where it stands with radiation.*
- Osteoid Osteoma ~ sclerosis around a **central clearing**
  - It's not malignant. It's sclerosis around a clearing.
  - Tx: NSAIDs and surgery

Osteosarcoma

- Mesenchymal cancer cells exhibit osteoblastic differentiation → **malignant osteoid** → aggressive malignancy
- Most common primary bone cancer
- ~ Rb, Li-Fraumeni Syndrome, Paget's Disease

- **Li-Fraumeni** AD
  - **P53** tumor suppressor gene mutation → many cancers of many different types
    - *[Great example of why naming medical conditions after people is a bad idea.]*

Ewing's Sarcoma

- t(11;22): Patrick Ewing wore #33 (11 + 22)
  - *James Ewing may have described it first, but Patrick Ewing helped me the most on Step 1.*
    - *Patrick Ewing eating an onion and bouncing a small, blue ball.*
- Cancer cells in bone or soft tissue.
  - Malignant, small, round, **blue cell tumor.**
  - Pelvis, femur, humerus, ribs or clavicle.
- Extreme bone pain w/ symptoms of an inflammatory systemic illness:
  - Intermittent fevers, anemia, leukocytosis, inc ESR
  - That basically what the onion skinning is from.

Bone Tumors Summary

- Osteosarcoma ~ **sunburst**
  - ~ retinoblastoma (Rb), radiation, **Li-Fraumeni** (mut **p53)**
  - Sclerotic, malignant osteoid → spread
  - Tx: Chemo + surgery
- Ewing Sarcoma ~ **onion skin**, t(11;22), blue cell tumor
  - **Lytic** in the lamina of the bone → onion skin → spread
  - Tx: Radiation + surgery
- Osteoid Osteoma ~ sclerosis around a **central clearing**
  - It's not malignant. It's sclerosis around a clearing.
  - Tx: NSAIDs and surgery

Peds – Endocrine 1

Who's a Big Boy?

Infants of Diabetic Mothers

- Hypoglycemia, hypocalcemia, hypomagnesemia
  - **Maternal hyperglycemia → fetal hyperinsulinemia**
    - **Thus, placental separation → fetal hypoglycemia**
      - all the extra insulin drives the glucose into cells and system goes through transient period of hypoglycemia that can be life threatening
- Macrosomia (ie. LGA)
  - Insulin is the major fetal GH → inc size of all organs except brain
  - Polycythemia → hyperviscosity & hyperbilirubinemia → jaundice
    - Hyperviscosity → renal vein thrombosis
    - Hyperbilirubinemia → jaundice
- Congenital anomalies
  - Cardiac: VSD, ASD, transposition
    - Cardiomegaly due to asymmetric septal hypertrophy
  - Small left colon syndrome: Transient delay in development.
  - Caudal regression syndrome

Infants of Diabetic Mothers 2

- Maternal hyperglycemia → fetal hyperinsulinemia
  - Placental separation → fetal hypo -glycemia, -Ca, -Mg
- Macrosomia (ie. LGA) (**Insulin is the major fetal GH**)
  - Polycythemia
    - Hyperviscosity → renal vein thrombosis
    - Hyperbilirubinemia → jaundice
- Congenital anomalies
  - Caudal regression syndrome
  - Cardiac
  - Transient delay in left colon development.

IGF-1 = Insulin-like Growth Factor 1

- aka. **somatomedin C**
- Nonsuppressible insulin-like activity
  - Structure similar to insulin.
- Produced in liver, stimulated by GH
- Produced throughout life
  - Highest amount in pubertal growth spurts.
  - Lowest in infancy and old age
  - Important role in childhood growth and has anabolic effect in adults
- 98% bound to IGF-BP (IGF binding proteins). Only free IGF-1 is active.
  - **IGFBP-1 is regulated by insulin**
  - **IGF-1 regulated by GH**
- IGF-1 levels don't fluctuate greatly throughout the day, therefore IGF-1 is used as a screening test
  - Growth hormone deficiency, Growth hormone excess (ie. acromegaly/gigantism)
  - **Wide normal range and variations based on age, sex, and pubertal stage make this more of a monitoring tool than a diagnostic one**

- Mecasermin, a synthetic analog is used to treat growth failure

IGF-1 More Focused

- Nonsuppressible insulin-like activity
  - Structure similar to insulin
- Highest amount in pubertal growth spurts.
  - Important role in childhood growth
- 98% bound to IGF-BP (IGF binding proteins). Only free IGF-1 is active.
  - IGFBP-1 is regulated by **insulin**. IGF-1 regulated by **GH**
- IGF-1 levels don't fluctuate, but normal range varies across many fields
  - Better as a screening or monitoring tool than diagnostic

- **Mecasermin**: a synthetic analog is used to treat growth failure

Hyperpituitarism

- Generally from a pituitary adenoma.
  - More common in adults.
- Causes growth disruption in kids
- Results in oversecretion of prolactin, ACTH, GH
  - Excess prolactin, ie. **prolactinoma**
    - Headaches, visual, growth failure
    - Puberty: Suppression of gonadotropin secretion —> hypogonadism
  - Excess ACTH, ie. **Cushing's Disease**
    - Wt gain, hirsutism, premature adrenarche, acne, fatigue/depression
  - Excess GH, ie **Gigantism**
    - Severity depends on if epiphyseal plat is open

Infant of DM Mom Summary

- **Infants of Diabetic Mothers**
  - Maternal hyperglycemia → fetal hyperinsulinemia → fetal hypo -glycemia, -Ca, -Mg
  - Macrosomia, Polycythemia → renal vein thrombosis, jaundice
  - Congenital anomalies: Caudal regression, Cardiac, Left colon

IGF-1 and Hyperpituitarism Summary

- IGF-1
  - Nonsuppressible insulin-like activity
  - 98% bound to IGF-BP (IGF binding proteins). Only free IGF-1 is active.
    - **IGFBP-1 is regulated by insulin. IGF-1 regulated by GH**
  - IGF-1 levels **don't fluctuate**, however the vary across many fields
    - Screening tool and monitoring tool. Not really a diagnostic tool
  - **Mecasermin**
    - a synthetic analog is used to treat growth failure
- Hyperpituitarism
  - ~ Pituitary adenoma
  - Inc prolactin, ACTH, GH
    - Excess prolactin, ie. **prolactinoma**
      - Headaches, visual, **growth failure**
      - **Puberty**: Suppression of gonadotropin secretion —> **hypogonadism**
    - Excess ACTH, ie. **Cushing's Disease**
    - Excess GH

Peds – Endocrine 2

MEN2

Lets Go Over Something Simple

- When you read **"hyperplasia"** or **"hypertrophy"**, your first thought should be "makes a lot more of whatever it normally makes".
  - This isn't always true, but it's true a LOT
- When **cancer** is inferred, this is usually the case as well.
- So, before you get into what is going on, take a second to ask, **"what was this thing originally producing"**?
  - Even epithelial cells produce something

Example: MEN II

- MEN IIA
  - Adrenal medullary hyperplasia +
  - Thyroid hyperplasia +
  - Parathyroid hyperplasia
- MEN IIB = Mucosal Neuroma Syndrome
  - Adrenal medullary hyperplasia +
  - Medullary Thyroid Carcinoma +
  - **Multiple neuromas**
- **Note**:
  - MENIIA often states thyroid hyperplasia while MENIIB often states thyroid carcinoma.
  - They both have the symptom of **hyperthyroidism.**
    - [Not to cloud the point, but **calcitonin** secretion is often the issue]

Example: MEN II

- So, you could interpret these as
  - (and would make them simpler to remember)
- MEN IIA
  - Pheochromocytoma + Hyperthyroidism (esp. calcitonin) +
  - Parathyroid hyperplasia
- MEN IIB = Mucosal Neuroma Syndrome
  - Pheochromocytoma + Hyperthyroidism (esp. calcitonin) +
  - **Multiple neuromas**
- Therefore:
  - MENIIA and MENIIB have all the same features, but MENIIA has hyperPTH and MENIIB has neuromas.
    - ie. MENIIA has bone/calcium/phosphorous/kidney issues
    - ie. **MENIIB has a bunch of neural tumors**

MEN IIB
Mucosal Neuroma Syndrome

- Child < 10yo, tall & lanky, elongated face and protruding, blubbery lips.
  - Benign tumors in mouth, eyes, and submucosa of almost every organ by 10yo.
- ie. The **man to be** is 10yo Mic Jagger
  - Tall & lanky w/ elongated face and protruding, blubbery lips.
  - He's really hyperactive like he's on something. Maybe its epinephrine or norepinephrine. Maybe its free T4.
    - Whatever, he's moving around everywhere with those big lips and lanky movements.
  - That is the man to be – 10yo Mic Jagger
    - MEN2B ~ 10yo Mic Jagger

MEN IIA

- Acts a lot like the man to be, but he doesn't look like the man to be. He is just **A** man with Stones, Bones, Groans, Thrones, and Psychic Overtones.
  - hyperPTH → hyperCa

MEN II Summary

- The man to be is 10yo Mic Jagger
  - MEN IIB = Mucosal Neuroma Syndrome
    - Pheochromocytoma + Hyperthyroidism (esp. calcitonin) +
    - **Multiple neuromas**
- Just A man w/ stones, bones, groans, thrones, and psychic overtones
  - MEN IIA
    - Pheochromocytoma + Hyperthyroidism (esp. calcitonin) +
    - Parathyroid hyperplasia

Peds – Endocrine 3

CAH to Cushing **Syndrome**

The Story of CAH

- My friends call me **CAH**. I'm **21**, and I'm always **stressed** out, and that causes me to **lose a lot of sweat**. I used to be **17**. **OH** do you remember being **17**. Lots and lots and lots of **17**. My female parts **look like guy parts**, but my internal sex organs are still there. If I'd been a guy, I'd been sprouting pubes really, really early.
- The real test is, do I still think about being **17** after some **ACT**ing classes.

CAH = **Congenital Adrenal Hyperplasia**

- My friends call me CAH. I'm 21 (**21-hydroxylase deficiency**), and I'm always stressed out (**dec cortisol → inc ACTH**), and that causes me to lose a lot of sweat (**salt wasting,** <u>not in all cases</u>). I used to be 17 (**17-OH progesterone**). Boy do you remember being 17. Lots and lots and lots of 17. My female parts look like guy parts (shunting to androgen synthesis → **masculinization of external genitalia**), but my internal sex organs are still there. If I'd been a guy, I'd been sprouting pubes really, really early.
- The real test is, do I still think about being 17 after some acting classes (**ACTH bolus → inc 17-OH progesterone**).
- If you know how to treat me, you'll give me cortisol, or the manufactured pseudo equivalent **hydrocortisone**.
  - If patient is salt wasting, and not all do, give **fludrocortisone**.
- Females need surgery.

CAH = Congenital Adrenal Hyperplasia

- **21-Hydroxylase deficiency**
  - → accumulation of **17-OH progesterone**
  - → the over accumulation forces biochemical **shunting** down the **androgen synthesis pathway** → overproduction of androgens
  - → **masculinization**
- 21-hydroxylase is required for **cortisol** production
  - Cortisol is secreted in response to stress and low blood glucose
  - **Hydrocortisone is the medicine version of cortisol.**
  - **Fludrocortisone is cortisol for salt wasters.**
- Dx:
  - **ACTH bolus challenge**: if inc in 17-OH progesterone is noted, then you can't go down the 21-hydroxylase pathway
- Tx: guys might live with it, but women need surgery

(Compare CAH to Cushing Syndrome**)**

Cushing Syndrome

- Prolonged glucocorticoid exposure
- Endogenous
  - Infant: Adrenocortical tumor
  - Adult: Cushing Disease
    - pituitary adenoma → excess ACTH
- Exogenous
  - Steroids
    - ie. bodybuilders and long-term prednisone for medical reasons
- Symptoms:
  - Moon facies, buffalo hump, truncal obesity, abdominal striae
  - Steroid SE:
    - osteoporosis, hyperglycemia, masculinization, HTN, amenorrhea
- Dx: Dexamethasone Suppression Test

CAH Summary

- **21-Hydroxylase deficiency**
  - Inc **17-OH progesterone**
  - Masculinization
  - Dec cortisol
    - Tx: **Hydrocortisone**
      - **Fludrocortisone** if salt wasting
  - Dx: **ACTH bolus challenge**
    - if inc in 17-OH progesterone is noted, then you can't go down the 21-hydroxylase pathway

Cushing **Syndrome** Summary

- Prolonged glucocorticoid exposure
- Symptoms:
  - Moon facies, buffalo hump, truncal obesity, abdominal striae
  - Steroid SE:
    - osteoporosis, hyperglycemia, masculinization, HTN, amenorrhea
- Dx: **Dexamethasone Suppression Test**

Peds – Endocrine 4

Dexamethasone Suppression Test
Interpretation

Cushing **Syndrome** Review

- Prolonged glucocorticoid exposure
- Symptoms:
  - Moon facies, buffalo hump, truncal obesity, abdominal striae
  - Steroid SE:
    - osteoporosis, hyperglycemia, masculinization, HTN, amenorrhea
- Dx: **Dexamethasone Suppression Test**

Dexamethasone-Suppression Test

1. Low dose: suppresses cortisol in normal people
2. High dose: negative feedback to pituitary → dec ACTH production

Dexamethasone-Suppression Test Physiology

- Stress triggers synthesis of ACTH which stimulates cortisol production and secretion.
- Cortisol is produced in the adrenal glands.
- Low dose dexamethasone just affect the <u>adrenal glands</u>
  - ie. low-dose suppresses adrenal production/secretion of cortisol.
- High dose dexamethasone suppresses pituitary production of <u>ACTH **and** adrenal glands</u>

Dexamethasone-Suppression Test Interpretation

1. ACTH: Are they super-high (>100)? [ACTH ref < 60]
   - Yes = **Ectopic ACTH Syndrome**
     I. Pituitary tumor
        - get a CT head
     II. Chest or abdominal tumor producing ACTH
        - get a CT chest & abdomen
     - I then II. I is much more likely and reasons exist not to expose someone to CT.

Dexamethasone-Suppression Test Interpretation

2. Dexamethasone suppression test
   I. Low-dose given and cortisol is unchanged = no negative feedback sensing at adrenals
      - ACTH is not super-abundant to override the negative feedback of the dexamethasone. You ruled that out in step 1.
   II. High-dose given
      - Cortisol goes down (and ACTH is normal or slightly elevated)
        - **Cushing Disease**
          » Pituitary still retains some feedback control. Get an MRI to confirm.
      - Cortisol doesn't change (and ACTH is low)
        - Cushing Syndrome = Primary Hypercortisolism
          » Pituitary responded to negative feedback but adrenals didn't. Therefore, adrenals are doing this all on their own.

Dexamethasone-Suppression Test Summary

1. ACTH >100 = **Ectopic ACTH Syndrome**
    - MRI brain, then possible chest/abdomen CT
2. Low-dose given and cortisol is unchanged.
3. High dose given and
    I.   Cortisol goes down (ACTH is normal or slightly elevated)
       - **Cushing Disease**
         - ie. Pituitary functioning a little
    II. Cortisol is unchanged (and ACTH is low)
       - **Cushing Syndrome** = Primary Hypercortisolism
         - ie. The problem is with the adrenals

Peds – Endocrine 5

The Significance of Cortisol

Cortisol

- Biological stress → inc pituitary production of ACTH → inc production/secretion of cortisol by adrenals
  - Cortisol is the bodies defense for stress (and hypoglycemia)
    - Therefore, cortisol plays a part in liver breakdown of glycogen & TGs.
    - Actually, it affects glucagon production (which affects the liver), and it activate glycogen phosphorylase.
    - *Kind of hits it from both ends.*
  - When we get stressed, we need the available resources to respond to the stress. So, might part of "stressing out" be that you have too many resources available and certain system synapses are firing like crazy?

Cortisol Suppresses the Immune System

The immune system is not necessary for immediate survival, eg. running away from a tiger or fighting with your spouse. If you ramp up your immune system now or a bit later, you'll probably be fine, but if you don't say that one hurtful thing to your spouse immediately, how are you ever going to live to regret it.

Cortisol is more of a resource distributor than an immune suppressor.

- Cortisol acts as a diuretic.
  - GFR increases, RPF increases, sodium is retained and potassium is excreted.
    - Another way to say this, is cortisol increases blood pressure and get the blood flowing.
    - You've got to run away from that tiger. Oxygen demands may be critical!
- Cortisol levels go up in the day and down at night.
  - When do you need your resources? When your species is normally most active. During the day.

Cortisol Increases **Flash-Bulb Memories**

But, long-term cortisol damages cells in the hippocampus → long-term memory damage (decreased learning).

- If you did something stupid that directly resulted in your life being at risk, you better remember it. Like taking an indelible picture. But drugs may help for a while, but they are destructive long-term.

Cortisol, The Fetus & Mom

- Fetus going to need increased resources to become a neonate.
  - Going to need to pump own oxygen through the body, therefore going to need some surfactant.
  - Doesn't it make sense that cortisol is the stimulant for surfactant production (and that **betamethasone** would mimic it)?
    - Before delivering a child before 36w, treat with betamethasone to help mature the lungs
- Mom needs to redistribute resources too.
  - *That's a whole other discussion.*

Cortisol Summary

- Biological stress → inc pituitary production of ACTH → inc production/ secretion of cortisol by adrenals
  - Cortisol is the bodies defense for stress (and hypoglycemia)
- More appropriate to say, cortisol is a resource distributer.
  - Sure, it suppresses the immune system, but isn't that freeing up resources that are more time critical?
    - Do you need T-cells or to outrun the tiger?
  - Sure, it works as a diuretic, but increasing GFR and RBF ends up increasing systemic blood flow and pressure.
    - Primes the pump for action.
  - Frees up energy: Increases glucagon → glycogen & TGs breakdown
    - Also, cortisol activates glycogen phosphorylase to help
  - Cortisol levels go up in the day and down at night.
    - When our species is most active.
- Cortisol increases **flash bulb memories**, but long-term use damages long-term memories.
- Also: Cortisol is the stimulant for surfactant production in the fetus

Cortisol Re-Summary

- Cortisol is a resource distributer and protector.
  - Increases available resources:
    - Increases glucagon → glycogen & TGs breakdown
      - Also, cortisol activates glycogen phosphorylase to help
    - Suppresses the immune system
      - Not critical for immediate survival
    - Increasing GFR and RBF → inc systemic blood flow and pressure.
      - Primes the pump for action.
    - Cortisol levels go up in the day and down at night.
      - When our species is most active.
    - Cortisol is the stimulant for surfactant production in the fetus
      - The lungs are a resource the neonate will need.
  - Some mistakes should never be made again
    - Cortisol increases **flash bulb memories**
      - but long-term use damages long-term memories.

Cortisol: Resources & Protection Turned Pathologic

- Cushing disease:
  - Pituitary adenoma still has some feedback mechanism
- Ectopic ACTH Syndrome:
  - Pituitary adenoma has no feedback mechanism or the tumor is in the chest or abdomen
- Cushing Syndrome = Primary Hypercortisolism
  - The adrenals aren't listening to anyone.
- Steroid Abuse:
  - Mr. Muscles or someone with a chronic autoimmune disease is self-administering steroids.

- Store the resources in your abdomen or torso, maybe some fat-pads in your shoulders/neck
- Maybe its so bad your face is swollen up, glucose is coursing through your body, your BP is high all the time, your not getting a period, hair is popping out everywhere.
- Keep it up and your bones will be brittle.

NEUROLOGY & PSYCHOLOGY CENTRIC

Neuro – Early Assessment

This One is Short

- A couple of simple things that people just don't get.

Subcortical vs. Brainstem Lesions

- **Subcortical Lesions**
  - Internal capsule, cerebral peduncles, thalamus, and pons
  - All the structures being controlled by the cerebral cortex are dispersed across a wide area. In subcortical area, they are all coming together. Therefore, a lesion here takes out a chunk of the same side of the body.
    - ie. One doesn't lose the use of an arm. They lose the use of an arm, a leg, and the ipsilateral face.
- **Brainstem Lesions**
  - Corticospinal tract, dorsal columns and spinothalamic tracts cross, but cranial nerves do not
  - Look for deficits of ipsilateral face and contralateral body

Glascow Coma Scale

Get your coma certified at the Glasgow EMV

- **E**ye opening
- **M**otor response
- **V**erbal reasoning

- *The Glascow Score is really important to get down. How can you communicate the deterioration or improvement of a patient without sharing a solid frame of reference.*
- *Many students just give it a rough guess, and that doesn't work.*

Glascow Coma Scale

- Eye opening
  - None 1
  - Opens to pain: 2
  - Opens to voice: 3
  - Opens spontaneously: 4

Glascow Coma Scale

- Motor Response
  - None 1
  - **Decerebrate posture** 2
    - ie. extensor posturing
  - **Decorticate posturing** 3
    - ie. elbows, wrists, and fingers flexed
  - Withdraws from pain 4
  - Localizes pain stimulus 5
  - Obeys commands 6

Glascow Coma Scale

- Verbal Response
  - None 1
  - Incomprehensible sounds 2
  - Inappropriate words 3
  - Appropriate but confused 4
  - Appropriate and oriented 5

Glascow Coma Scale

Get your coma certified at the Glasgow EMV

- Eye opening
  - None: 1 → Opens to pain: 2 → Opens to voice: 3
  - Opens spontaneously: 4

- Motor Response
  - None: 1 → Decerebrate posture: 2 → Decorticate posturing: 3
  - Withdraws from pain: 4 → Localizes pain stimulus: 5
  - Obeys commands: 6

- Verbal Response
  - None: 1 → Incomprehensible sounds: 2 → Inappropriate words: 3
  - Appropriate but confused: 4 → Appropriate and oriented: 5

Summary

- Subcortical vs. Brainstem Lesions
  - **Subcortical Lesions**:
    - One doesn't lose the use of an arm. They lose the use of an arm, a leg, and the ipsilateral face.
  - **Brainstem Lesions**:
    - Ipsilateral face and contralateral body
- **Glascow Coma Scale** (EMV)
  - Eye opening
    - None: 1 → Opens to pain: 2 → **Opens to voice**: 3
    - Opens spontaneously: 4
  - Motor Response
    - None: 1 → **Decerebrate posture**: 2 → **Decorticate posturing**: 3
    - Withdraws from pain: 4 → **Localizes pain stimulus**: 5
    - Obeys commands: 6
  - Verbal Response
    - None: 1 → Incomprehensible sounds: 2 → **Inappropriate words**: 3
    - Appropriate but confused: 4 → Appropriate and oriented: 5

Neuro – Spinal Cord Dz 1

Syringomyelia, Transient Myositis,
Brown-Séquard

Spinal Cord Diseases

- Syringomyelia
- Brown-Séquard Syndrome
- Transverse Myelitis
- Horner's Syndrome
- Hereditary Spastic Paraplegia
- Poliomyelitis

Syringomyelia

- Central cavitation of the cervical cord due to abnormal collection of fluid within the spinal cord parenchyma
  - ~ Postinfectious, trauma, intramedullary tumor, **Arnold-Chiari**, tethered cord
    - Arnold-Chiari Malformation
      - Downward displacement of the cerebellar tonsils and through the foramen magnum
    - Normally the spinal cord hangs loose in the spinal canal. Surrounded by buoyant CSF, the cord is free to move up or down, and even bend and stretch. A **tethered cord** is held taut at some point along the spinal canal → stretching and damage
      - ~ the closing of spina bifida
- Symptoms
  - Bilateral loss of pain and temp over shoulders in "**cape-like**" distribution
    - ie. lateral spinothalamic tract
  - Touch is preserved but muscle atrophy of the hands may be noted

Transverse Myelitis

- Affects tracts across the horizontal aspect of the spinal cord. Normally thoracic.
- Idiopathic or postviral. Progression is rapid
- Motor, sensory and bowel deficits below level of the lesion

Brown-Séquard Syndrome

- Spinal cord hemisection, often cervical
- Symptoms
  - **Contralateral loss of pain and temp**
    - Spinothalamic tract
    - Two vertebrae below the level of the lesion
      - Spinothalamic tract crosses and then ascends. The other tracts ascend and then cross.
  - **Ipsilateral hemiparesis**
    - Corticospinal tract
    - Often flaccid paralysis of the muscles supplied by the nerve at the exact level of the lesion
  - **Ipsilateral loss of position/vibration**
    - Dorsal columns
    - Recovery is often complete
- Trauma site is often very narrow and neurons are able to reestablish the original tract.

Summary

- **Syringomyelia**
  - Central cavitation of the cervical cord due to abnormal collection of fluid within the spinal cord parenchyma
  - Cape-like loss of pain and temp over shoulders
  - Preserved touch, atrophied hands
- **Transverse Myelitis**
  - Horizontal separation of tracts in spinal cord.
    - Normally thoracic.
  - Idiopathic or postviral. Progression is rapid
  - Motor, sensory and bowel deficits below level of the lesion
- **Brown-Séquard Syndrome**
  - Spinal cord hemisection, often cervical
  - **Contralateral loss of pain and temp.** Pain and temp cross and ascend.
  - **Ipsilateral hemiparesis**
  - **Ipsilateral loss of position/vibration**

Neuro – Spinal Cord Dz 2

Horner, CNIII, Bell

Horner's Syndrome

- Lesion the interrupts the cervical sympathetic nerves
- Causes
  - Most commonly idiopathic
  - Trauma, tumor (esp. pancoast), brainstem stroke
- Symptoms:
  1. Ipsilateral ptosis = mild drooping of lid
  2. Ipsilateral miosis = pinpoint pupil
  3. **Ipsilateral anhidrosis** = dec sweating on forehead

- Note: this is a spinal cord lesion

Bell's Palsy

- Hemifacial weakness of muscles innervated by **CNVII**
- Causes may be any condition that can lead to infection/ swelling of the cranial nerve
  - ie. Herpes, URI, Lyme
    - If Lyme is suspected, you can **NOT** use steroids
- Symptoms:
  - Acute onset of unilateral facial weakness.
  - **Both upper and lower parts of face affected**
- Tx:
  - Generally self-resolving in 1m, but pt should wear eye patch at night to prevent corneal abrasions
  - Surgical decompression may be necessary if condition worsens

Horner's Syndrome vs. CNIII Palsy vs. Bell's Palsy

- Levator palpebrae superioris & superior tarsal muscles raise your eyelid.
  - Sympathetic innervation damage in Horner's → no superior tarsal muscle innervation
  - CNIII Palsy → no levator palpebrae innervation.
  - Both lead to drooping of the eyelid.
- Orbicularis oculi closes the eyelid and tenses the area around the eye.
  - Damage to CNVII, as in Bell's Palsy → the area around the eye droops, but the actual eyelid does not.

- These conditions look very much alike. So how do you tell the difference?
  1. Have the pt close and open their eyes. If the lid moves up and down, then you are not dealing with Bell's Palsy.
  2. Shine a light in the eye. Does the pupil constrict? If it does, you aren't dealing with CNIII Palsy.

Summary

- Horner's Syndrome:
  - **Cervical sympathetic nerve lesion**
  1. Ipsilateral ptosis = mild drooping of lid
  2. Ipsilateral miosis = pinpoint pupil
  3. **Ipsilateral anhidrosis** = dec sweating on forehead
- Bell's Palsy:
  - **CNVII swelling**
    - Causes: Herpes, URI, Lyme (no steroids w/ Lyme)
  - Acute onset of unilateral facial weakness.
  - **Both upper and lower parts of face affected**
  - Self-resolving, nighttime eye patch, possible decompression needed

Horner's vs. CNIII Palsy vs. Bell's Palsy Summary

1. ## Lid moves up and down
   - CNVII is working, so this isn't Bell's

2. ## Pupil constricts to light
   - CNIII is working, so this isn't CNIII Palsy.

3. ## This is Horner's
   - the only one of these which is a spinal cord lesion

Neuro – Spinal Cord Dz 3

HSP, Polio

Hereditary Spastic Paraplegia (**HSP**)

- Progressive axonal degeneration of descending & ascending neural tracts
  - Neuron bodies are preserved, no demyelination
  - Inheritance varies by affected SPG gene (1-31)
- Types
  - Type I: onset < 35yo. Spasticity of lower limbs > weakness
  - Type II: onset > 35yo. Weakness, sensory loss, urinary incontinence
    - Unlike most conditions, the later onset Type II is the worse Dx, evolves rapidly.

  Normal life expectancy
- Not a form of cerebral palsy!

Hereditary Spastic Paraplegia (**HSP**)

- Not a form of cerebral palsy!
- Symptoms
  - Progressive stiffness and spasticity in the lower limbs
    - Though some of the anti-spastic meds used for spastic cerebral palsy are used to treat HSP
  - Cataracts
    - Caused by optic nerve and retina damage
  - Deafness
  - Ataxia, peripheral neuropathy
  - Epilepsy, cognitive decline

Poliomyelitis

- Generally eradicated in the Western world, but it's still active in the rest of the world.
- 95% show no symptoms. 5% have cold-like symptoms w/ myalgia.
  - 0.5% result in an inability to move 1+ muscles, of which 15% die
- Affects the anterior horn cells and motor neurons and brainstem.
- Asymmetric muscle weakness, legs are most common
- Bulbar involvement → respiratory & CV impairment

HSP & Poliomyelitis Summary

- Hereditary Spastic Paraplegia (**HSP**) (Not a form of cerebral palsy!)
  - Progressive axonal degeneration of descending & ascending neural tracts
    - Neuron bodies are preserved, no demyelination
  - Type 1: onset < 35 → LE spasticity > weakness
  - Type 2: onset > 35 → Weakness, sensory loss, urinary incontinence
    - Evolves rapidly
  - Symptoms
    - Progressive stiffness and spasticity in the lower limbs
    - Cataracts, Deafness
    - Ataxia, peripheral neuropathy
    - Epilepsy, cognitive decline
- Poliomyelitis
  - Affects the **anterior horn cells and motor neurons and brainstem.**
  - Asymmetric muscle weakness, legs are most common
  - Bulbar involvement → respiratory & CV impairment

Spinal Cord Dz Summary

- **Syringomyelia**
  - Central cavitation of the cervical cord due to abnormal collection of fluid within the spinal cord parenchyma
  - Cape-like loss of pain and temp over shoulders.
  - Preserved touch, atrophied hands
- **Transverse Myelitis**
  - Horizontal separation of tracts in spinal cord.
  - Motor, sensory and bowel deficits below level of the lesion
- **Brown-Séquard Syndrome**
  - Spinal cord hemisection, often cervical
  - **Contralateral loss of pain and temp**. Pain and temp cross and ascend.
  - **Ipsilateral hemiparesis & loss of position/vibration**
- **Horner's Syndrome**
  - Cervical sympathetic nerve lesion
  1. Ipsilateral ptosis = mild drooping of lid
  2. Ipsilateral miosis = pinpoint pupil
  3. **Ipsilateral anhidrosis** = dec sweating on forehead

Spinal Cord Dz Summary

- Hereditary Spastic Paraplegia (**HSP**) (Not a form of cerebral palsy!)
  - Progressive axonal degeneration of descending & ascending neural tracts
    - Neuron bodies are preserved, no demyelination
  - Progressive stiffness and spasticity in the lower limbs
  - Cataracts, Deafness
- Poliomyelitis
  - Affects the **anterior horn cells and motor neurons and brainstem.**
  - Asymmetric muscle weakness, legs are most common
  - Bulbar involvement → respiratory & CV impairment

Spinal Cord Dz Summary

- Syringomyelia:
  - **Central cavitation** of the cervical cord due to fluid
  - **Cape-like** loss of pain and temp over shoulders.
- **Transverse Myelitis**: Horizontal separation of tracts in spinal cord.
- Brown-Séquard Syndrome:
  - Spinal cord hemisection, often cervical
  - **Contralateral loss of pain and temp.**
  - Ipsilateral hemiparesis & loss of position/vibration
- Horner's Syndrome:
  - Ipsilateral ptosis, **miosis, and anhidrosis**
- Hereditary Spastic Paraplegia
  - **Progressive axonal degeneration** of descending & ascending neural **tracts**
- Poliomyelitis: **anterior horn cells** and motor neurons and brainstem.
  - Asymmetric muscle weakness, legs are most common
  - Bulbar involvement → respiratory & CV impairment

ANS Drugs 1

PNS, SNS, Receptors

Autonomic Nervous System

- Parasympathetic (PNS) ~ "fight or flight"
- Sympathetic (SNS) ~ "rest and relax"

Adrenergic-agonists = Sympathomimetics

- Mimic the effects of SNS nt's (neurotransmitters)
  - Epinephrine (EPI) & Norepinephrine (NE)
  - Dopamine (DA)
- Very-oversimplified
  - Alpha-receptors respond to NE
  - Beta-receptors respond to EPI
  - Dopaminergic-receptors respond to DA

Adrenergic-agonists = Sympathomimetics

- Actual response potential (and probably doesn't help to think of it this way)
  - alpha1 (A,B,D): NE > EPI
  - alpha2 (A,B,C): EPI ≥ NE
  - beta1: EPI = NE
  - beta2: EPI >> NE
  - beta3: NE > EPI

- I'm sure that didn't make things clearer for you.
  - Beta3 enhances lipolysis and promotes relaxation of detrusor muscle in the bladder
    - (Not really that useful to know, maybe even as a urologist)

Adrenergic-agonists = Sympathomimetics

- Instead, focus on trends, focus on organ systems.
- For example
  - During exercise beta2-receptors dominate alpha1-receptors initially, but with heavy workouts, the alpha1-receptors begin to dominate. The result is, vasodilation when you are first using a muscle helps blood to pump in for the increased metabolic needs, but with large effort blood supply decreases → anaerobic use → acid buildup within the muscle.

Summary

- SNS ~ "rest and relax"
- **Sympathomimetics** = Adrenergic-agonists
- Receptor Types
  - Alpha-receptors respond to NE
  - Beta-receptors respond to EPI
  - Dopaminergic-receptors respond to DA
- Focus on trends. Focus on organ systems.
  - Don't focus on individual receptors.
  - Example
    - Begin of workout, beta2-receptors dominate → inc BF
    - During a heavy workout, alpha1-receptors begin to dominate
      → dec BF → anaerobic use → acid buildup within the muscle.

ANS Drugs 2

Alpha Receptors

Alpha-Receptors

- Alpha1 receptors are located on postsynaptic effector cells
  - Effector cells effect a change.
    - A presynaptic cell releases nt's that bind to receptors on postsynaptic effector cells. The effector cell then performs an action.
- Alpha2 receptors are on the presynaptic nerve terminals
  - These control the release of nt's

- In general, alpha-adrenergic agonists vasoconstrict or stimulate the CNS

Alpha-Receptor, Summary

- Alpha-Receptors
  - Alpha1: Located on postsynaptic effector cells
  - Alpha2: Presynaptic nerve terminals controlling the release of nt's
  - In general, alpha-adrenergic agonists vasoconstrict or stimulate the CNS

Alpha-Adrenergic Stimulation of Smooth Muscle

- Vasoconstricts blood vessels
- Relaxes GI smooth muscles
- Contracts uterus and bladder
- Male ejaculation
- Decreases insulin release
- Dilates pupils
  - Contraction of ciliary muscles

Summary

- Alpha-Receptors
  - Alpha1: Located on postsynaptic effector cells
  - Alpha2: Presynaptic nerve terminals, control release of nt's
  - **Alpha-adrenergic agonists vasoconstrict or stimulate the CNS**
- Alpha-Adrenergic Stimulation of Smooth Muscle
  - Vasoconstricts blood vessels & relaxes GI smooth muscles
  - Contracts bladder & uterus. Stimulates male ejaculation
  - Decreases insulin release
  - Dilates pupils by contracting ciliary muscles

Ophthalmic Agents

- Topical application to the eye surface stimulates alpha receptors on small arterioles → dec conjunctival congestion
- Naphazoline
  - alpha-agonist, ie. Clear Eyes & Naphcon
- Tetrahydrozoline
  - alpha-agonist, ie. Visine

ANS Drugs 3

Beta, Dopa. System responses.

Beta-Receptors

- Beta Receptors are postsynaptic
  - Beta1 ~ heart, kidney, and saliva
    - Heart beats faster and harder.
    - Kidneys secrete more renin (inc BP).
    - You drool.
  - Beta2 ~ smooth muscle of bronchioles, arterioles, and visceral organs
    - Bronchial tree, GI, and uterine smooth muscles relax
  - Beta-receptors also make energy available through glycogenolysis.

Dopaminergic Receptors

- DA → dilation of cerebral, coronary, renal, and mesenteric blood vessels → **inc BF**

Summary

- Beta Receptors are postsynaptic
  - **Beta1** ~ heart, kidney, and saliva
    - **Heart beats faster and harder.**
    - **Kidneys secrete more renin (inc BP).**
    - You drool.
  - **Beta2** ~ smooth muscle of **bronchioles, arterioles,** and visceral organs
    - Bronchial tree, GI, and uterine smooth muscles relax
  - Beta receptors also stimulate glycogenolysis.
- Dopaminergic Receptors
  - DA ~ dilation of cerebral, coronary, renal, and mesenteric blood vessels → **inc BF**

Cardiovascular Response

- Cardiac muscle, AV node, SA node
  - **beta1**: inc contractility & HR
- Sphincters
  - alpha1: dec motility
- Blood vessels
  - alpha1: constrict
  - beta2: dilate
- Skeletal muscle
  - beta2: inc BF
- Respiration: bronchial muscles
  - **beta2**: dilation/relaxation

GU Response

- Bladder sphincters
  - alpha1: constrict
- Penis
  - alpha1: ejaculate
- Uterus
  - alpha1: contraction
  - beta2: relaxation

Response Summary

- Cardiovascular
  - Cardiac ~ **beta1**: inc contractility & HR
  - Blood vessels: alpha1 constricts, beta2 dilates
  - Skeletal muscle, Bronchial muscles
    - **beta2**: dilation/relaxation → inc BF and air exchange
- GU
  - Bladder sphincters ~ alpha1: constrict
  - Penis ~ alpha1: ejaculate
  - Uterus: alpha1 contracts, beta2 relaxes

Summary

- Beta Receptors are postsynaptic
  - **Beta1** ~ heart, kidney, and saliva
    - **Heart beats faster and harder.**
    - **Kidneys secrete more renin (inc BP).**
    - You drool.
  - **Beta2** ~ smooth muscle of **bronchioles, arterioles,** and visceral organs
    - Bronchial tree, GI, and uterine smooth muscles relax
  - Beta receptors also stimulate glycogenolysis.
- Dopaminergic Receptors
  - DA ~ dilation of cerebral, coronary, renal, and mesenteric blood vessels → **inc BF**

Response Summary

- Cardiovascular
  - Cardiac ~ **beta1**: inc contractility & HR
  - Blood vessels: alpha1 constricts, beta2 dilates
  - Skeletal muscle, Bronchial muscles
    - **beta2**: dilation/relaxation → inc BF and air exchange
- GU
  - Bladder sphincters ~ alpha1: constrict
  - Penis ~ alpha1: ejaculate
  - Uterus: alpha1 contracts, beta2 relaxes

ANS Drugs 4

Response Review, Direct vs Indirect

Response Review

- Cardiovascular
  - Cardiac ~ **beta1**: inc contractility & HR
  - Blood vessels: alpha1 constricts, beta2 dilates
  - Skeletal muscle, Bronchial muscles
    - **beta2**: dilation/relaxation → inc BF and air exchange
- GU
  - Bladder sphincters ~ alpha1: constrict
  - Penis ~ alpha1: ejaculate
  - Uterus: alpha1 contracts, beta2 relaxes

Direct vs Indirect Sympathomimetics

- Direct-acting Sympathomimetic:
  - Binds to the receptor → physiologic response
- Indirect-acting Sympathomimetic:
  - Causes the release of catecholamine from the storage sites in the nerve endings
    - The catecholamine then binds to the receptors → physiologic response
  - With an Indirect-acting sympathomimetic, if the storage site is exhausted, it is ineffective.
- Mixed-acting Sympathomimetic
  - Direct + Indirect

Nasal Decongestants

- Topical, intranasal application → constriction of dilated arterioles and reduction of nasal BF → dec congestion
  - Epinephrine
  - Ephedrine
    - indirect-sympathomimetic for NE and DA
    - direct-effect is not determined
  - Pseudoephedrine (alpha & beta2 agonist, ic. Sudafed)
  - Both ephedrine and pseudoephedrine are used in the making of street-methamphetamine

Ophthalmic Agents

- Topical application to the eye surface stimulates alpha receptors on small arterioles → dec conjunctival congestion
- Naphazoline
  - alpha-agonist, ie. Clear Eyes & Naphcon
- Tetrahydrozoline
  - alpha-agonist, ie. Visine

Response Summary

- Cardiovascular
  - Cardiac ~ **beta1**: inc contractility & HR
  - Blood vessels: alpha1 constricts, beta2 dilates
  - Skeletal muscle, Bronchial muscles
    - **beta2**: dilation/relaxation → inc BF and air exchange
- GU
  - Bladder sphincters ~ alpha1: constrict
  - Penis ~ alpha1: ejaculate
  - Uterus: alpha1 contracts, beta2 relaxes

Sympathomimetic Summary

- Direct-acting: bind directly to the receptor
- Indirect-acting:
  - cause release of catecholamine from the storage sites in the nerve endings

- Nasal Decongestants
  - Topical: constriction of arterioles → nasal BF → dec congestion
  - Systemic:
    - Epinephrine
    - Ephedrine (indirect-sympathomimetic for NE and DA)
    - Pseudoephedrine (alpha & beta2 agonist)
- Opthalmic
  - Topical: stimulates alpha receptors on small arterioles → dec conjunctival congestion
  - Alpha-agonists
    - Naphazoline, Tetrahydrozoline

ANS Drugs 5

Adrenergic-Agonist SE

Alpha-Agonist Adrenergic SE

- CNS:
  - headache, insomnia
  - restlessness, excitement, euphoria
- CV:
  - dysrhythmia, tachycardia, vasoconstriction → HTN
- GI:
  - anorexia, dry mouth, n/v

Beta-Agonist Adrenergic S

- CNS:
  - headache, mild tremors, nervousness, dizziness
- CV:
  - dysrhythmias, tachycardia, fluctuant BP
- GI:
  - n/v
- Systemic
  - Sweating, muscle cramps

Agonist SE

- Notice alpha & beta-agonist adrenergics have similar SE.
- Differentiate by
  - CNS: euphoria and insomnia = alpha
  - CV: non-fluctuant HTN = alpha
  - GI:
    - anorexia & dry mouth = alpha
  - Systemic sweating & muscle cramps = beta

Agonist SE Summary

- Alpha
  - euphoria and insomnia
  - non-fluctuant HTN
  - anorexia & dry mouth
- Beta
  - sweating & muscle cramps

ANS Drugs 6

Adrenergic-Antagonists
Alpha-Blockers

Alpha-Blocker Uses

- Antihypertensives
  - Dilate arterial and venous → dec PVR and BP
- BPH (Benign Prostatic Hyperplasia)
  - Dec resistance to urinary outflow by reducing unitary obstruction

Prazosin

- Alpha-blocker
- Uses:
  - Urinary hesitancy from BPH
  - HTN
  - PTSD and kids w/ severe nightmares

Ergot Alkaloids

- Alpha-blockers
- Migraines
  - Constrict carotid arteries
    - also inhibits trigeminal signaling
- Postpartum bleeding
  - Induce vasoconstriction in uterus → contractions

Phentolamine

- Reverses the potent vasoconstrictive effects of vasopressors such as NE or EPI
  - Restores BF preventing necrosis
- Used for HTN emergency
  - Possibly due to pheochromocytoma
- 2nd line for cocaine-induced CV complications
  - Can't use beta-blockers, would lead to unopposed alpha-adrenergic mediated coronary vasoconstriction → worsening myocardial ischemia and HTN
  - 1st line: benzodiazepines, nitroglycerin, and CCBs

Alpha-Blocker Summary

- Main Uses
  - HTN: Dilate arterial/venous → dec PVR and BP
  - BPH
- Prazosin
  - Uses: Urinary hesitancy from BPH
- Ergot Alkaloids
  - Migraines:
    - Constrict carotid arteries & inhibit trigeminal signaling
- Phentolamine
  - Reverses vasopressors such as NE or EPI
  - Used for HTN emergency

ANS Drugs 7

Alpha-Blockers
Naturopathic and SE

Alpha-Blocker Review

- Main Uses
  - HTN: Dilate arterial/venous → dec PVR and BP
  - BPH
- Prazosin
  - Uses: Urinary hesitancy from BPH
- Ergot Alkaloids
  - Migraines:
    - Constrict carotid arteries & inhibit trigeminal signaling
- Phentolamine
  - Reverses vasopressors such as NE or EPI
  - Used for HTN emergency

Yohimbine

- **Alpha2**-selective blocker
- Marketed as a naturopathic remedy for erectile dysfunction, an aphrodisiac, for migraines, postpartum, and as a dietary supplement
- West African > Asian usage
- Small amounts → HTN, but large amounts → very, very low BP
  - Therapeutic index is small, so it is very easy to move from HTN to hypotension
- Other SE
  - Hallucinations or paralysis
  - Panic attack symptoms

Alpha-Blocker SE

- CNS:
  - Headache, dizziness/vertigo
  - Anxiety/depression, drowsy/fatigue, weak/numb
- CV:
  - Dysrhythmia, tachycardia, CP, orthostatic hypotension, edema
- GI: n/v/c/d, abdominal pain
- Head:
  - Tinnitus, rhinitis/epistaxis, dry mouth, pharyngitis
- GU: incontinence

Alpha-Blocker Summary

- Yohimbine (**Alpha2**-selective blocker)
  - Marketed for erectile dysfunction, aphrodisiac, migraines, and as a diet supplement
    - West African > Asian usage
  - Small amounts → HTN, but large amounts → severe **hypo**tension
    - Also: Hallucinations or paralysis, Panic attack symptoms
- Alpha-Blocker SE
  - CNS:
    - Headache, dizziness/vertigo
    - Anxiety/depression, drowsy/fatigue, weak/numb
  - Head: Tinnitus, rhinitis/epistaxis, dry mouth, pharyngitis
  - CV: Dysrhythmia, tachycardia, CP, orthostatic hypotension, edema
  - GI: n/v/c/d, abdominal pain
  - GU: incontinence

Not Quite Major Depression

Is this Depression?

A day care worker regularly ignores a child, and when asked about it replies, "She wants to be left alone." Which of the following defense mechanisms best explains her response?

- A. Rationalization
- B. Isolation of affect
- C. Intellectualization
- D. Projection
- E. Depression

Projection

- D — The day care worker wants to be left alone, but she projects her feelings onto the child.
    - Rationalization (A) is making excuses for your behavior.
        - ie. "I was building the lesson-plan for tomorrow"
        - ie. "I'm teaching her to be more independent"

Is this Depression?

- A father comes into the ER holding the lifeless body of his son. He shows absolutely no emotion.

Defense Mechanisms

- Isolation = separation of an idea from the affect that accompanies it

- Depression is not a defense mechanism.
  - Depression is a disturbance in neurotransmitters → known symptoms that can be diagnosed
    - and most-likely treated.
- Depression is not a mental weakness.
  - It is not how a manipulative relative controls family members.
  - It is a sickness that can be treated.

Grief (Bereavement) vs Depression

- Symptoms:
  - **wax and wane** vs. pervasive and unremitting
  - can last **up to 1y** vs. can last much longer than 1y
- Return to Baseline Functioning:
  - w/in **2 months** vs. never
- With Depression:
  - shame and guilt more common
  - threaten suicide more often
- Treatment
  - **supportive psychotherapy** vs. antidepressants

Postpartum:
Blues vs. Depression vs. Psychosis

An inexperienced mother is more likely to have a severe psychiatric reaction postpartum.

- Child #
  - A mother may become blue after the birth of any child, but psychosis is something that occurs after the first child.
  - **Depression is more common after the 2nd child.**
- Onset
  - Blues occur w/in 2w, depression and psychosis may take up to a month to become apparent
- Mother cares for baby?
  - A blue-mother cares for her kid, while a depressed or psychotic mom may not.
- Level of depression
  - **mild** vs. **severe** vs. **severe + psychotic**
- Treatment
  - self-limited vs. antidepressants vs. antidepressants + mood stabilizers or antipsychotics

Postpartum:
Psychosis vs. Depression vs. Blues

- Child #
  - 1st vs 2nd vs any
- Onset
  - < 1m vs < 1m vs < 2w
- Mother cares for baby?
  - may hurt baby vs. thoughts of hurting baby vs. yes
- Level of depression
  - severe + psychotic vs severe vs mild
- Treatment
  - antidepressants + mood stabilizers or antipsychotics
  - vs antidepressants
  - vs self-limited

Depression is One of the 5 Stages of Dying

- Shock and denial
- Anger
- Bargaining
- Depression
- Acceptance

- Occur in any order

Major Depression 1

Dispel the Notion and Define the nt's

Depression is not Weakness

- Depression is not a defense mechanism. It is a disturbance in neurotransmitters which result in known symptoms that can be diagnosed, and, for the most part, treated.
- Depression is not a mental weakness. It is not how a manipulative relative controls family members. It is a sickness that can be treated.

Depression Neurotransmitter Targets

- Neurotransmitters
  1. Serotonin
  2. Norepinephrine
  3. Dopamine
  - In that order

Neurotransmitters

- Neurotransmitters
  - serotonin, norepinephrine, dopamine (in that order)
- This explains the order of preferred treatment agents
  - 1st: SSRIs (-pram, -tine)
    - → increases serotonin
  - 2nd: SNRIs (-pran, -xine)
    - → increases serotonin & increases norepinephrine
  - Think SSRI first, then SNRI if SSRI's fail
    - **-pram or –tine, then –pran or –xine**

Neurotransmitters

- Neurotransmitters
  - serotonin, norepinephrine, dopamine (in that order)
- This explains the order of preferred treatment agents
  - 1st: SSRIs (-pram, -tine) → +serotonin
  - 2nd: SNRIs (-pran, -xine)→ +serotonin & +norepinephrine
  - 3rd: atypicals: bupropion, mirtazapine
  - 4th: serotonin modulators (-azodone) → +serotonin, -others
  - 5th: TCAs (-tryptyline, -pramine) → +serotonin & +NE
    - *tryp as is triple*
  - 6th: all else fails, MAOIs (phenelzine, selegiline) → +all

Treatment Summary

- **Think SSRI first, then SNRI if SSRI's fail**
  -pram or –tine, then –pran or –xine
- Depressed and worried about wt gain?
  - bupropion
- Depressed and anorexic?
  - mirtazapine
- Having trouble sleeping?
  - Trazodone, nefazodone (SE: priapism)
    - 'z' is for sleep

Treatment Summary

- Is depression refractory to treatment, or is patient dealing with chronic neuropathic pain?
  - TCAs (tryptyline, -pramine)
    - <u>Three</u> times I <u>pray mine</u> neuro pain and depression will stay fine.
- Pt drank red wine or ate cheese and BP went sky high?
  - Selegiline, phenelzine (hypertensive crisis)
    - Bud <u>Selig</u> was in <u>Phoenix</u> and blew up at a <u>wine & cheese</u> party.

Treatment Re-summary

- **-pram or –tine, then –pran or –xine**
- Depressed
  - & obese: Rx **bupropion**
  - & anorexic: Rx **mirtazapine**
  - & need sleep: Rx t**razodone**, nefazodone
    - SE: priapism
    - 'z' is for sleep

- Refractory or chronic neuropathic pain?
  - TCAs (-tryptyline, -pramine)
    - <u>Three</u> times I <u>pray mine</u> neuro pain and depression will stay fine.

- Bud <u>Selig</u> was in <u>Phoenix</u> and blew up at a <u>wine & cheese</u> party.

Major Depression 2

Review the Drugs & Special Cases

Treatment Review

- Think SSRI first, then SNRI if SSRI's fail
  -pram or –tine, then –pran or –xine
- Depressed and worried about wt gain?
  – bupropion
- Depressed and anorexic?
  – mirtazapine
- Having trouble sleeping?
  – Trazodone, nefazodone (SE: priapism)
    - 'z' is for sleep

Treatment Review

- Is depression refractory to treatment, or is patient dealing with chronic neuropathic pain?
  - TCAs (-tryptyline, -pramine)
    - <u>Three</u> times I <u>pray mine</u> neuro pain and depression will stay fine.
- Pt drank red wine or ate cheese and BP went sky high?
  - Selegiline, phenelzine (hypertensive crisis)
    - Bud <u>Selig</u> was in <u>Phoenix</u> and blew up at a <u>wine & cheese</u> party.

Treatment Re-review

- -pram or –tine, then –pran or –xine
- Depressed
  - & obese: Rx **bupropion**
  - & anorexic: Rx **mirtazapine**
  - & need sleep: Rx t**razodone**, nefazodone
    - SE: priapism
    - 'z' is for sleep

- Refractory or chronic neuropathic pain?
  - TCAs (-tryptyline, -pramine)
    - <u>Three</u> times I <u>pray mine</u> neuro pain and depression will stay fine.

- Bud <u>Selig</u> was in <u>Phoenix</u> and blew up at a <u>wine & cheese</u> party.

Dx Depression

- At least 5 for at least 2 weeks

- **S** leep changes (inc during day, dec at night)
- **I** nterest loss
- **G** uilt (worthlessness)
- **E** nergy (lack of)
- **C** ognition/Concentration
- **A** ppetite (significant wt loss or gain)
- **P** sychomotor (agitation, retardation)
- **S** uicide/death preoccupation

Special Notes on D

- Elderly are less likely to complain of depressed mood and more likely to complain about somatic issues, worthlessness, be hypochondriacs, or manifest psychotic delusion
- Psychotic features = worse prognosis
- Must treat worst symptom first
  - ie. treat psychosis before underlying D.
  - **This is why elderly often get <u>haloperidol</u> or <u>risperidone</u> first**.

Indications for ECT

- Unipolar major D
    - Refractory or resistant to antidepressant therapy
    - Need exist for rapid treatment response, such as in pregnancy, persistent suicidal intent, or food refusal leading to dehydration or nutritional compromise
    - Medical comorbidities prevent the use of antidepressant meds
    - Previous response to ECT
    - Psychotic creatures (eg. delusions or hallucinations)
    - Catatonia
    - Persistent suicidal intent
- Bipolar depression or mania

Personalities

more like disorders

Personality Disorders

- Defined: pervasive, inflexible, and maladaptive personality patterns
- Cluster A:
  - Peculiar thought processes, inappropriate affect
- Cluster B:
  - Mood lability, dissociative symptoms, preoccupation w/ rejection
- Cluster C:
  - Anxiety, preoccupation w/ criticism or rigidity

Cluster A

- Paranoid PD:
  - Distrust and suspiciousness
- Schizoid PD:
  - Detachment and restricted emotionality
- Schizotypal PD:
  - Discomfort w/ social relationships
  - Thought distortion
  - Eccentricity

Cluster B

- Histrionic PD
  - Flamboyant, dramatic, and needs to be looked at.
  - Sexually seductive
  - Must be center of attention
- Borderline PD
  - Unstable w/ mood swings and impulsive
  - Unstable relationships. Main defense mechanism is **splitting**
  - Often empty and bored w/ recurrent suicidal behaviors. **A cutter.**
  - Disturbed identity and inappropriate anger. If stressed → psychotic
- Antisocial PD
  - began by 15yo & pt > 18yo
- Narcissistic PD

Cluster C

- Avoidant PD
  - Inhibited, inadequate, and hypersensitivity
  - Feelings of inadequacy → few friendships
    - Lonely and substandard, preoccupied w/ rejection
- Dependent PD
  - Submissive and clinging
  - Need to be taken care of.
- OCPD
  - Perfectionist. Preoccupied w/ orderliness and control.
  - Consumed by details and lose overall goals
  - Hesitant to delegate.
  - Indecisive
  - Miserly and unable to give up possessions.
  - *Don't confuse w/ OCD*

Review the Clusters

Cluster A

- I prefer to be alone → Okay, I'll be around people, but I don't trust them → I'm around people but I don't think like they do

Cluster B

- Everyone look at me → If you're not with me, your against me → Screw you. I hate you → I'm the best. Worship me.

Cluster C

- Everything has to be perfect → I'm uncomfortable there. They'll criticize me → Please don't leave me!

OCPD vs. OCD

- Chronic, maladaptive pattern of dealing w/ life
  vs
- Anxiety disorder w/ recurrent obsessions and compulsions

- Perfection who needs control
  vs
- Obsessive & Compulsive
  - Obsessive = thoughts, images or ideas that won't go away
  - Compulsive = behaviors that you must carry out over and over
    - **Aimed at getting rid of your anxiety**

The 'P' stands for Perfectionist vs. Obsessive & Compulsive

Sleep 1

Normal

Non-REM vs REM

- **Brain inactive, body active** vs **brain active, body inactive**
- Slowing of EEG rhythms vs. aroused EEG patterns
- High muscle tone vs. generalized atony & sexual arousal
- Absence of eye movement vs saccadic eye movement
- Thought-like mental activity vs dreams

- In REM, body is paralyzed but brain is active (eyes are part of brain).
    - A paralyzed body is relaxed.
    - A relaxed body feeds blood to sex organs → sexual arousal.
    - In REM, we dream (or have nightmares)

Stages of Sleep

- Stage 1:
  - Dec alpha waves, increase <u>theta</u>   5%
- Stage 2:
  - <u>K</u> complexes + **sleep spindles**   45%
- Stage 3 + 4:
  - **Delta** waves   12% + 13% = 25%
- REM:
  - Bursts of **saw-toothed** waves   25%

Stages of Sleep

- Stage 1: dec alpha waves, increase <u>theta</u>   5%
- Stage 2: <u>K</u> complexes + <u>sleep</u> spindles   45%
  - **Longest** of all sleep stages
- Stage 3 + 4: **delta** waves   12% + 13% = 25%
  - Hardest to arouse
  - Tends to vanish in the elderly
- REM: bursts of **saw-toothed** waves   25%
  - Easiest to arouse
  - Lengthens in time as night progresses
  - Increased during the 2nd half of the night

Latency

- Sleep latency
  - Time needed before you actually fall asleep
    - Typically < 15 min
- REM latency
  - Typically 90 min
  - Shortened during depression, narcolepsy, ...

Infancy to Geriatric

- Total sleep time decreases
- REM % decreases
- Stage 3 & 4 vanish

Neurotransmitters of Sleep

- **S** → SAn → D → awake
  - "sand" as in sandman
  - **<u>S</u>erotonin** initiates sleep

  - <u>S</u>erotonin & <u>A</u>cetylcholine increase during sleep
  - <u>n</u>orepinephrine decreases during sleep
    - ACh and NE are linked to REM sleep

  - **<u>D</u>A increases toward end of sleep**
    - linked to arousal and wakefulness

Sleep 2

Altered

Review: Stages of Sleep

- 5%   Stage 1: theta
- 45%   Stage 2: k-complexes + sleep spindles
  - longest of all sleep stages
- 25%   Stage 3 + 4: **delta** waves
  - hardest to arouse
  - tends to vanish in the elderly
- 25%   REM: bursts of **sawtooth** waves
  - easiest to arouse
  - lengthens as night progresses → inc in 2nd half

Review: Neurotransmitters of Sleep

- Increasing Serotonin → sleep
- inc ACh + dec NE = stay asleep
- inc DA → waking up

SSSSSleep → SAn + DDDD → awake

Chemicals

- Tryptophan increases total sleep time
  - *eat turkey*

- Suppresses Stage 3 & 4
  - Benzodiazepine
    - sometimes used for sleep terror disorder (night terrors) & sleepwalking, though normally condition is self-limited
    - chronic use → inc sleep latency
- Suppress REM
  - Alcohol and barbiturate intoxication
    - withdrawal results in REM rebound
  - TCAs
    - sometimes used for dream anxiety disorder (nightmares), though normally condition is self-limited

Sleep and Major Depression

- Shortened REM latency w/ increased REM time
- suppresses delta

  a disturbed sleep w/ early rising

Parasomnias

- All stages
  - Sleeptalking
- Stages 3 & 4
  - *[inactive brain, active body = don't remember]*
  - Sleepwalking
  - Night terrors = sleep terror disorder
  - usually don't treat either, but may consider BZD
- REM
  - *[active brain, inactive body = remember]*
  - Nightmares = dream anxiety disorder
    - usually don't treat, but can suppress REM w/ TCAs

Narcolepsy

- **Cataplexy** = sudden loss of muscle tone w/o LOC which may have been precipitated by a loud noise or intense emotion
  - Usually young. Is not syncope or bp abnormality
- Narcolepsy Treatment
  - Preferred: forced naps at regular times
  - Pharm: psychostimulants
  - If cataplexy is present, TCAs are preferred
  - GHB improves quality of nighttime sleep

CARDIAC CENTRIC

PCI, Stents, and Antiplatelet Therapy 1

Stent Type & Thrombus Risk

PCI

- Obstructed coronary arteries require clearing of the blockages
  - aka. **PCI = Percutaneous Coronary Intervention**
- PCI includes **balloon angioplasty**.
  - A **balloon catheter** is passed into the narrowed locations and then inflated to a fixed size using water pressure. Once maximal effect is achieved, the balloon is deflated and withdrawn.
  - A **stent** may or may not be inserted at the time of ballooning to ensure the vessel remains open.

Stents

- BMS = Bare Metal Stents
- DES = Drug-Eluting Stents
  - consist of a metallic stent backbone, an antiproliferative drug, and a polymer that serves as the vehicle for the drug and also controls the drug release rate. The drug inhibits excessive growth of neointima, a major cause of restenosis.
  - 1st gen: Sirolimus stents, Paclitaxel stents
    - most common
  - 2nd gen: Everolimus stents, Zotarolimus stents

BMS vs. DES

- In most studies, DES outperform BMS with regard to the need for repeat revascularization and there is no difference in long-term mortality.

- BMS is better than DES in patients who require long-term anticoagulation

PCI Summary

- PCI = Percutaneous Coronary Intervention
  - Balloon angioplasty.
  - Stent
- Stents
  - BMS = Bare Metal Stents
  - DES = Drug-Eluting Stents
    - 1st gen: Sirolimus stents, Paclitaxel stents
      - most common
  - BMS vs DES
    - DES outperforms w/ regards to repeat revascularization
      - No difference in long-term mortality.
    - BMS in patients who require long-term anticoagulation

Stent Thrombosis Summary

- Stent thrombosis may lead to sudden death or MI
- 6 month mortality with successful repeat revascularization is high

Defining Stent Thrombosis

- Definite:
  - When thrombosis is found within 5mm of stent, or in the stent
- Probable:
  - With events within 30 days
    - aka. acute or subacute stent thrombosis
- Possible:
  - With events after 30 days
    - aka. late stent thrombosis

PCI, Stents, and Antiplatelet Therapy 2

Stent Thrombus and Therapy

Stent Thrombosis Summary

- Stent thrombosis may lead to sudden death or MI
- 6 month mortality with successful repeat revascularization is high

Defining Stent Thrombosis

- Definite:
  - When thrombosis is found within 5mm of stent, or in the stent
- Probable:
  - With events within 30 days
    - aka. acute or subacute stent thrombosis
- Possible:
  - With events after 30 days
    - aka. late stent thrombosis

Default Post-Stent Therapy

- Long-term **DAPT (dual antiplatelet therapy)**
  - STARS trial
  - Always: Aspirin 75-100mg Daily
  - Plus: Clopidogrel 75mg Daily for 12 months
    - can use Prasugrel or Ticagrelor instead
- Minimum duration of uninterrupted therapy
  - BMS: 4 weeks
  - DES: 6 months

Patient Scheduled for PCI

- If on aspirin therapy, continue
  - If not on aspirin therapy, give Aspirin 325mg 2 hours before procedure
- Clopidogrel is contraindicated in most cases, but with a high-risk of thrombosis, it can be used
- All patients get Heparin or Bivalirudin

Emergency PCI

- If time does not allow for adequate pretreatment w/ aspirin and/or clopidogrel, give a glycoprotein IIb/IIIa inhibitor
  - Abciximab (ReoPro)
  - Eptifibatide (**Integrillin**)
  - Tirofiban (Aggrastat)

PCI w/o Stent Placement

- If patient receives PCI w/ balloon angioplasty and no stenting, and the patient is not at high risk of bleeding or planned surgery within 30 days
  - Give **DAPT (aspirin + clopidogrel) for 30 days** post-procedure

Summary

- PCI includes balloon angioplasty +/- stent
- Prior to procedure,
  - Get patient on **aspirin**
    - If high-risk for thrombosis, add **clopidogrel**
  - If patient can't get proper pretreatment, give
    - Abciximab (ReoPro) or Eptifibatide (**Integrillin**)
  - All patients get Heparin (or Bivalirudin)
- Use DES unless long-term anticoagulation is expected

Summary

- To prevent thrombosis after stenting, DAPT
  - STARS trial
  - 75mg Aspirin Daily forever + 75mg Clopidogrel Daily for one year
  - BMS can't be interrupted for 4 weeks
  - DES can't be interrupted for 6 months
- If patient got PCI w/o stenting,
  - DAPT for 30 days

Big Points

- DES over BMS unless expected to be on anticoagulation therapy for the future
- Aspirin and Heparin before surgery
  - In specific cases, add Clopidogrel
- DAPT (reference **STARS trial**)
  - Post procedure w/ stent:
    - Aspirin 75mg Daily; Clopidogrel 75mg Daily for 1y
  - Post procedure w/o stent:
    - 30 days

Tachycardia 1

Above the Node Drugs

Sinus Tachy:
Know Your Drugs

- Rate Control
  1. Beta-blockers
     - Cardio-selective BB's: **metoprolol**, atenolol, acebutolol, **esmolol**
     - Also, inhibit renin secretion → dec BP
     - This is the go to for most cardiac issues.
  - CCBs (**diltiazem**, verapamil)
    - Vasodilator and strongly depress the AV node
  - Digoxin
    - Strongly depress the AV node
  - *Learn 'DVD': Diltiazem, Verapamil, Digoxin*
    - *This is the order of preference very often.*
    - *If one isn't available on the test, go to the next one*
- **Procainamide**
  - Blocks Na-channels → dec conduction velocity and inc refractory period.
  - Primarily used for WPW
  - SE: **lupus-like**

Sinus Tachy:
Know Your Drugs

- Cardioversion (ie. Afib)
  - **Amiodarone**
    - Lots of known SE, but it's so useful that we just learn to care for the SE and beware of the contraindications
    - Works like a beta-blocker and a K-channel blocker on SA and AV nodes → inc refractory period, slows intra-cardiac conduction
    - SE (generally with chronic use)
      - Development of interstitial lung disease
      - Structural similar to thyroxine → abnormal thyroid function
      - Corneal micro-deposits → optic dick swelling and reversible vision defects
      - Blue-grey skin, Peripheral neuropathies
    - Contraindications: pregnancy or nursing. Monitor closely w/ lung issues
      - Given w/ digitalis toxicity can be lethal.
  - Flecainide

Sinus Tachy:
Know Your Drugs

- **Adenosine**
  - Causes a transient heart block
  - Used for **paroxysmal SVT**
    - Works therapeutically and diagnostically
  - **Lethal w/ WPW**
    - Always r/o WPW before giving adenosine.

Sinus Tachy:
Know Your Drugs Summary

- Rate Control
  - Beta-blockers (most often)
    - Cardio-selective BB's: **metoprolol**, atenolol, acebutolol, **esmolol**
  - CCBs (**diltiazem**, verapamil), Digoxin
    - *'DVD': Diltiazem, Verapamil, Digoxin*
- **Procainamide** ~ WPW
  - SE: **lupus-like**
- Cardioversion
  - **Amiodarone**
    - SE (generally w/ chronic use)
      - **Interstitial lung disease, Abnormal thyroid**
      - **Blue-grey skin**, Vision problems, Peripheral neuropathies
    - Contraindications: pregnancy/nursing. Lung issues
      - **Given w/ digitalis toxicity can be lethal.**
  - Flecainide
- **Adenosine** ~ paroxysmal SVT
  - Causes a transient heart block
  - **Lethal w/ WPW**

Read the EKG

1. Rate
   - **Sinus Tachycardia = > 100bpm**
2. Rhythm
   a. P before each QRS
   b. PR interval (AV blocks, WPW)
   c. QRS interval (for BBB)
3. Axis
4. Hypertrophy (check V1)
   a. P-wave for atrial hypertrophy
   b. R-wave for right ventricular hypertrophy
   c. S-wave depth in V1 + R-wave height in V5 for left ventricular hypertrophy
5. Infarction
   a. ST-segment elevation/depression
   b. Inverted T-waves
   c. Scan for Q-waves

Tachycardia 2

Above the Node Tachy Types

Sinus Tachy:
Know Your Drugs Review

- Rate Control
  - Beta-blockers (most often)
  - CCBs (**diltiazem**, verapamil), Digoxin
    - *'DVD': Diltiazem, Verapamil, Digoxin*
- **Procainamide** ~ WPW
- Cardioversion
  - **Amiodarone**
    - SE (generally w/ chronic use)
      - **Interstitial lung disease, Abnormal thyroid**
      - **Blue-grey skin**, Vision problems, Peripheral neuropathies
    - Contraindications: pregnancy/nursing. Lung issues
      - **Given w/ digitalis toxicity can be lethal.**
  - Flecainide
- **Adenosine** ~ paroxysmal SVT
  - Causes a transient heart block
  - **Lethal w/ WPW**

Read the EKG

1. Rate
   - **Sinus Tachycardia = > 100bpm**
2. Rhythm
   a. P before each QRS
   b. PR interval (AV blocks, WPW)
   c. QRS interval (for BBB)
3. Axis
4. Hypertrophy (check V1)
   a. P-wave for atrial hypertrophy
   b. R-wave for right ventricular hypertrophy
   c. S-wave depth in V1 + R-wave height in V5 for left ventricular hypertrophy
5. Infarction
   a. ST-segment elevation/depression
   b. Inverted T-waves
   c. Scan for Q-waves

If Tachy From Above The AV Node, Rule Out the Unusual Ones

- **Atrial Flutter** (saw-tooth wave pattern)
  - Is patient hypotensive?
  - If unstable, **cardioversion**

- **Multifocal Atrial Tachycardia**
  - Is the p-wave changing form?
    - Then it's coming from many different spots.
    - If rate was under 100bpm, this would be Wandering Pacemaker
  - Generally seen w/ COPD pt w/ respiratory failure
  - Tx: **diltiazem**, verapamil, or digoxin
    - Diltiazem is a potent vasodilator which strongly depresses the AV node
      - ie. Inc BF + slows down the rate
    - NOTE: avoid beta-blockers due to lung disease

HR: Normal to 200 in a Blink
(Avg. Rate Between 150-250bpm)

- Rates that jump from normal to over 200 rapidly are generally either due to an accessory pathway (ie. WPW) or nodal-reentrant SVT.
  - Automaticity-type SVT is a more gradual increase and decrease due to an area in the heart generating its own electrical signal.
  - The common treatment for suspected SVT is both therapeutic and diagnostic, but if given to a pt with WPW, it can be lethal.
  - **Therefore, r/o WPW before all else.**

WPW

1. r/o accessory pathways, ie. WPW
   - **WPW**: short PR & delta wave (wave mixed into the R-wave)
     - If positive for WPW, this is a hemodynamically unstable condition suggesting immediate synchronized cardioversion
     - When stable, give **procainamide**
       - Procainamide blocks particular Na-channels → → decreased conduction velocity and increased refractory period
     - Later, surgical ablation
     - Avoid: digoxin and CCBs → inc tachycardia due to inhibition of normal conduction pathway causes increased use of accessory pathway, ie. no AV node control
       - **Adenosine is deadly**

Paroxysmal SVT

2. Treat paroxysmal SVT w/ **adenosine**
   - Causes a transient heart block that is both therapeutic and diagnostic.

AFib

- r/o WPW. Rates over 200 suggest WPW
- **CHADS score**
  - Risk of stroke and need for anticoagulation
  - **C**HF, **H**TN, **A**ge > 75yo, **D**iabetes, prior **S**troke (or TIA)
    - 1pt for each. Stroke gets 2pts
  - 0: ASN → 1: ASN or warfarin → ≥ 2: warfarin
- **Ventricular rate control**
  - BB, CCB, or Digoxin
- **Pharmacologic cardioversion**
  - Amiodarone (or flecainide)
  - Same drugs used to **maintain sinus rhythm**

Supraventricular Summary

- **Atrial Flutter** (saw-tooth wave pattern)
- **Multifocal Atrial Tachycardia** (Is the p-wave changing form?)
  - Generally seen w/ COPD pt w/ respiratory failure, so <u>NO beta-blockers</u>
  - Tx: **diltiazem**
1. r/o accessory pathways, ie. WPW
   - **WPW**: short PR & delta
     - Unstable: synchronized cardioversion → Stable: **Procainamide** → ablation
     - Avoid: CCBs and digoxin. Especially avoid adenosine. **Adenosine is deadly**
2. Treat paroxysmal SVT w/ **adenosine** (Therapeutic and diagnostic)
3. Afib
   - **CHADS score**: **C**HF (1), **H**TN (1), **A**ge > 75yo (1), **D**iabetes (1), **S**troke (2)
     - 0: ASN → 1: ASN or warfarin → ≥ 2: warfarin
   - **Ventricular rate control**: BB, CCB, or Digoxin
   - **Pharmacologic Cardioversion & Sinus Rhythm Maintenance**:
     - Amiodarone (or flecainide)

Tachycardia 3

Below the Node Tachy Types

Ventricular Tachycardia

- QRS > 0.12s
  - r/o WPW
- Check for pulse. If no pulse, treat as VF.
- If unstable, sedate and synchronized cardioversion
  - If don't synchronize to the heartbeat can devolve into Vfib
  - O2 → sedation → cardiovert 100J → 200J → 300J → 360J
    - *if at first you don't succeed, crank it up higher and try again*
- If stable, pharmacologically cardioversion
  - **O2 → amiodarone → lidocaine until VT resolves → procainamide until VT resolves → cardiovert**
    - If amiodarone is contraindicated, just straight to lidocaine
    - Lidocaine is a class 1b and procainamide is a class 1a, so you try 'b', and if that fails, you crank it up to 'a'

V Fib

- Check rhythm. Is it shockable?
  - Not shockable: Asystole (ie. PEA)
    - PEA = pulseless electrical activity
    - **CPR for 5 cycles → Epi 1mg q 3min → check rhythm**
      - May give 1 dose of vasopressin 40 units to replace 1st or 2nd dose of Epi
        - » vasopressin = AVP = ADH
  - Shockable
    - Give 1 shock → CPR for 5 cycles → check rhythm
      → 1 shock → CPR → Epi 1mg every 3min → check rhythm
      → 1 shock → CPR → antiarrhythmic: amiodarone or lidocaine (consider Mg for TdP) → CPR for 5

Torsade de Pointes (**TdP**)

- Causes
  - Vulnerable person w/ a long QT can be set off by sound
  - Antiarrhythmics: quinidine, procainamide, disopyramide;
  - Psychotropics: phenothiazines, thioridazine, TCAs, Li
- Tx:
  - **Lidocaine**
    - increase the refractory period
  - If unstable, may try cardioversion, but dysrhythmia often returns
  - **Check for hypokalemia and hypoMg →** correct
  - Cardiac pacing or isoproterenol infusion may suppress in emergency

Ventricular Tachycardia/Fib Summary

- V Tach (QRS > 0.12s)
  - If no pulse, treat as VF. If unstable, sedate and synchronized cardioversion
  - If stable, pharmacologically cardioversion
    - **O2 → amiodarone → lidocaine until VT resolves → procainamide until VT resolves → cardiovert**
- V Fib: Check for rhythm
  - Not shockable: Asystole (ie. PEA)
    - **CPR for 5 cycles → Epi 1mg q 3min → check rhythm**
  - Shockable
    - 1 shock → CPR for 5 cycles → check rhythm
    - → 1 shock → CPR → Epi 1mg every 3min → check rhythm
    - → 1 shock → CPR → antiarrhythmic: amiodarone or lidocaine (consider Mg for TdP) → CPR for 5
- Torsade de Pointes (**TdP**)
  - **Lidocaine.** If unstable, may try cardioversion, but dysrhythmia often returns
  - **Check for hypokalemia and hypoMg →** correct
  - Cardiac pacing or isoproterenol infusion may suppress in emergency

INFECTION-SPECIFIC ANTIBIOTICS

Infection-Specific Abs 1

Gram-Pos:

PCN's and a preview of Cephalosporin

Gram Pos Cocci

- PCNs
  - Penicillins (PCN)
  - Beta-lactamase-resistant PCNs
  - Semisynthetic PCNs
- Cephalosporins
- Macrolides
- Fluoroquinolones
- Clindamycin

Gram-Pos Cocci: Penicillin

- Stept
- Staph
- Clostridium
- Listeria

Gram-Pos Cocci:
Beta-lactamase Resistant PCNs

- Naf Ox Clox Diclox -cillins
- Nafcillin, Oxacillin, Cloxacillin, Dicloxacillin
  - aka. anti-staphylococcal penicillins
  - also good for Strept

Gram-Pos Cocci: Semisynthetic PCNs

- PCN G, PCN VK, ampicillin, amoxicillin
  - useful with Gram-neg (ie. Neisseria)
  - Strept (not Staph)
    - for Staph coverage, combo with β-Lactamase inhibitor
      - ampicillin-sulbactam, amoxicillin-clavulanate
- Enterococci and Listeria
  - ampicillin, amoxicillin
- E. coli
  - ampicillin

Summary: Staph, Strept, and Some

- Staph (, Strept):
  - nafcillin, oxacillin, cloxacillin, dicloxacillin
- Strept, Clostridium, Listeria:
  - PCN G, PCN VK, ampicillin, amoxicillin
  - + Enterococci: ampicillin, amoxicillin
  - + E. coli: ampicillin
- Strept, Staph, Clostridium, Listeria, Enterococci:
  - ampicillin-sulbactam, amoxicillin-clavulanate

Preview: Cephalosporins

- Came Coverage as Semisynthetic PCNs:
  - Strept (not staph)
- And some gram-neg:
  - 1st gen: Moraxella, E. coli
  - 2nd gen: + some G- bacilli:
    - Haemophilus, Klebsiella, Citrobacter, Morganella, Proteus, Providencia
- 1st-gen: the cefa's
  - cefazolin, cefadroxil, cephalexin
- 2nd-gen: *fox fur fight'n prozac*
  - cefoxitin, cefuroxime, cefotetan, cefprozil

Infection-Specific Abs 2

Gram-Pos:

Cephalosporins

Review: Staph, Strept, and Some

- Staph (, Strept):
  - nafcillin, oxacillin, cloxacillin, dicloxacillin
- Strept, Clostridium, Listeria:
  - PCN G, PCN VK, ampicillin, amoxicillin
  - + Enterococci: ampicillin, amoxicillin
  - + E. coli: ampicillin
- Strept, Staph, Clostridium, Listeria, Enterococci:
  - ampicillin-sulbactam, amoxicillin-clavulanate

Gram-Pos Cocci: Cephalosporins

- 1st-gen: the cefa's
  - <u>cefa</u>zolin, <u>cefa</u>droxil, <u>cepha</u>lexin
- 2nd-gen: *fox fur fight'n prozac*
  - cefoxitin, cefuroxime, cefotetan, cefprozil

Cephalosporins

- Same Coverage as Semisynthetic PCNs:
  - Strept (not staph)
- And some gram-neg:
  - 1st gen: Moraxella, E. coli
  - 2nd gen: + Haemophilus, Klebsiella, Citrobacter, Morganella, Proteus, Providencia
- If a gram-pos bug, generally answer 1st-gen
  - Gram-pos gets Cefa

Cephalosporin with a PCN Allergy

- If PCN causes a rash, you can still use
- If PCN causes anaphylaxis, no cephalosporins
  - minor infection, use macrolide or fluoroquinolone
    - m**AC**rolid**E**: **A**zithromycin, **C**larithromycin, **E**rythromycin
      - not for Staph
    - Fluoroquinolone: Fluoro flox flox floxacin (LeGeMo)
      - levo**floxacin**, gemifloxacin, moxifloxacin
      - excellent for Strept
  - serious infections:
    - Vanc, Linezolid, Daptomycin

Summary: Staph, Strept, and Some

- Staph (, Strept):
  - nafcillin, oxacillin, cloxacillin, dicloxacillin
- Strept, Clostridium, Listeria:
  - PCN G, PCN VK, ampicillin, amoxicillin
  - + Enterococci: ampicillin, amoxicillin
  - + E. coli: ampicillin
- Strept, Staph, Clostridium, Listeria, Enterococci:
  - ampicillin-sulbactam, amoxicillin-clavulanate

Summary: Gram-Pos Cephalosporins (or not)

Strept (not Staph)

- 1st: the cefa's: cefazolin, cefadroxil, cephalexin
    - + Moraxella, E. coli
- 2nd: fox fur fight'n prozac: cefoxitin, cefuroxime, cefotetan, cefprozil
    - + Moraxella, E. coli + some gram-neg bacilli:
        - Haemophilus, Klebsiella, Citrobacter, Morganella, Proteus, Provedencia
- With PCN-allergy resulting in rash: use it anyway
- With PCN-allergy resulting in anaphylaxis:
    - minor wound: macrolide or fluoroquinolone
        - mACrolidE: Azithromycin, Clarithromycin, Erythromycin
        - Fluoroquinolone: levo**flox**acin, gemi**flox**acin, moxi**flox**acin (LeGeMo)
    - serious wound: vanc, linezolid, daptomycin

Infection-Specific Abs 3

Gram-Pos:

VRE & MRSA

Review: Staph, Strept, and Some

- Staph (, Strept):
  - nafcillin, oxacillin, cloxacillin, dicloxacillin
- Strept, Clostridium, Listeria:
  - PCN G, PCN VK, ampicillin, amoxicillin
  - + Enterococci: ampicillin, amoxicillin
  - + E. coli: ampicillin
- Strept, Staph, Clostridium, Listeria, Enterococci:
  - ampicillin-sulbactam, amoxicillin-clavulanate

Review: Gram-Pos Cephalosporins (or not)

Strept (not Staph)
- 1st: the cefa's: cefazolin, cefadroxil, cephalexin
  - + Moraxella, E. coli
- 2nd: fox fur fight'n prozac: cefoxitin, cefuroxime, cefotetan, cefprozil
  - + Moraxella, E. coli + some gram-neg bacilli:
    - Haemophilus, Klebsiella, Citrobacter, Morganella, Proteus, Providencia
- With PCN-allergy resulting in rash: use it anyway
- With PCN-allergy resulting in anaphylaxis:
  - minor wound: macrolide or fluoroquinolone
    - mACrolidE: Azithromycin, Clarithromycin, Erythromycin
    - Fluoroquinolone: levofloxacin, gemifloxacin, moxifloxacin (LeGeMo)
  - serious wound: vanc, linezolid, daptomycin

Gram+
Life-threatening PCN Allergy or VRE

- PCN allergy and a serious infections:
  - **Vanc, Linezolid, Daptomycin**
  - Need oral: **Linezolid**
- VRE: Linezolid, Daptomycin, quinupristin/dalforpristin

MRSA

- Minor skin infection can be treated orally:
  - Linezolid, TMP/SMX, Clindamycin, Doxycycline
    - Of these, **only linezolid is used for MRSA bacteremia**

- Major infections: Vancomycin

MRSA: Alternative

- MRSA: Vanc → → linezolid, tigercycline, ceftaroline, telavancin, daptomycin
  - Ceftaroline is the only cephalosporin to cover MRSA
    - don't use if sensitive to methicillin

Review: Staph, Strept, and Some

- Staph (, Strept):
  - nafcillin, oxacillin, cloxacillin, dicloxacillin
- Strept, Clostridium, Listeria:
  - PCN G, PCN VK, ampicillin, amoxicillin
  - Enterococci, Listeria: ampicillin, amoxicillin
  - E. coli: ampicillin
- Strept, Staph, Clostridium, Listeria, Enterococci:
  - ampicillin-sulbactam, amoxicillin-clavulanate

Review: Gram-Pos Cephalosporins (or not)

Strept (not Staph)
- 1st: the cefa's: cefazolin, cefadroxil, cephalexin
  - + Moraxella, E. coli
- 2nd: fox fur fight'n prozac: cefoxitin, cefuroxime, cefotetan, cefprozil
  - + Moraxella, E. coli + some gram-neg bacilli:
    - Haemophilus, Klebsiella, Citrobacter, Morganella, Proteus, Provedencia
- With PCN-allergy resulting in rash: use it anyway
- With PCN-allergy resulting in anaphylaxis:
  - minor wound. macrolide or fluoroquinolone
    - mACrolidE: Azithromycin, Clarithromycin, Erythromycin
    - Fluoroquinolone: levofloxacin, gemifloxacin, moxifloxacin (LeGeMo)
  - serious wound: vanc, linezolid, daptomycin

Review: PCN-allergy, MRSA, VRE

- Life-threatening PCN Allergy:
  - vanc, linezolid, daptomycin
  - oral: linezolid
- MRSA: Vancomycin
  - alt: linezolid, tigercycline, ceftaroline, telavancin, daptomycin
  - oral: linezolid, TMP/SMX, clindamycin, doxycycline
    - only linezolid for MRSA bacteremia
- VRE: linezolid, daptomycin, quinupristin/dalforpristin

Infection-Specific Abs 4

Gram-Neg bacilli: PCN and
Cephalosporin (3rd, 4th)

Gram-Neg Bacilli

- Enterobacteriaceae:
  - Enterobacter, Citrobacter,
  - E. coli, Haemophilus, Klebsiella,
  - Moraxella, Morganella, Proteus, Serratia
- Pseudomonas

Gram-Neg Bacilli: PCNs

- Piperacillin, ticarcillin, mezlocillin
  - Enterobacteriaceae & Pseudomonas
  - To cover Staph, combine with beta-lactamase inhibitor
    - pipercillin/tazobactam, ticarcillin/clavulanate
      - ampicillin/sulbactam & amoxicillin/clavulanate won't cover Pseudomonas

Gram-Neg Bacilli: Cephalosporins

- 3rd-gen: ceftazidime, cefotaxime, ceftriaxone
  - "cefta", "cefota", "ceftria"
- 4th-gen: cefepime
- All cover Enterobacteriaceae
  - Ceftazidime and cefepime: Pseudomonas
    - cefepime will also cover Staph
  - Ceftriaxone and cefotaxime: PCN-insensitive pneumococci-causing meningitis or pneumonia

Gram-Neg Bacilli Summary:
PCN & Cephalosporins (3rd, 4th-gen)

- PCNs: piperacillin, ticarcillin, mezlocillin:
  - Enterobacteriaceae & Pseudomonas
  - combo for Staph: pipercillin/tazobactam, ticarcillin/clavulanate
    - ampicillin/sulbactam & amoxicillin/clavulanate don't cover Pseudomonas
- 3rd & 4th gen cephalosporins cover Enterobacteriaceae
  - 3rd: (**ceft**azidime, **cefota**xime, **ceftria**xone)
  - 4th: cefepime
  - ceftazidime & cefepime cover Pseudomonas
  - cefepime also covers Staph
  - cefotaxime & ceftriaxone for meningitis or pneumonia

Infection-Specific Abs 5

Gram-Neg bacilli:
Quinolones, Aminoglycosides,
Monobactam

Gram-Neg Bacilli

- Enterobacteriaceae:
  - Enterobacter, Citrobacter,
  - E. coli, Haemophilus, Klebsiella,
  - Moraxella, Morganella, Proteus, Serratia
- Pseudomonas

Gram-Neg Bacilli Review:
PCN & Cephalosporins (3rd, 4th-gen)

- PCNs: piperacillin, ticarcillin, mezlocillin:
  - Enterobacteriaceae & Pseudomonas
  - combo for Staph: pipercillin/tazobactam, ticarcillin/ clavulanate
    - ampicillin/sulbactam & amoxicillin/clavulanate don't cover Pseudomonas
- 3rd & 4th gen cephalosporins cover Enterobacteriaceae
  - 3rd: (**cefta**zidime, **cefota**xime, **ceftria**xone)
  - 4th: cefepime
  - ceftazidime & cefepime cover Pseudomonas
  - cefepime also covers Staph
  - cefotaxime & ceftriaxone for meningitis or pneumonia

Gram-Neg Bacilli: Quinolones

- All Quinolones cover Enterobacteriaceae
  - Ciprofloxacin, ofloxacin,
  - Levofloxacin, gemifloxicin, moxifloxacin
- Ciprofloxacin covers Pseudomonas
- Levofloxacin, gemifloxicin, moxifloxacin (LeGeMo) also works w/ gram-pos clusters, esp. Strept pneumo

Gram-Neg Bacilli:
Aminoglycosides & Monobactams

- Aminoglycosides:
  - Gentamycin, Amikacin, Tobramycin
  - Synergistic w/ PCN for Staph coverage
- Monobactam: Aztreonam
- Both give coverage for Enterobacteriaceae & Pseudomonas

Gram-Neg Bacilli Summary:
Quinolones, Aminoglycosides, Monobactam

- Aminoglycosides, Aztreonam, & Ciprofloxacin
  - Cover Enterobacteriaceae & Pseudomonas
- All other Quinolones
  - Cover Enterobacteriaceae
  - Fluoroquinolines cover gram-pos clusters
    - Levofloxacin, gemfiloxicin, moxifloxacin (LeGeMo)

Gram-Neg Bacilli Summary: Enterobacteriaceae & Pseudomonas

- Enterobacteriaceae & Pseudomonas
  - piperacillin, ticarcillin, mezlocillin
  - ceftazidime
  - gentamycin, amikacin, tobramycin; aztreonam
  - ciprofloxacin
- Enterobacteriaceae & Pseudomonas + Staph
  - pipercillin/tazobactam, ticarcillin/clavulanate
  - cefepime

Gram-Neg Bacilli Summary: Enterobacteriaceae (no Pseudomonas)

- Enterobacteriaceae only
  - cefotaxime, ceftriaxone
    - 1st-line for meningitis or pneumonia
  - ofloxacin
- Enterobacteriaceae + Staph
  - ampicillin/sulbactam & amoxicillin/clavulanate
  - levofloxacin, gemifloxicin, moxifloxacin

Infection-Specific Abs 6

Anaerobes + Gram-Neg bacilli

Gram-Neg Bacilli Review:
Enterobacteriaceae & Pseudomonas

- Enterobacteriaceae & Pseudomonas
  - piperacillin, ticarcillin, mezlocillin; ceftazidime
  - gentamycin, amikacin, tobramycin; aztreonam
  - ciprofloxacin
- Enterobacteriaceae & Pseudomonas + Staph
  - pipercillin/tazobactam, ticarcillin/clavulanate; cefepime

Gram-Neg Bacilli Review: Enterobacteriaceae (no Pseudomonas)

- Enterobacteriaceae only
  - cefotaxime, ceftriaxone
    - 1st-line for meningitis or pneumonia
  - ofloxacin
- Enterobacteriaceae + Staph
  - ampicillin/sulbactam & amoxicillin/clavulanate
  - gemifloxicin, levofloxacin, moxifloxacin

Gram-Neg Bacilli: Carbapenems

- Doripenem, imipenem, meropenem, ertapenem
  - Enterobacteriaceae, Pseudomonas
    - ertapenem doesn't cover Pseudomonas
  - Excellent Staph and anaerobic
    - equal to metronidazole in anaerobic coverage

Anaerobes

- Clindamycin above diaphragm, Metronidazole below
  - Clindamycin good w/ anaerobic Strept in mouth
- Carbapenems almost as good
  - dorpenem, imipenem, meropenem, ertapenem
- PCN combo will work:
  - G+: amoxicillin/clavulanate
  - G-: piperacillin/tazobactam, ticarcillin/clavulanate

Gram-Neg Bacilli Summary: Enterobacteriaceae & Pseudomonas

- Enterobacteriaceae & Pseudomonas
  - piperacillin, ticarcillin, mezlocillin; ceftazidime
  - gentamycin, amikacin, tobramycin; aztreonam
  - ciprofloxacin
- Enterobacteriaceae & Pseudomonas + Staph
  - pipercillin/tazobactam, ticarcillin/clavulanate; cefepime
- Enterobacteriaceae & Pseudomonas + Staph + Anaerobes
  - Imipenem (ertapenem doesn't cover Staph)

Gram-Neg Bacilli Summary: Enterobacteriaceae (no Pseudomonas)

- Enterobacteriaceae only
  - cefotaxime, ceftriaxone
    - 1st-line for meningitis or pneumonia
  - ofloxacin
- Enterobacteriaceae + Staph
  - ampicillin/sulbactam & amoxicillin/clavulanate
  - levofloxacin, gemifloxicin, moxifloxacin
- Enterobacteriaceae + Staph + Anaerobes
  - ertapenem

Anaerobes Summary

- Anaerobes
  - Clindamycin above diaphragm, Metronidazole below
- Anaerobes + Gram-Pos
  - G+: amoxicillin/clavulanate
- Anaerobes + Gram-Neg
  - G-: piperacillin/tazobactam, ticarcillin/clavulanate

B. Ellis Myers

HEMATOLOGY CENTRIC

Alpha-Thalassemia

People Can Do Pretty Good

w/ One α -Chain

Hgb Barts

- This is the worst type of alpha-thalassemia.
- No α -chains.
- So bad, most fetuses die
- Hydrops fetalis
- The few newborns are stillbirths

Overall

- Two alpha-chains plus two beta-chains constitute HbA.
  - HbA is 97% of the total adult Hgb
- Two alpha-chains plus two delta-chains constitute HbA-2
  - HbA-2 +HbF (fetal hemoglobin) is the other 3% of adult Hgb

Adult Hgb

- Protein View
  - 97%: 2 α + 2 β = HbA
  - 3%:
    - 2 α + 2 γ = HbA-2
    - HbF
- Genetic View
  - (everyone has two of each non-sex chromosome)
  - chr16: α/α, α/α
  - chr11: β/β, β/β

Alpha-Thalassemia

- A deletion in chr 16p ➜ bad α-protein

How many of the chromosomes are effected determines the level of effect

- $-/\alpha$, α/α = α-thal minima
- $-/-$, α/α = α-thal minor-cis (Asian)
- $-/\alpha$, $-/\alpha$ = α-thal minor-trans (African)
- $-/-$, $-/\alpha$ = HgH Disease
- $-/-$, $-/-$ = Hb Barts

Alpha-Thalassemia

- Deletion in chr 16p
- α-thalassemia
  - minima: $-/\alpha$, α/α
  - minor-cis: $-/-$, α/α
    - Asian
  - minor-trans: $-/\alpha$, $-/\alpha$
    - African
- HgH Disease: $-/-$, $-/\alpha$
- Hb Barts: $-/-$, $-/-$

Decrease in α-Chains

- Leads to an increase in beta-chains (adults)
  - increase in delta-chains (newborns)
- Beta-chains form unstable tetramers
- $\gamma 4$ in fetus = Hb Barts ➜ hydrops fetalis or stillbirth
- HbH disease
  - target cells, Heinz bodies
  - hepatosplenomegaly
  - first noted in child or adult

Decrease in α-Chains

- α-thalassemia minor
  - Mild microcytic, hypochromic anemia
  - Often mistaken for iron-deficiency anemia
    - pretty common
- α-thalassemia minima
  - "Silent carriers"
  - Slight decrease MCV & MCH

Summary

- Alpha-thalassemia is a decrease in alpha-proteins due to deletion in 16p
  - Results in more delta-chains in fetus/newborn
  - Results in more beta-chains in adult
  - β-chains and γ-chains form unstable tetramers
- *As long as a person has some alpha-chains, they can do okay*

Summary 2

- Hb Barts = $\gamma 4$ in fetus ➔ hydrops fetalis
- HbH disease (may not be noted until an adult)
  - Target cells, Heinz bodies, hepatosplenomegaly
- α-thalassemia minor (pretty common)
  - Looks like iron-deficiency anemia
    - mild microcytic, hypochromic anemia
- α-thalassemia minima (silent carriers)
  - Slight decrease MCV & MCH

Summary 3

- Hb Barts = $\gamma 4$
- HbH dz = $\alpha 1 \beta 3$
- α-thal minor = $\alpha 2 \beta 2$
  - Appears as iron-deficiency anemia
- α -thal minima = silent carriers: $\alpha 3 \beta 1$

Splenomegaly 1

What causes it?

You Palpate an Enlarged Spleen

- What causes splenomegaly?
  - Acronym?

You Palpate an Enlarged Spleen

- What causes splenomegaly?
  - SPLEEN
    - What's it stand for?

You Palpate an Enlarged Spleen

- What causes splenomegaly?
- **SPLEEN**
  - **S**equestration
  - **P**roliferation due to chronic inflammation
  - **L**ipid deposition
  - **E**ndowment
  - **E**ngorgement
  - i**N**vasion

Spleen

- **Sequestration:**
  - Hereditary Spherocytosis
  - Congenital or Acquired Hemolytic Anemias
- P
- L
- E
- E
- N

Spleen

- S
- **Proliferation due to chronic inflammation**
  - SLE, RA
  - Endocarditis
  - Viral, bacterial, fungal and parasitic infections
- L
- E
- E
- N

Spleen

- S
- P
- **Lipid deposition**
  - Gaucher, Nieman-Pick
- E
- E
- N

Spleen

- S
- P
- L
- **Endowment:**
  - Congenital splenic hemangioma, hamartoma, or cysts
- E
- N

Spleen

- S
- P
- L
- E
- **Engorgement:**
  - Splenic trauma w/ intracapsullar hematoma
  - Sequestration crisis in SC, CHF
  - Peds only: Portal vein thrombosis
- N

Spleen

- S
- P
- L
- E
- E
- **iNvasion:**
  - Granulomas, Histiocytes
  - Lymphoproliferation, Malignant hematologic diseases

Review: SPLEEN

- **S**equestration
- **P**roliferation due to chronic inflammation
- **L**ipid deposition
- **E**ndowment
- **E**ngorgement
- i**N**vasion

Review: **SPLEEN**

- **S**equestration:
  - spherocytosis, hemolytic anemias
- **P**roliferation due to chronic inflammation
- **L**ipid deposition:
  - Gaucher, Neiman-Pick
- **E**ndowment:
  - Congenital hemangioma, hamartoma, cysts
- **E**ngorgement:
  - trauma, sequestration crisis in SC/CHF
  - Peds only: portal vein thrombosis
- i**N**vasion:
  - granulomas, histiocytes, lymphocytes

Splenomegaly 2

What to ask?

Review: Causes

- **SPLEEN**
  - **S**equestration
  - **P**roliferation due to chronic inflammation
  - **L**ipid deposition
  - **E**ndowment
  - **E**ngorgement
  - i**N**vasion

Review: **SPLEEN**

- **S**equestration: spherocytosis, hemolytic anemias
- **P**roliferation due to chronic inflammation
- **L**ipid deposition:
  - Gaucher, Neiman-Pick
- **E**ndowment:
  - Congenital hemangioma, hamartoma, cysts
- **E**ngorgement: trauma, sequestration crisis in SC/CHF
  - Peds only: portal vein thrombosis
- i**N**vasion: granulomas, histiocytes, lymphocytes
  - leukemia, lymphoma

Questions to Ask

- **PAM HUGS FOSS**
  - **P**MHx, **A**llergies, **M**eds
  - **H**ospitalizations/surgical, **U**rology, **G**I, **S**leep
  - **F**Hx, **O**b/gyn, **S**exual, **S**ocial

Questions to Ask: **PAM**

- **P**MHx
  - Recent colds/infections?
  - B-signs: fever, night sweats, wt loss?
  - Hx of bruising, bone pain, or frequent infections?
  - Hx of trauma?
  - Congenital heart diseases? Storage diseases? Liver diseases? Bleeding disorders?
- **A**llergies
- **M**edicines

Questions to Ask: **HUGS**

- **H**ITS
  - Hospitalization, Injuries, Trauma, Surgery
- **U**rology
- **G**astrointestinal
- **S**leep

Questions to Ask: **FOSS**

- **F**Hx
  - Autoimmune diseases: SLE, RA?
  - Storage diseases? Cancers?
  - Family ethnicity?
- **O**b/gyn
  - Pregnancy uneventful?
  - Post-delivery persistent jaundice?
- **S**exual
- **S**ocial
  - Recent travel?

Thrombocytopenia 1

Gotta Start Somewhere

Important Specifics

- Always examine the blood smear

- 100, 10-20, <10

- Why are these numbers significant?

Important Specifics

- Plts > **100**-150:
  - Normal platelets, low end
- Plts **10-20**:
  - Concern for spontaneous bleeds
- Plts < **10**:
  - Think autoimmune

- 100, 10-20, <10
- Always examine the blood smear

Causes

- Major
  - decreased production
  - increased destruction
- Minor
  - platelet sequestration
    ~ splenomegaly
  - hemodilution

Isolated Thrombocytopenia

- Define
- What is the most common cause?

Isolated Thrombocytopenia

- Define
  - low plts
  - w/o abnormal RBC or WBC
  - w/o symptoms

Isolated Thrombocytopenia is most commonly ITP

Isolated Thrombocytopenia

- ITP = Idiopathic Thrombocytopenic Purpura
  - = Immune Thrombocytopenic Purpura
  - = Immune Thrombocytopenia
  - = Primary Immune Thrombocytopenia
  - = Autoimmune Thrombocytopenia

Immune Thrombocytopenic Purpura (ITP)

- *Idiopathic = don't know where it came from*
- *Immune = immune system is attacking plt's*
- *Thrombocytopenia = low platelets*
- *Purpura = bruising*

- *Don't know where it came from.*
- *It's probably immune-related.*
- *My platelets are low, so I'm bruising easily.*

Immune Thrombocytopenic Purpura

- ITP in a child is generally self-resolving
- ITP in an adult is generally chronic

ITP is a Diagnosis of Exclusion

- U/S abdomen:
  - Liver and spleen: r/o enlargement
- CXR:
  - r/o: "silent" mediastinal lymph nodes
  - r/o: "silent" TB
- Labs:
  - Antiplatelet antibodies
  - ITP vs DITP
    - What is DITP?

ITP

- Most common: **recent viral infection**
  - Including HIV, HepC, and CMV
- Could be H. pylori
  - Do you suspect ulcers?
- Vaccinations
  - *You really did need to ask about vaccinations this time*

DITP

- Drug-induced ITP
  - Don't forget foods qualify as drugs in this case
    - walnuts
    - cow's milk
    - cranberry juice
    - tonic water (quinine)
    - herbal intake

Summary

- 100, 10-20, <10
- Always examine the blood smear
- Do you think it's decreased production or increased destruction?
- Any hepatospenomegaly? Maybe it's sequestration
- Receiving fluids? Maybe it's hemodilution

Summary

- Are the plt's low but the RBC and WBC are normal?
  - Is the patient mostly free of symptoms?
    - ITP

Summary

- Child who recently had a cold or got some meds
  - Probably self-resolving ITP
- Adult
  - Think about autoimmune diseases
  - Think about liver diseases
- Elderly
  - Think about bowel disorders

Thrombocytopenia 2

ITP

Review

- Are the Plt's low but the RBC and WBC are normal? Is the patient mostly free of symptoms?

ITP

(a diagnosis of exclusion)

ITP vs DITP

- ITP
  - An infection made the immune system malfunction
- DITP
  - It wasn't an infection. It was a food or drug

ITP

- Most common: recent viral infection
  - including HIV, HepC, and CMV
- Could be H. pylori
  - Do you suspect ulcers?
- Vaccinations
  - *You really did need to ask about vaccinations this time*

DITP - It Was a Drug

- Abx, NSAIDs, food, -ine/-dine, furosemide
  - APLS: Antibiotics/Penicillin/Linezolid/Sulfas
  - Pain: NSAIDs or Gold
    - gold is used to treat arthritis
- Food: nuts, milk, cranberry juice
  - -ine & -dine: Quinine/Quinidine/Ranitidine
    - tonic water/malaria/Zantac
- Furosemide

ITP
(that's right, I'm repeating it)

- Most common: recent viral infection
  - including HIV, HepC, and CMV
- Could be H. pylori
  - Do you suspect ulcers?
- Vaccinations
  - *You really did need to ask about vaccinations this time*

Thrombocytopenia 3

Beyond the Land of ITP

It Wasn't ITP or DITP

- If it wasn't ITP or DITP, go back to the basics.
  - Decreased production
  - Increased destruction

Decreased Production

- Congenital thrombocytopenia
  - Absence of megakaryocytes in bone marrow and low plt's
- Myelodysplastic syndrome
  - Dysplasia = Ineffective production of cell lines

Increased Destruction

- Autoimmune conditions
  - SLE
  - RA
  - Antiphospholipid syndromes
- Common variable immunodeficiency
  - Greatly decreased immunoglobulins
  - Lots of infections. Takes time to heal
  - Deal with all kinds of cell-line issues

Where Did You See the Patient

- Outpatient
- Inpatient
  - Multi-system Illness/ICU
  - Cardiac
- Pregnancy/Post-partum

Outpatient

- Increased destruction
  - ITP or DITP
  - Connective Tissue disorders
- Decreased production
  - Congenital thrombocytopenia
  - Myelodysplastic syndrome

Outpatient

- Increased destruction
  - ITP
    - viral: recent cold, HIV, HepC, CMV
    - vaccinations
    - H. pylori
  - DITP
    - Abx, NSAIDs, -ine/-dine, furosemide
    - Food: nuts, milk, cranberry juice
  - Connective Tissue disorders
    - SLE, RA, antiphospholipid syndrome

Outpatient

- Decreased production
  - Congenital thrombocytopenia
    - Absence of megakaryocytes in bone marrow and low plt's
  - Myelodysplastic syndrome
    - Dysplasia = Ineffective production of cell lines

Thrombocytopenia 4

Inpatient

Inpatient

- Multisystem Illness/ICU
- MICU, PICU, NICU
- Cardiac

Inpatient

- Multisystem Illness/ICU
  - ITP/DITP
  - HIT
  - TTP
  - HUS
  - Liver Dz, Bowel Disorder

Inpatient

- Increased destruction
  - ITP
    - viral, vaccinations, H. pylori
  - DITP
    - Abx, NSAIDs, -ine/-dine, furosemide
    - Food: nuts, milk, cranberry juice
  - **HIT = heparin-induced thrombocytopenia**
    TTP = thrombotic thrombocytopenia purpura
  - **HUS = hemolytic-uremic syndrome**

Heparin Induced Thrombocytopenia

- Most common symptom:
  - Enlargement of a previously diagnosed blood clot or develop new blood clot elsewhere
    - arterial or venous thrombosis
- Systemic reaction: infusion starts, and then
  - fever/chills, HTN, tachycardia, SOB, CP
  - ± skin rash

Don't forget the necrotic looking fingers this condition is so famous for

Thrombotic Thrombocytopenic Purpura

- Extensive microscopic clots in the small blood vessels → organ damage (kidney, heart, brain)
  - Most due to inhibition of **ADAMTS13**
    - ADAMTS13 can't cleave vWF multimers → multimers float around and bind to platelets → clots
    - RBCs can't pass clots → **schistocytes** & anemia
  - Tx: plasma exchange
    - With relapse, Tx: immunosuppressants
      - glucocorticoids, rituximab, cyclophosphamide, vincristine, or cyclosporine

TTP Summary

- Inhibit ADAMTS13
  - vWF multimers bind to platelets → clots
  - RBCs can't pass clots → schistocytes & anemia
- Tx: plasma exchange
  - Relapse, Tx: immunosuppressants
    - glucocorticoids, rituximab, cyclophosphamide, vincristine, or cyclosporine

HUS = Hemolytic-Uremic Syndrome

- **HUS** is defined by **HUT**
1. **H**emolytic anemia
   - ie. anemia by destruction of RBCs
2. **U**remia ← **AKF** (acute kidney failure)
3. **T**hrombocytopenia
- Endothelial damage leads to
  - Widespread inflammation:
    - leukocyte activation, platelet activation
  - TMA (thrombotic microangiopathy)
    - multiple thromboses in small blood vessels
      - organ damage

HUS = Hemolytic-Uremic Syndrome

- Predominantly children
- 10% mortality
- E. coli O157:H7
  - or Shigella, Campylobacter or virus
  - Most common cause of acquired ARF in child
- 5%: pneumococcal HUS
  - Streptococcus pneumoniae
- atypical hemolytic uremic syndrome (**aHUS**)
  - genetic, chronic uncontrolled complement activation

HUS Summary

- HUS = HUT
  - **H**emolytic anemia, **U**remia (from ARF), **TP**
- Children
- **Endothelial damage** → inflammation → TMA
  - TMA = Thrombotic MicroAngiopathy
- Caused by
  - Most: E. coli O157:H7
    - or Shigella, Campylobacter or virus
  - 5%: pneumococcal HUS
  - atypical-HUS (genetic)
    - chronic uncontrolled complement activation

ITP vs HIT vs TTP vs HUS

- ITP: post-immune activation (probably virus)
  - DITP: post-drug or food immune activation (probably Abx)
- HIT
  - Clot getting bigger or new clot elsewhere
  - Is he having a heart attack?
    - CP, tachycardia, HTN, SOB, fevers/chills
  - Necrotic looking fingers?
- TTP
  - Clots + hemolysis
    - schistocytes, anemia
  - Tx: plasma exchange. If relapse: immunosuppressants
    - glucocorticoids, rituximab, cyclophosphamide, vincristine, or cyclosporine
- HUS (= HUT)
  - **H**emolytic-anemia, **U**remia (from AKF), **T**hrombocytopenia
  - Endothelial damage → inflammation → TMA (thrombotic microangiopathy)
  - Caused by E. coli O157:H7 (, Shigella, Campylobacter or virus), 5% Staph pneumo
    - **aHUS** = atypical HUS: genetic, chronic, uncontrolled complement activation

Thrombocytopenia 5

Inpatient 2

Review: ITP vs HIT vs TTP vs HUS

- ITP: post-immune activation (probably virus)
  - DITP: post-drug or food immune activation (probably antibiotic)
- HIT
  - Clot getting bigger or new clot elsewhere
  - Is he having a heart attack?
    - CP, tachycardia, HTN, SOB, fevers/chills
  - Necrotic looking fingers?
- TTP
  - Clots + hemolysis
    - schistocytes, anemia
  - Tx: plasma exchange. If relapse: immunosuppressants
    - glucocorticoids, rituximab, cyclophosphamide, vincristine, or cyclosporine
- HUS (= HUT)
  - **H**emolytic-anemia, **U**remia (from AKF), **T**hrombocytopenia
  - Endothelial damage → inflammation → TMA (thrombotic microangiopathy)
  - Caused by E. coli O157:H7 (, Shigella, Campylobacter or virus), 5% Staph pneumo
    - **aHUS** = atypical HUS: genetic, chronic, uncontrolled complement activation

Review: ITP vs HIT vs TTP vs HUS

- ITP: post-immune activation (probably virus)
  - DITP: post-drug or food immune activation (probably antibiotic)
- HIT: post-Heparin. Activated clotting
  - Bigger/new clot, "Is it a heart attack?", Necrotic fingers
- TTP: Clots w/ signs of hemolysis (schistocytes, anemia)
  - Tx: plasma exchange. Tx relapse: immunosuppressants
- HUS (= HUT)
  - Hemolytic-anemia, Uremia (from AKF), Thrombocytopenia
  - 5% Staph pneumo; aHUS = genetic, complement activation

Review: ITP vs HIT vs TTP vs HUS

- Isolated thrombocytopenia:
  - Immune destruction of platelets
  - ITP/DITP
  - Thrombocytopenia + Clots
- HIT: clots getting bigger, got Heparin
- TTP:
  - Clots + hemolytic anemia (schistocytes & anemia)
- HUS:
  - Clots + hemolytic anemia + uremia (kidney damage)

Cardiac Patients

- Cardiac pts get thrombocytopenia from
  - Surgery
  - Medications
  - Fluids

Inpatient - Cardiac

- Surgery
  - Cardiac bypass
- Medications
  - DITP, HIT
  - GPIIb/GPIIIa inhibitor
    - abciximab, eptifibatide (Integrilin), tirofiban
- Fluids
  - Dilutional

Inpatient Summary

- Multisystem/ICU (MICU, PICU, NICU)
  - Isolated thrombocytopenia: immune destruction of platelets
    - ITP/DITP
  - Thrombocytopenia + Clots
    - HIT: clots getting bigger, got Heparin
    - TTP: clots + hemolytic anemia (schistocytes & anemia)
    - HUS: clots + hemolytic anemia + uremia (kidney damage)
- Cardiac
  - Surgery: Cardiac bypass
  - Medications
    - DITP, HIT
    - GPIIb/GPIIIa inhibitor
      - abciximab, eptifibatide (Integrilin), tirofiban
  - Fluids: Dilutional

Thrombocytopenia 6

Pregnancy

Pregnancy/Post-Partum

- ITP, TTP, HUS
  - *Just like everyone else*
- Gestational Thrombocytopenia (GT)
  - benign condition
- Preeclampsia
- Abruptio Placentae = Placental Abruption
- HELLP Syndrome

Gestational Thrombocytopenia (GT)

- 5 criteria
    1. mild and asymptomatic thrombocytopenia
    2. no evidence of fetal thrombocytopenia
    3. development late in pregnancy
    4. no history of thrombocytopenia outside of pregnancy
    5. spontaneous resolution once the child is delivered

Preeclampsia

- Preeclampsia = HTN + protein in urine
    - Abnormal placenta can cause preeclampsia, and preeclampsia can cause placental abruption
        - Abnormal placenta may require increased pressure to maintain sufficient nutrient flow to fetus resulting in HTN
            - Chronic HTN causes kidney damage → the degree of kidney damage leads to the degree of proteinuria
        - Abruptio placenta
            - Early separation of the placenta from the uterine wall
            - Inc risk with HTN, further increased with chronic HTN

Worsening Preeclampsia

- HELLP syndrome
  - Most severe preeclampsia
  - Vascular endothelial damage results in
    - microangiopathic **H**emolytic anemia
    - **E**levated **L**iver enzymes
    - thrombocytopenia
- **H**emolysis
- **E**levated **L**iver-enzymes
- **L**ow **P**latelets

HELLP Syndrome

- 10% of all pregnancies have HTN
- 10% of all pre-eclampsias → HELLP
- 20% of all thrombocytopenia in pregnancy are due to HELLP
- **HELLP really means that HTN → hemolysis**
  - Schistocytes, total bili >1.2, LDH >600
  - Elevated LFT's
  - Plt's < 100k

Preeclampsia Gradient

- Pregnant and develop HTN
- Pre-eclampsia:
  - HTN damaged kidneys and protein is escaping in urine
- Pre-eclampsia caused abruptio placentae
  - or maybe abruptio placentae caused pre-eclampsia
- HELLP syndrome
  - Pre-eclampsia at most severe:
    - HTN damaged kidneys, and now its damaging the vascular endothelium
    - RBCs are bursting, liver is working to make protein and cleanup, platelets are being used up
  - Hemolysis, Elevated Liver-enzymes, Low Platelets

Thrombocytopenia Testing 1

Begin With a Blood Smear

Blood Smear

- See clumping
- See giant platelets
- See tiny platelets
- See no platelets

Clumping

- This is artificial thrombocytopenia.
  - Why are you seeing clumps?
    - Too many options to cover here

Giant Platelets

- Hereditary Thrombocytopenia =
- Hereditary Macrothrombocytopenia =
  - "Macro" = large; "thrombocyte" = platelet

  - If gray on Wright-Giemsa stain
    - Gray Platelet Syndrome
  - If bleeding tendency
    - Autosomal Dominant Macrothrombocytopenia

Small Platelets

- Test the **WAS** gene
  - (as in what's up **W**iskott-**A**ldrich **S**yndrome)
  - X X X X X X X **X-linked** X X X X X X X X
  - Major: Wiskott-Aldrich Syndrome
  - Minor: X-linked Thrombocytopenia
    - from a mutation
- Small platelets + thrombocytopenia =
  - WAS gene: X-linked:
    - Major Wiskott-Aldrich
    - Minor mutation

Variable Size Platelets

- If variable size & **hypo**granular
  - Myelodysplasia syndromes

Giant vs Small Platelet Thrombocytopenia

- Giant is **Hereditary**
  - **Gray** on Wright stain: Gray Platelet Syndrome
  - Bleeding is **Autosomal Dominant**
- Small platelets + thrombocytopenia =
  - WAS gene: **X-linked**:
    - Major **Wiskott-Aldrich**
    - Minor mutation
- Variable size & **hypo**granular
  - **Myelodysplasia** syndromes

Thrombocytopenia Testing 2

True TCP (no platelets on smear)

What Do You See?

- Normal looking, but no platelets
- Lymphocytosis
- Schistocytes
- Immature cells or Dacryocytes
- Microspherocytes + clumping

Think Of

- **Normal looking, but no platelets**
  - Isolated thrombocytopenia: ITP/DITP, HIT, DIC, GT
- Lymphocytosis
  - Infection
- Schistocytes
  - TTP, HUS, DIC
- Immature cells or Dacryocytes
  - Bone Marrow disorder
- Microspherocytes + clumping
  - Evan's syndrome

Normal Looking, but No Plts

- This is called Isolated Thrombocytopenia
- Think ITP/DITP, HIT, DIC, GT
  - What's the clinical eval?

ITP

- Most common: recent viral infection
  - Probably a respiratory infection in a child
  - Could be any viral infection
    - including HIV, HepC, and CMV
- Could be H. pylori
  - Do you suspect ulcers?
- Vaccinations
  - *You really did need to ask about vaccinations this time*

DITP

- Drug-induced ITP
  - Probably an antibiotic
  - Don't forget foods qualify as drugs in this case
    - walnuts
    - cow's milk
    - cranberry juice
    - tonic water (quinine)
    - herbal intake

Big Groups

- Child who recently had a cold or got some meds
  - Probably self-resolving ITP
- Adult
  - Think about autoimmune diseases
  - Think about liver diseases
- Elderly
  - Think about bowel disorders

Special Cases

- Did the patient just get heparin?
  - HIT = Heparin-Induced Thrombocytopenia
    - Any large clots getting bigger? Necrotic fingers?
    - "Does it look like a heart attack?"
- Really sick?
  - DIC = Disseminated Intravascular Coagulopathy
    - small-vessels clotting, failing organs (incl. skin)
- Pregnant and asymptomatic?
  - GT = Gestational Thrombocytopenia

Investigation

- No simple answer
- Testing is based upon the clinical assessment

Thrombocytopenia Testing 3

Lymphocytosis, Schistocytes

Review: Blood Smear Shows

- Normal looking, but no platelets
  - Think: Isolated thrombocytopenia: ITP/DITP, HIT, DIC, GT
- **Lymphocytosis**
  - Think: Infection
- Schistocytes
  - Think: TTP, HUS, DIC
- Immature cells or Dacryocytes
  - Think: Bone Marrow disorder
- Microsphcrocytcs + clumping
  - Think: Evan's syndrome

Lymphocytosis

- Terms within this field
  - Neutrophilia
  - Atypical lymphocytes
  - Toxic granulations
  - Probably not Eosinophilia
    - this is generally asthma
      - or maybe parasitic infestation

Lymphocytosis Testing

- CXR and/or imaging specific to symptom-organ
- Blood culture (BCx), Virology
- ESR, CRP
- Suspected bacterial: **Procalcitonin**
- Suspected UTI: UA

Review: Blood Smear Shows

- Normal looking, but no platelets
  - Think: Isolated thrombocytopenia: ITP/DITP, HIT, DIC, GT
- Lymphocytosis
  - Think: Infection
- **Schistocytes**
  - Think: TTP, HUS, DIC
- Immature cells or Dacryocytes
  - Think: Bone Marrow disorder
- Microspherocytes + clumping
  - Think: Evan's syndrome

Schistocytes

- TTP (Thrombotic Thrombocytopenic Purpura)
  - clots + hemolytic anemia
- HUS (Hemolytic-Uremic Syndrome)
  - clots + hemolytic anemia + uremia (kidney damage)
- DIC (Disseminated Intravascular Coagulation) = Consumptive Coagulopathy
  - clots + hemolytic anemia + multiple organ damage
  - *This is a complication of some other condition*

Schistocytes Testing

- LDH, bili
- Haptoglobin, PT/PTT
- D-dimer, fibrinogen

Thrombocytopenia Testing 4

Immature Cells, Microspherocytosis

Descriptions That Confuse

- "Atypical lymphocytes" ~ viral
- **"Toxic granulations"**
  - dark course granules in neutrophils
  - ~ sepsis
- "Hypolobulated neutrophils = **Pelger-Huet**
  - nuclear envelope even messed up
    - **laminopathy**
  - myelodysplastic syndrome
- "Abnormal WBC" ~ leukemia

Atypical vs. Abnormal

- **"Atypical** lymphocytes"
  - This is probably a **viral** infection
- "Abnormal WBC"
  - This may be leukemia
- Neutrophils have lots of lobules
  - So, if it's "<u>hypolobulated</u>", it's being produced wrong
    - It's <u>myelodysplastic</u>. This is a problem at the nucleus, therefore <u>lamin</u> is involved
- "Toxic granulations"
  - *Neutrophils are spewing like crazy because of sepsis*

Review: Blood Smear Shows

- Normal looking, but no platelets
  - Think: Isolated thrombocytopenia: ITP/DITP, HIT, DIC, GT
- Lymphocytosis
  - Think: Infection
- Schistocytes
  - Think: TTP, HUS, DIC
- **Immature cells or Dacryocytes**
  - Think: Bone Marrow disorder
- Microspherocytes + clumping
  - Think: Evan's syndrome

Bone Marrow Disorders

- Blasts
- Nucleated RBCs
- Pelger-Huet (laminopathy)
  - lamin = gene coding nuclear envelope
- Dacryocytes (poikocyte shaped like teardrop)
  - Poikocyte = abnormal shaped RBC
  - Dacrocytes ~ myelofibrosis & myelophthisic anemia

Bone Marrow Disorder Testing

- Bone marrow aspirate
- Biopsy

Review: Blood Smear Shows

- Normal looking, but no platelets
  - Think: Isolated thrombocytopenia: ITP/DITP, HIT, DIC, GT
- Lymphocytosis
  - Think: Infection
- Schistocytes
  - Think: TTP, HUS, DIC
- Immature cells or Dacryocytes
  - Think: Bone Marrow disorder
- **Microspherocytes + clumping**
  - Think: Evan's syndrome

Evan's Syndrome

- Autoimmune
- Antibodies attack own RBCs and Plts
- ie. autoimmune hemolytic anemia + ITP

Evan's Syndrome Testing

- DAT = direct agglutination test
- Reticulocytes
- LDH, bili

GI CENTRIC

GI Bleed 1

What to do first

Always Think Treatment First

- 80% stop spontaneously w/ appropriate fluids
- 5% the source will never be determined

1. Fluid resuscitation w/ NS or LR
2. CBC, PT, type and cross-match
3. If PT is elevated → fresh frozen plasma (FFP)
4. If Plt < 50k & active bleed, transfuse platelets
5. If Hx of cirrhosis, add octreotide
   1. decreases portal HTN

Nasogastric Tube

- It has no therapeutic benefit
- Saline or ice water lavage through tube has no benefit.

NG tube helps to determine bleeding site and guide endoscopy.

Acute Bleed

- Maintain hematocrit (Hct)
  - If older, maintain Hct > 30%
  - If younger, maintain Hct > 20%
- Control Gastric Acid
  - with gastritis or possible ulcerative disease
  - empiric PPIs
    - omeprazole, pantoprazole, lansoprazole, esomeprazole
    - H_2 blockers are of no use here

Esophageal Varices

1. Give octreotide to lower portal pressure
2. If fails → endoscopy to band bleeding varices
   - sclerotherapy works, but more complications
3. If fails → TIPS
   - **T**ransjugular **I**ntrahepatic **P**ortosystemic **S**hunting
     - catheter placed into jugular vein and guided by IR through liver to form shunt between systemic circulation in the hepatic vein and portal circulation in the portal vein
     - **TIPS can worsen hepatic encephalopathy**

Long-term Management of Portal HTN

- **Propranolol** decreases frequency of bleeding
  - Everyone with varices from portal HTN and cirrhosis should be on a β -blocker

Summary

- Treatment First
    - NS or LR → CBC, PT, type & crossmatch
    - If PT elevated, FFP
    - If Plt < 50k & active bleed, transfuse platelets
    - If cirrhotic, **octreotide**
- NG Tube to find bleed & assist with endoscopy

Summary 2

- Maintain hematocrit (Hct)
    - Older: > 30%; Younger: > 20%
- Control Gastric Acid (w/ gastritis or ulcer)
    - **PPI**: omeprazole, pantoprazole, lansoprazole, esomeprazole

Summary 3

- Esophageal Varices
  - **octreotide** → banding → TIPS
    - TIPS can worsen hepatic encephalopathy

- Everyone with varices from portal HTN and cirrhosis should be on a β-blocker
  - **propranolol**

Full Summary

- Treatment First
  - NS or LR → CBC, PT, type & crossmatch
    - If PT elevated, FFP
    - If Plt < 50k & active bleed, transfuse platelets
  - If cirrhotic, **octreotide**
  - NG Tube to find bleed & assist with endoscopy
    - Esophageal Varices: **octreotide** → banding → TIPS
      - TIPS can worsen hepatic encephalopathy
- Maintain
  - Maintain Hct: Older: > 30%; Younger: > 20%
  - Control Gastric Acid (PPI, ie –prazole)
  - Everyone with varices from portal HTN and cirrhosis should be on a β-blocker
    - **propranolol**

GI Bleed 2

Roughly, how much and where

How Significant is the Blood Loss

- Orthostasis
  1. Pt goes from supine to standing or sitting
  2. Wait at least a minute to measure to allow autonomic discharge accommodation
  - If rise in pulse > 10 (or) drop in SBP > 20
    - > 15% blood loss
  - If pulse > 100 (or) SBP < 100
    - > 30% blood loss

Rectum Blood Rules

- The darker the blood, the higher the bleed
  - Heavy upper GI bleeds can be red at rectum
- The darker the stool from a upper GI bleed, the larger the bleed
  - More oxidation occurs
  - Brown Stool vs. Melena
    - brown stool: <10mL of blood loss
      - includes coffee-ground emesis
    - melena: > 100mL blood loss

Upper GI Bleed

- Above the ligament of Treitz
  - Separates the duodenum from the jejunum
- Most common, in order
  - Ulcer, gastritis,
  - Mallory-Weiss, esophagitis
  - Gastric cancer
- Special cases
  - with cirrhosis, think portal HTN: variceal bleeding
  - with AAA repair in past year: aortoenteric fistula

Lower GI Bleed

- Most common
  - Diverticulosis
  - Angiodysplasia = AVM = vascular ectasia
  - Hemorrhoids
  - Cancer
  - IBD

Summary

- Orthostasis
  - Rise in pulse > 10 (or) drop in SBP > 20
    - > 15% blood loss
  - Pulse > 100 (or) SBP < 100
    - > 30% blood loss
- Stool Color
  - The brighter the red, the closer to the rectum.
  - Brown stool < 10mL
  - Melena > 100mL

GI Bleed 3

Dx

The Likelihood of Bleed Location

- Most GI bleeds are in the upper GI tract.
- The older you get, the more likely the bleed is from the lower GI tract.
- Upper is always more likely unless evidence to the contrary is present.

1. Endoscopy

- Endoscopy is most accurate assessment of GI bleed
  - Upper endoscopy → lower endoscopy
    - upper is more likely, unless you have evidence to contrary
    - Upper endoscopy = Esophagogastroduodenoscopy
      = EGD = panendoscopy = PES
    - Lower endoscopy = colonoscopy
  - Endoscopy can also be used to treat

2. Capsule Endoscopy

- Upper endoscopy only goes to ligament of Treitz
- Lower endoscopy only reaches ileocecal valve
- **Capsule endoscopy** is used for the in-between

3. Nuclear Bleeding Scan

- If endoscopy fails, do nuclear bleeding scan

Angiography

- Angiography only useful for large bleeds
  - May use prior to embolization or hemicolectomy
  - Can also guide local vasopressin injection

Virtual Endoscopy

- Don't use it. It's a CT scan that doesn't help with diagnosis

Summary

- Upper GI tract bleed is more likely.
- Endoscopy is the best test
- Dx
  - Upper endoscopy → lower endoscopy → capsule endoscopy → nuclear bleeding scan
- Angiography is only for large bleeds.
  - Specifically for embolization, hemicolectomy, or for a local vasopressin injection

IBD 1

The Big Picture

INFLAMMATORY Bowel Disease

- IBD is NOT IBS (IRRITABLE Bowel Syndrome)
- Inflammation is brought about by cytokines and an immune response
- Irritable is a vague term. It is a response to <u>some</u> stimulation. The response and the stimulation are not exactly defined.
- Crohn's and Ulcerative Colitis are <u>inflammatory</u>. The stimulation and response are defined.

Inflammatory Bowel **DISEASE**

- Disease = a health condition that has a clearly defined reason behind it
  - Crohn's **Disease** (CD), Ulcerative Colitis (UC) have
    - recognized etiologic agents (cause)
    - identifiable group of signs/symptoms
    - consistent anatomic alterations
- Syndrome = may produce a number of symptoms without an identifiable cause
  - CD and UC have a cause, therefore they are <u>diseases</u>

<u>Inflammatory</u> Bowel <u>Disease</u> (IBD)

Crohn's Disease (CD)

Ulcerative Colitis (UC)

Treatment of Disease vs Syndrome

- With disease, we attack the cause
- With syndromes, we treat the symptoms

It's the Helper Cells

Review: Helper cells, TH_1 and TH_2, CD4 binding to MHCII on APCs

- It's alphabetical. $\underline{C}$D is $TH_{\underline{1}}$. $\underline{U}$C is $TH_{\underline{2}}$
- TH_1: cell mediated vs. TH_2: humoral
  - Activates macrophages and CD8+ cell vs. helps B-cells make antibodies (IgE > IgG)
  - Response to intestinal bacteria vs. autoimmune
  - Granulomas vs. ulcers (hence **Ulcer**ative Colitis)
- CD ~ granulomas vs. UC ~ autoimmune

Treatment: Big Picture

- These are diseases. The cause is immune response. Treatment is to attack the immune response
  - Anti-immune = Anti-inflammatories
    - mesalamine, azathioprine, 6MP
      - *IBD - Messing around with me, in AZ, were 6 MPs*
    - Acute exacerbations: budesonide (high-dose steroid)

Summary

IBD = Inflammatory Bowel Disease
- CD = Crohn Disease
  - TH1, cell mediated (macrophages & CD8+ cell), responding to bacteria, forming granulomas
- UC = Ulcerative Colitis
  - TH2, humoral (B-cells making Abs, IgE > IgG), autoimmune, ulcers
- Treatment:
  - *IBD - Messing around with me, in AZ, were 6 MPs*
    - mesalamine, azathioprine, 6MP
    - Acute exacerbation: budesonide

Summary 2

- It's all alphabetical
    - CD < UC
    - TH1 < TH2
    - cell-mediated < humoral
    - granulomas < ulcers

IBD - Messing around with me, in AZ, were 6 MPs

IBD 2

Recognize

Review 1

- It's all alphabetical
  - CD < UC
  - TH1 < TH2
  - cell-mediated < humoral
  - granulomas < ulcers

IBD - Messing around with me, in AZ, were 6 MPs

Review 2

IBD = **Inflammatory** Bowel **Disease**
- CD = Crohn's Disease
  - TH1, cell mediated (macrophages & CD8+ cell), responding to bacteria, forming granulomas
- UC = Ulcerative Colitis
  - TH2, humoral (B-cells making Abs, IgE > IgG), autoimmune, ulcers
- Treatment:
  - *IBD - Messing around with me, in AZ, were 6 MPs*
    - mesalamine, azathioprine, 6MP
    - Acute exacerbation: budesonide

What We Feel and See w/IBD

- Inflammatory Bowel Disease has extraintestinal symptoms. All inflammatory.
  - Eye: episleritis, scleritis, iritis
  - Skin: erythema nodosum & pyoderma gangrenous
    - **Legs**: inflamed nodules & necrotic ulcers
  - Joint pain

What We Feel and See: CD & UC

- Granulomas are hard nuggets. Skip lesions form bumps. Therefore, **CD may be palpable**
- CD involves entire GI tract, so you may see signs in the mouth or perianal
- UC is a mucosal disease. The mucosa is the top layer. When it bleeds, nothing keeps it in. **UC <u>always</u> shows blood.**
  - CD <u>might</u>

What We See on X-Ray (XR)

- CD can attack any portion of the GI tract
  - It is a response to intestinal bacteria, and bacteria are everywhere
  - CD in the small intestine after drinking barium may look like a string of beads = **"string sign"**

- UC =Ulcerative **Colon**itis (inflammation of the colon)
  - It starts at the rectum and progresses up the <u>colon</u>
  - UC is non-stop ulcerations from the rectum and up the colon. It looks like a **"lead pipe"**

CD has Some Complications

- Crohn's affects absorption in small intestine
  - Kidney stones: calcium oxalate renal calculus
  - Gallstones: cholesterol cholelithiasis
  - Diarrhea
    - UC may also have diarrhea (often bloody diarrhea)
  - Elevated PT

CD Complications: Causes

- It's all malabsorption
  - Kidney stones: calcium oxalate renal calculus
    - low calcium and increased oxalate absorption
  - Gallstones: cholesterol cholelithiasis
    - fat malabsorption
  - Diarrhea
  - Elevated PT
    - vitamin K malabsorption

Colon Cancer

- Big question – Does it involve the colon?
  - Both CD and UC can lead to colon cancer after 10y, **but** <u>CD doesn't always involve the colon.</u>
- Ulcerative Colitis is only in the colon (and rectum). Therefore, you remove the colon and you are cured.
  - 60% will require surgery in 5y
  - CD not so much. Disease reoccurs at site of anastomosis.
    - and it's not just in the colon

Summary 1

- IBD may also show inflammation of the eyes, skin, and joints. In particular, inflamed nodules & necrotic ulcers in leg.
  - erythema nodosum & pyoderma gangrenous
- CD: may palpate in abdomen. May see inflammation around mouth or perianal.
- Both may give you diarrhea. CD might have some blood. UC always has some blood. UC may be a bloody diarrhea.

Summary 2

- On XR
  - CD w/ barium ~ string-sign
  - UC w/o ~ lead pipe
- CD may lead to malabsorption in small intestine
  - kidney stones, gallstones, and elevated PT
- Colon cancer after 10y is possible
  - CD doesn't always involve the colon.
- Surgery
  - Not a good idea for CD
  - For UC, it is curative.
    - 60% of UC pt's will require surgery in 5y.

IBD 3

Dx and Tx

Review

- It's all alphabetical
  - CD (Crohn's Disease) < UC (Ulcerative Colitis)
  - TH1 < TH2
  - cell-mediated < humoral
  - granulomas < ulcers

IBD - Messing around with me, in AZ, were 6 MPs

Diagnose

- **"ASCA ANCD you will receive"** *(Ask and you will receive)*
  - *It's all alphabetical*
  - CD ~ ASCA = anti-saccharomyces cerevisiae
    - Malabsorptive diseases tend to get yeast infections and therefore have antibodies for them. CD happens to have a LOT more than anything else of this antibody
  - UC ~ ANCA = anti-neutrophil cytoplasmic antibody
- Biopsy:
  - CD has granulomas
  - UC has ulcerations and is anchored to rectum

Treatment: Big Picture

- IBD = <u>Inflammatory</u> Bowel Disease
- Anti-inflammatories
  - Mesalamine, azathioprine, 6MP
    - *IBD - Messing around with me, in AZ, were 6 MPs*
  - Acute exacerbations: budesonide (high-dose steroid)

Tx: too much information

- Mesalamine = mesalazine
  - These are all mesalazine. **PAR** for the course
  - CD:
    - **P**entasa is released in upper and lower bowel
  - UC:
    - **A**sacol is only released in large bowel
    - **R**owasa is exclusively for **R**ectal disease

    - UC can also use balsalazide and olsalazine

Tx: extended

- CD is associated with intestinal infections
  - Tx: ciprofloxacin & metronidazole
- CD – if fistula formed or refractory
  - Get a PPD
    - if neg, infliximab
    - if pos, isoniazid
      - Infliximab can reactivate TB

Tx: SE

- Mesalamine
  - sulfa SE: rash, AIN, infertility in men, leukopenia
- Azathioprine and 6MP:
  - drug-induced pancreatitis
- Infliximab
  - arthralgias

Summary 1

- Dx
  - ASCA ANCD you will receive
  - Biopsy: CD ~ granulomas, UC ~ ulcers and anchored to rectum
- Tx Inflammatory Bowel Disease w/ anti-inflammatories
  IBD - Messing around with me, in AZ, were 6 MPs
  - Mesalamine, Azathioprine, 6MP
  - Acute exacerbations: Budesonide

Summary 2

- **PAR** for the course
  - CD: **P**entasa
  - UC: **A**sacol
  - **R**ectal only: **R**owasa
- CD Intestinal Infections:
  - ciprofloxacin & metronidazole
- CD w/ fistula or refractory:
  - inflixamab or isoniazid
    - w/o TB or w/ TB

Diarrhea, Infectious 1

What to do first and a few special bugs

What to Do First

- **First, evaluate for hypovolemia**
  - A person can die from hypotension.
- If hypovolemic + fever + abdominal pain, hospitalize + IV fluids + Abx
- If blood in stool,
  - Make the Abx **ciprofloxacin ± metronidazole**
  - If suspect HUS, don't give any Abx or platelets
    - HUS takes >5d after diarrhea starts to develop
    - Need to check stool for toxin

Infectious Diarrhea

- Always assume this first, then r/o
  - Are there white cells, ova, or parasites in the stool?
  - Clostridium difficile toxin?
  - Giardia-antigen?

Agents: Most Common

- Sickle cell and achlorhydria:
  - Campylobacter and Salmonella
    - Campylobacter also seen w/ reactive arthritis and preceding Guillain-Barre
- HIV+ w/ CD4 < 100:
  - Cryptosporidia, Isospora
- Daycare, No systemic manifestation, No blood or white cells:
  - Virus

Agents: Water

- Camping, unfiltered water:
  - Giardia
    - No blood in stool
    - Abd fullness, bloating, gas.
    - Simulates celiac dz: fat malabsorption
- Unfiltered water in Mexico:
  - Entamoeba histolytica = amebiasis
    - bloody diarrhea, RUQ pain, liver abscess (flask-shaped ulcer)
    - can have blood diarrhea in under a day

Agents: Food

- Refried Chinese food: Bacillus cereus
  - VOMITING
  - NO blood
  - short incubation: 1-6h
- Picnic, potato salad: S. aureus
  - short incubation: 1-6h
- E. coli 0157:H7
  - HUS takes >5d after diarrhea starts to develop
  - HUS happens when organism dies, that is why Abx are contraindicated.
  - Plt transfusions contraindicated, they make it worse

D Initial Summary

1. Evaluate for hypovolemia
2. If hypovolemic with fever & abd pain → in-hospital IV fluids + Abx
   a. if blood in stool, Abx = ciprofloxacin ± metronidazole
   b. If suspect HUS, NO Abx or platelets
      • HUS takes >5d after diarrhea starts to develop

Differentiate Summary

- Special situation
  - Sickle cell or achlorhydria ~ Campylobacter and Salmonella
  - HIV+ w/ CD4 < 100 ~ Cryptosporidia, Isospora
  - Daycare: think virus first
- Been on a trip
  - Camping ~ Giardia
  - Mexico, flask-shaped ulcer ~ amebiasis

Diarrhea, Infectious 2

Some more special bugs

Review

- Special situation
  - Sickle cell or achlorhydria ~ Campylobacter and Salmonella
  - HIV+ w/ CD4 < 100 ~ Cryptosporidia, Isospora
  - Daycare: think virus first
- Been on a trip
  - Camping ~ Giardia
  - Mexico, flask-shaped ulcer/liver abscess ~ amebiasis
    - also, bloody diarrhea in under a day

Agents: Fish

- Scombroid:
  - Organism releases histamine into flesh of fish → vomit, diarrhea, flushing, wheezing w/in minutes.
- Raw shellfish: mussels, oysters, clams: Vibrio
  - Pt's usually have underlying disease
  - V. parahaemolyticus is severe
  - V. vulnificus ~ w/ liver dz and hemochromatosis
    - skin bullae
- Large reef fish (grouper, red snapper, barracuda): Ciguatera-toxin
  - Incubation 2-6h
  - Neuro: parasthesia, weakness, reversal of heat and cold

Agents of Liver Diseases

- Vibrio vulnificus and Yersinia common with hemochromatosis or iron overload
  - Vibrio is from uncooked shelf fish → skin bullae
  - Yersinia can mimic appendicitis
- Entamoeba histolytica
  - liver abscess
  - flask-shaped ulcer
  - can get bloody diarrhea in under a day

Fast Acting Agents

- As little as an hour or two, no longer than six
- Bacillus cereus ~ refried Chinese food
- S. aureus ~ potato salad
- Ciguatera-toxin ~ large reef fish

Special Diagnostic Points

- Bloody diarrhea takes 24-36h except for Entamoeba histolytica.
  - Think Salmonella, Shigella, E. coli, Campylobacter, Yersinia, Vibrio
- Dx Cryptosporidiosis by modified acid-fast test
  - not ova or parasite exam (unreliable)
- Giardia: best is ELISA test of stool
  - stool for ova/parasite is a close 2nd

Differentiate Summary

- Special pt condition
  - Sickle cell or achlorhydria ~ Campylobacter and Salmonella
  - HIV+ w/ CD4 < 100 ~ Cryptosporidia, Isospora
  - Hemochromatosis ~ Vibrio & Yersinia
    - Vibro ~ uncooked shellfish
    - Yersinia ~ mimic appendicitis
- Been on a trip
  - Camping ~ Giardia
  - Mexico, flask-shaped ulcer ~ amebiasis
- Was eating seafood
  - Scombroid releases histamine into flesh of fish → anaphylaxis look in human
  - Vibro ~ uncooked shellfish
  - Ciguatera-toxin ~ reef fish and neuro symptoms (reverse heat and cold)

Special Diagnostic Test Summary

- Cryptosporidiosis
  - requires a <u>modified acid-fast test</u>
- Giardia
  - best test is ELISA test of stool

Diarrhea, Infectious 3

How to deal

Review

- Special pt condition
  - Sickle cell or achlorhydria ~ Campylobacter and Salmonella
  - HIV+ w/ CD4 < 100 ~ Cryptosporidia, Isospora
  - Hemochromatosis ~ Vibrio & Yersinia
    - Vibro ~ uncooked shellfish
    - Yersinia ~ mimic appendicitis
- Been on a trip
  - Camping ~ Giardia
  - Mexico, flask-shaped ulcer ~ amebiasis
- Was eating seafood
  - Scombroid releases histamine into flesh of fish → anaphylaxis look in human
  - Vibrio ~ uncooked shellfish
  - Ciguatera-toxin ~ reef fish and neuro symptoms (reverse heat and cold)

Special Diagnostic Test Summary

- Cryptosporidiosis
  - requires a <u>modified acid-fast test</u>
- Giardia
  - best test is ELISA test of stool

Treatment Review

- With high-volume stools, dehydration, abd pain, blood and fever, don't wait on stool culture
  - Tx: ciprofloxacin ± metronidazole
    - or other fluoroquinolone
  - Unless blood started 5 days after diarrhea started, suspect HUS and don't give Abx or platelets.

Specific Abx Needs

- Isospora: TMP/SMX
- Vibrio: doxycycline
- Traveler's diarrhea: **rifaximin**
  - mild loose stools w/o fever or blood: Loperamide
  - if worse, fluoroquinolone or azithromycin
  - ❖Never give prophylactic Abx for Traveler's D

Horribly Bad Abx Mnemonics

- **Vibrio** – it's the Gonorrhea of diarrhea
  - because you can treat them both with **doxycycline**
- **Isospora** – the non-Cryptosporidia
  - If HIV poop Is So Porous, maybe it's Isopora.
  - TeMPorary SMacking of toilet bowel water, treated w/ **TMP/SMX**
- To be a traveler, requires a river crossing at minimum. Rifa X i Min → **rifaximin**
  - When it's at its worst, it can leave you on the Floor Alone in AZ
- If worse, **fluoroquinolone or azithromycin**

Antibiotic-Associated Diarrhea

- Treatment of C. diff
  - Metronidazole
    - May use **oral** <u>vanc</u> (not IV, won't pass bowel wall)
  - Fidaxomicin
    - decreases number of reoccurrences
- Erythromycin causes increased GI motility
  - don't confuse w/ C. difficile

Diarrhea, Infectious 4

Malabsorption Diarrhea

Lactose Intolerance

- Gas and bloating
  - NEVER bloody or w/ leukocytes
  - NO wt loss
  - If malabsorption is present, think pancreatic insufficiency, celiac sprue, bacterial overgrowth
- Easiest Dx
  - remove all milk products from diet for 36h and observe for resolution
    - vs. Celiac Dz, which can take weeks to resolve
- Harder Dx
  - increased osmolar gap (> 50)
  - Mg & polyethylene glycol in stool

Malabsorption Syndromes

- Fat malabsorption
    1. celiac dz   2. chronic pancreatitis......
    ..... 3. tropical sprue   4. Whipple dz
    - all have wt loss (fat has highest caloric content)
    - dec ADEK, Ca → easy bruising and inc PT
    - if in duodenum → iron deficiency

Other Things to Look For

- Celiac Dz
    - Usually presents with <u>iron deficiency anemia</u>
    - Dermatitis herpetiformis
- Chronic pancreatitis
    - episodes from alcohol or <u>gallstones</u>
- Tropical Sprue ~ tropical country
- Whipple (rarest)
    - arthralgias, ophthalmoplegia, <u>dementia</u> (10%)
        - *Remember how the Rock wrapped that demented thugs <u>whip</u> around his <u>wrist</u> in The Rundown? I couldn't believe my <u>eyes</u>.*

Dx Celiac Dz

- GET your Abs first
  - anti-**G**liadin
  - anti-**E**ndomysial
  - anti-**T**ranslutaminase
- Then a small bowel biopsy
  - flattened villi
    - to exclude small bowel lymphoma
- ❖ Stopping gluten isn't accurate. Abs will be circulating for <u>weeks</u>.

Dx: Chronic Pancreatitis

- XR or CT for calcifications
- Most accurate: secretin test or low trypsin
  - secretin → huge bicarb (and other enzyme) release into duodenum
  - Secretin test: Place NG tube into duodenum and inject secretin into blood, pancreas won't release
    - rarely done
- D-xylose testing not done anymore
  - used to differentiate celiac from chronic panc.

Dx/Tx: Tropical Sprue and Whipple Dz

- Bowel-wall biopsy → PCR
  - Tropheryma whippelii also shows foamy macrophages
- Tx
  - Tropical sprue: TMP/SMX or doxycycline for 6m
  - Whipple dz: TMP/SMZ or ceftriaxone for 1y

Summary 1

- Lactose ~ gas and bloat.
  - No blood or wt loss.
- With fat malabsorption, expect bruising and inc PT
- To Dx Celiac, **GET** your Abs first:
  - anti-**G**liadin
  - anti-**E**ndomysial
  - anti-**T**ranslutaminase
    - stopping gluten is not a test

Summary 2

- With chronic pancreatitis,
  - XR or CT
  - secretin test is most accurate
  - D-xylose testing outdated
- Treat Tropical sprue or Whipple w/
  - TMP/SMX or
    - Tropical sprue w/ doxy for 6m
    - Whipple w/ ceftriaxone for 1y

Liver Disease and Cirrhosis 1

Liver function and Cirrhosis
dysfunction

Specific Liver Functions

- Synthesis
- Energy
- Detox
- Assist in Maintaining Gradients

Specific Liver Functions: Synthesis

- Serum proteins that act as hormone carriers
- Immune substances, such as gamma globulin
- Testosterone and the **estrogen** hormones
- Bile to break down fats

Synthesis And Beyond

- All clotting factors are made in the liver except **VIII** and **von Willebrand factor**
  - They are made in endothelial cells

- 70% of liver function must be lost for the synthetic capacity of the liver to be diminished

Specific Liver Functions: Energy

- Converting fats, proteins and carbohydrates to energy and nutrients
- Storing sugars as fuel (glycogen) for future use
- Storing vitamins and minerals, such as iron
- Storing extra blood for quick release

Specific Liver Functions: Detox

- Filtering blood
- Eliminate fat-soluble toxins, including excess hormones
  - Regulating sex hormone levels and eliminating excess hormones.
- Removing harmful chemicals, bacteria, and excesses
- Metabolizing drugs and breaking down alcohol

Cirrhosis

- Common failures leading to symptoms
  - Synthetic failure
    - low albumin level → peripheral edema
    - low clotting factors → elevated PT
  - Detox failure
    - Inc estrogen: palmar erythema, spider angiomata
    - Inc ammonia: asterixis, encephalopathy
  - Portal HTN → ascites, esophageal varices

Liver Function Summary

- Synthesis of proteins, testosterone, estrogen, and bile
- Convert fats, proteins, and carbs to energy
- Store glycogen, vitamins/minerals, blood
- Filter blood. Eliminate toxins. Manage hormones.
- Assist in maintaining gradients

(Cirrhosis)
Liver Dysfunction Summary

- Synthetic failure → peripheral edema, inc PT
- Detox failure
  - Inc estrogen → palmar erythema, spider angiomata
  - Inc ammonia → asterixis, encephalopathy
- Portal HTN → ascites, esophageal varices

Liver Disease and Cirrhosis 2

What the ascites tells us, and what we
do then

Cirrhosis (Liver Dysfunction) Review

- 70% of liver function must be lost for the synthetic capacity of the liver to be diminished
- Synthetic failure
  - low albumin level → peripheral edema
  - low clotting factors → elevated PT
    - *All clotting factors are made in the liver except VIII and von Willebrand factor. They are made in endothelial cells*
- Detox failure
  - Inc estrogen: palmar erythema, spider angiomata
  - Inc ammonia: asterixis, encephalopathy
- Portal HTN → ascites, esophageal varices

Ascites

- Paracentesis
  - needle though anterior abdominal wall
- What matters clinically
  - SAAG
    - ie. Serum-Ascites Albumin Gradient
  - White cell count
  - Neutrophils

SAAG

- Transudates are a result of increased pressure in the hepatic portal vein due to portal hypertension
  - low protein, low LDH, high pH, normal glucose.
- Exudates are actively secreted fluid due to inflammation or malignancy
  - high protein, high LDH, low pH (<**7.30**), a low glucose, inc WBC
- Serum-Ascites Albumin Gradient
  - Serum should have more albumin than ascites
  - **SAAG > 1.1** = low gradient ~ **portal HTN**
  - SAAG < 1.1 = high gradient ~ inflammation or cancer

SBP

- SBP = Spontaneous Bacterial Peritonitis
  - Density is low, so gram stain is not useful. Can't wait for culture
- If white cell count > 500 (or) neutrophils > 250, we have SBP
- Tx: **cefotaxime** or **ceftriaxone + albumin**
  - Albumin infusion decreases risk of hepatorenal syndrome

What to Do With Ascites

1. Perform paracentesis
2. Calculate SAAG
   - if SAAG > 1.1: portal HTN
   - if **SAAG < 1.1: cancer or infection**
3. If SAAG < 1.1
   - White cell count > 500 (or) neutrophils > 250: SBP
     - else malignancy
4. If SBP
   - Tx: cefotaxime or ceftriaxone + albumin infusion
   - else work up malignancy

Main Cirrhotic Issues

- Edema and fluid overload in third space
- Portal HTN and varices
- Encephalopathy and asterixis

Treatment

- Edema and fluid overload
  - diuretics, particularly **spironolactone**
- Portal HTN and varices
  - **propranolol** to prevent bleeding
- Encephalopathy and asterixis
  - **neomycin** and/or **lactulose**
    - Neomycin kills bacteria in the intestinal tract, keeping nitrogen levels low.
    - Lactulose a nonabsorbed disaccharide that bacteria metabolize in colon. This makes it more acidic. The acidity converts NH3 to NH4+ (ammonia to ammonium). Ammonium is not absorbed very well and is excreted from the body.

Listening to Ascites: Summary

1. Perform paracentesis
2. Calculate SAAG
   - if SAAG > 1.1: portal HTN
   - if SAAG < 1.1: cancer or infection
3. If SAAG < 1.1
   - White cell count > 500 (or) neutrophils > 250: SBP
     - Tx: cefotaxime or ceftriaxone + albumin infusion
   - else malignancy → workup

Dealing w/ Cirrhosis: Summary

- Edema and fluid overload: **spironolactone**

- Portal HTN and varices: **propranolol**

- Encephalopathy and asterixis:
  - **neomycin** and/or **lactulose**

Liver Disease and Cirrhosis 3

PBC vs PSC

Primary Biliary Cirrhosis (PBC)

- A fatigued and pruritic middle-aged woman with possible autoimmune disease history.
- PBC is an autoimmune condition associated with Sjögren's syndrome, RA, scleroderma
- Pt may not be pruritic
  - Bili doesn't elevate until advanced (5-10y)
  - 1/3 only have elevate ALP and no symptoms.

PBC: Dx

- Elevated ALP and GGTP
- Elevated total IgM
- Most specific: antimitochondrial Ab
- A biopsy is the best. May or may not be done

PBC: Tx

- Steroids are not helpful
- UV light can help with pruritus
- Ursodeoxycholic acid <u>may</u> help.
- Possible liver transplant in advanced stages.

Primary Sclerosis Cholangitis (PSC)

- Presentation and testing are same as PBC, except
  - PBC ~ Sjögren's syndrome, RA, scleroderma vs. PSC ~ IBD (UC > CD)
  - PSC is negative for antimitochondrial Ab

PSC: Dx & Tx

- Dx
  - ERCP or transhepatic cholangiogram
  - This is the only liver disease where liver biopsy isn't the most accurate test.
- Treatment same as PBC
  - UV light can help with pruritus
  - Ursodeoxycholic acid may help.
  - Possible liver transplant in advanced stages

PBC & PSC: Summary

- Primary Biliary Cirrhosis (PBC)
  - A fatigued and pruritic middle-aged woman with **autoimmune** disease history.
  - or elevated ALP, GGTP, and **antimitochondrial** Ab positive
  - Tx:
    - NO steroids (useless)
    - UV light + ursodeoxycholic acid → liver transplant
- Primary Sclerosis Cholangitis (PSC)
  - Same as above but
    - No autoimmune-Hx. Instead, expect a **IBD**-Hx
    - Antimitochondrial Ab negative
  - Diagnose and treat as above but
    - get a ERCP or a transhepatic cholangiogram

Liver Disease and Cirrhosis 4

The other diseases

Hemochromatosis

- Extrahepatic symptoms
  - Restrictive cardiomyopathy (15%)
  - Hyperpigmentation, hypogonadism, diabetes, and arthralgias
  - *A bronze diabetic with small testicles and a heart problem*
- Vibrio vulnificus and Yersinia infections occur more often because of their avidity for iron.

Hemochromatosis: Dx & Tx

- Dx
  - Liver biopsy or MRI
  - Abnormal C282Y gene
- Tx
  - Phlebotomy
  - If can't do phlebotomy,
    - deferoxamine or deferasirox

Wilson's Disease

- Copper builds up in the liver, brain and cornea
- Brain
  - Basal ganglia dysfunction → movement d/o
    - tremor and Parkinson's in 1/3 of pts
  - psychiatric disturbance (10%)
- Kidney (proximal tubule)
  - Fanconi syndrome
    - glucose, amino acids, uric acid, phosphate and bicarbonate are passed into the urine, instead of being reabsorbed
  - Type II (proximal) RTA
    - Failure of renal tubules to reabsorb bicarb → hypoK and hypoP
- High copper levels are toxic to RBC → hemolytic anemia

Wilson's: Tx & Dx

- Dx
  - Low ceruloplasmin & high Cu level
  - Liver biopsy is best
- Tx
  - Penicillamine or Trientine (copper chelators)
  - Oral zinc (interferes w/ copper absorption)
  - Liver transplant is curative
  - *Steroid will NOT help*

Alpha-1 Antitrypsin Deficiency

- AR
- Young person with cirrhosis and emphysema
- Tx: replacement enzyme

Chronic Hep B & C

- Define
  - persistence of hepB surface antigen for > 6m
  - Ab to hepC and elevation of viral load by PCR
- Treatment
  - HepB:
    - interferon, lamivudine, telbivudine, entecavir, or adelfovir
  - HepC:
    - **interferon + ribavirin + (boceprevir or telaprevir)**

Summary 1: The Metals

- Hemochromatosis
  - *A bronze diabetic w/ small testicles and a heart problem.*
  - Hx of **Vibrio** and **Yersinia**
  - Dx: Liver biopsy or MRI + abnormal **C282Y** gene
  - Tx: Phlebotomy or deferoxamine
- Wilson's
  - Movement disorder and kidney problems
  - Dx: Low **ceruloplasmin** and high Cu
  - Tx: **Penicillamine** and oral zinc → liver transplant
    - Steroids DON'T help

Summary 2: Enzymes and Viruses

- Alpha-1 Antitripsin
  - young person w/ cirrhosis and emphysema
- Chronic Hep B:
  - hepB surface antigen for > 6m
  - Tx: interferon, lamivudine, or entecavir
- Chronic Hep C:
  - anti-hepC antibody and elevation of viral load by PCR
  - Tx: interferon + ribavirin + (boceprevir or telaprevir)

REPRODUCTIVE CENTRIC

Reproduction 1

The Hormones

hCG

- $10 + 10 = 20$
  - Notable at **10**th day
  - Peaks at **10**th week
  - Falls to plateau at **20**w
- Maintains corpus luteum production of progesterone until placenta can take over
  - corpus luteum only: <u>7w</u> → <u>both</u> → <u>9w</u>: placenta only
- Regulates steroid biosynthesis
  - In placenta and fetal adrenal gland
- Stimulates testosterone production in fetal-male testes

Elevated hCG

- Expected if having twins, but is also high with
  - Hydatidiform mole
  - Choriocarcinoma
  - Embryonal carcinoma

hPL = Placental Lactogen

- Produced by syncytiotrophoblast
- Similar to HGH and prolactin
- hPL decreases insulin sensitivity
  - aka. antagonist to insulin
  - Reason for predisposition in pregnancy to glucose intolerance and diabetes
- If low
  - Threatened abortion
  - IUGR

Estrogen

- Estradiol: non-pregnant, reproductive years
  - CE in follicular theca cells → androgens → follicular granulosa cells (possess aromatase) → estradiol
- Estriol: during pregnancy
  - DHEAS produced by fetal adrenal glands → → estriol
- Estrone: menopause
  - peripheral adipose tissue conversion

- *No 'd' in pregnancy.*
- *Old women have soft <u>bones</u> as in estr<u>one</u>*

Progesterone is like a Good Host

- It gets the party going.
- Invites the guests in and protects them from harm while keeping the unwanted guests out.
- If the event isn't a hit, it leaves and the party stops.
- But, if the party is a success, it keeps the records spinning and the people dancing until the dawn

Progesterone

- Converts endometrium to secretory state preparing uterus for implantation
- Decreases maternal immune response allowing acceptance of sperm and guides sperm & decreases uterus contractility
- Makes vaginal epithelium and cervical mucus think preventing more sperm from entering
- If not pregnant, progesterone decreases → menstruation
- If pregnant, corpus luteum makes progesterone
    - Preventing menstruation & lactation
    - When ceases to be made → labor and lactation

Progesterone: The Good & Bad

- Along with prolactin, progesterone induces lobuloalveolar maturation of the breasts allowing for milk production
    - However, it's also involved in breast cancer.
- Decreases gastric motility → increased emptying time
    - Prone to aspiration pneumonia

Reproduction 2

The Changes with Pregnancy

The Signs

- Chadwick sign
  - Bluish/purplish vagina and cervix
    - Due to increased vascularity
- Chloasma
  - Blotchy pigmentation of nose and face
- Striae gravidarum = stretch marks
  - More likely to have birthing lacerations

CV changes

- Central venous pressure is unchanged
- Femoral venous pressure inc 2x-3x by 30w
- Plasma volume inc 50% by 30w
- Systolic murmurs are normal
  - <u>But</u> diastolic murmurs are never normal and must be investigated

Respiratory Changes

- Tidal volume inc 40%
  - Only lung volume that doesn't decrease
- Minute ventilation inc 40%
- Blood gasses:
  - dec P_{CO2} → inc pH = respiratory alkalosis

Renal Changes

- Kidneys get bigger, ureters expand, GFR inc
  - BUN, Cr, Uric acid decrease
  - Glucosuria increases
  - Proteinuria unchanged

Hormone Glands

- Pituitary: size increased 100%
  - *going to be lactating*
- Adrenals' size unchanged but <u>cortisol inc 3x</u>
  - *under a lot of stress (cortisol is the stress hormone)*
- Thyroid increased 15%

- Final 8 weeks, secrete colostrum

Reproduction 3

Good Pregnancy

Conception

- Normal pregnancy is 38 weeks
- Conception is 40 weeks from LMP
- Naegele's Rule:
  - Due date = LMP – 3m + 7d

This is normal

- 1st Trimester < 13w
  - Spotting and bleeding occur 20%
    - 50% will continue successfully
  - Avg wt gain: 8lbs
- 2nd Trimester 13-26w
  - Round ligament pain is common
  - Braxton-Hicks can start at 14w
  - Quickening at 18-20w (mom aware of movement)
  - Avg wt gain: 1lb/wk after 20w
- 3rd Trimester 26w-40w
  - Lightening = descent of fetal head into pelvis
    - Easier to breath but pelvic pressure

Common Complaints

- Migraines
- Epulis = bleeding gums; Nosebleeds
  - Due to inc blood flow
- Chloasma = mask of pregnancy
- Telogen effluvium = excessive shedding (1-5m)
- Carpal tunnel
  - 50% get wrist splint

Reproduction 4

Postconception

Week 1

- Intratubal phase:
    - Morula into uterine cavity → 8cell stage
- Intrauterine phase:
    - Morula into uterus (day 3), implant (day 6)

- Outer layer → trophoblast or placenta
- Inner mass → embryo

Week 2 & 3

- Week 2
    - 2 layer embryo
    - survive or die (an insult destroys)
- Week 3
    - 3 layer embryo
        - ectoderm, mesoderm, endoderm

Day 22-28

- Neural tube defects:
    - High risk women should take **4**mg of folic acid
    - All women should take **0.4**mg

Week 4-8

- Organs and organ systems formed
  - Ectoderm:
    - Central and peripheral nervous systems
    - Seeing and hearing
    - Integument
  - Mesoderm: muscles, cartilage, CV, urogenital
  - Endoderm: lining of GI and respiratory

After Week 9, Your Safe-ish

- Insults generally don't destroy embryo or mutate it. Most likely, insults will result in organ hypertrophy or hyperplasia

Reproduction 5

Y the Changes

Review: Estrogen

- In non-pregnant women in their reproductive years
  - Cholesterol in follicular <u>theca cells</u> → androgens → follicular <u>granulosa cells</u> (possess aromatase) → estradiol

- During pregnancy
  - DHEAS produced by fetal adrenal glands → → estriol
- During menopause
  - peripheral adipose tissue conversion → Estrone

Müllerian, Paramesonephric Duct

- By default, the paramesonephric duct develops into
  - Fallopian tubes
  - Corpus of uterus, Cervix
  - Proximal vagina
  - *Para = closely related to; Meso = in the middle:*
    - *close to the kidney but in the middle*
- Y-chromosome induces gonadal secretions of Mülerian inhibitory factor (MIF)
  - Sertoli cell → MIF → inhibits female
    - *Sertoli didn't want to be a woman*

Mesonephric (Wolffian) Duct

- In females, duct undergoes regression
- In males testosterone stimulates duct to become
  - Vas Deferens
  - Seminal vesicles
  - Epididymis
  - Efferent Ducts
  - *Meso = in the middle, or membrane supporting a part:*
    - *in the middle of the renal tract but supports a part*
      - *supports male reproduction*

Male External Genitalia

- DHT stimulation is required to develop penis and scrotum
- Leydig cell → testosterone → maintains Wolffian duct → stimulates 5α-reductase → DHT → male genitals

Sertoli vs Leydig

- Sertoli cell → MIF → inhibits female
  - *certain to be MIFfed and turn off the females*
  - (Sertoli, MIF)

  vs.

- Leydig cell → testosterone → → DHT → penis/scrotum
  - *lie and dig, test her patience, dhat guy's a penis (and a wolf)*

Embryology: Gonadal

- Germ cells
  - oogonia ~ spermatogonia
- Coelomic epithelium
  - granulosa cells ~ Sertoli cells
- Mesenchyme
  - theca cells ~ Leydig cells
- Mesonephros
  - rete ovarii ~ rete testis

Embryology: Ductal

- Paramesonephric (Müllerian)
  - F: fallopian tubes, uterus, part of vagina
  - M: Y-chr → MIF → testis hydatid
    - (vestigial remnant of paramesonephric duct)
- Mesonephric (Wolffian)
  - F: Gartner's duct
    - (vestigial remnant of mesonephric duct)
  - M: vas deferens, seminal vesicles, epididymis
- Mesonephric tubules
  - F: Epoophoron, Paraoophron
  - M: Efferent ducts

Reproduction 6

Checking on the Fetus

Review on Mom

- Direct Coombs test
  - Blood type and Rh
    - *"What blood-type are you" is a pretty direct question*
- Indirect Coombs test
  - atypical RBC Abs
    - "Are your RBS antibodies atypical" is an indirect way of asking if you're abnormal.

Review

- Pregnant moms get tested for
  - STD's: VDRL or RPR, ELISA for HIV
    - CDC recommend **Informed Refusal** (or Opt Out)
      - test unless she refuses
  - PPD
    - If positive, get CXR
      - If CXR is negative: **isoniazid + vit B6 for 9m**
      - If CXR is positive: get sputum Cx and begin triple meds
      - Antituberculosis drugs are **not** contraindicated in pregnancy

Non-Invasive Obstetric Procedures

- Dating in 1st Tri: Transvaginal U/S ($\pm$5d)
  - *it's small so you have to get closer*
- Dating in 2nd Tri: Transabdominal U/S ($\pm$10d)
- Doppler is used to check umbilical artery and MCA blood flow
- Genetic sonogram (18-20w):
  check anatomic markers of fetal aneuploidy

Nuchal Translucency

- 10-14 week
- Measures fetal **fluid** behind neck
- Combined with blood tests of free β hCG & PAPP-A in 1st trimester for aneuploidy screening

Chorionic Villus Sampling

- 10-12 week
- Carries a pregnancy loss rate of **0.7%**
- Needle is placed into placental tissue without entering amniotic cavity
- Can go in transcervical or transabdominal

Amniocentesis

- After 15 weeks
- Pregnancy loss rate is **0.5%**
- Used to check AFP and acetylcholinesterase
  - For neural tube defects
- Used to access
  - Chromosomal abnormalities
  - Fetal infections
  - Sex

Quad Screen

- 15-20 weeks
- AFP + estriol + hCG + inhibin-A
- T21 (Down's)
  - dec: AFP & estriol; inc: hCG & inhibin-A
    - perform amniocentesis for karyotype
- T18 (Edwards)
  - dec all four
    - perform amniocentesis for karyotype

PUBS
(percutaneous umbilical blood samples)

- After 20 weeks
- Pregnancy loss rate is < 2%
- Diagnostic uses
  - eg. blood gases, karyotype, IgG & IgM
- Therapeutic uses
  - eg. intrauterine transfusion with fetal anemia

Timing Review

- 10-14w
  - Nuchal Translucency
  - Chorionic Villus Sampling
- > 15w
  - Amniocentesis
  - Quad Screen
- 18-20w: Genetic sonogram
- >20w
  - PUBS (percutaneous umbilical blood samples)
  - Fetoscopy

Reproduction 7

Pregnancy Losses

How to Handle Abortions

- 1st Trimester
  - D&C < 13 weeks
  - Mifepristone + misoprostol < 2 months
- 2nd Trimester
  - D&E
    - Break it up and remove in pieces
  - Induce labor with prostaglandins
    - & Intracardiac inject a feticidal agent like KCl or digoxin
      - prevents live births

Most Common Early Pregn Losses

- Cytogenetic: chromosomal abnormality
- Mendelian: autosomal or X-linked or recessive

- Antiphospholipid syndrome
  - some women w/ SLE produce Abs against own vascular system and fetoplacental tissues
  - Tx: SQ heparin

Fetal Demise Evacuation

- Big threat is DIC
  - DIC usually not seen until 4 weeks after demise
  - If no DIC, can defer to allow for grief.
  - 90% spontaneous labor after 2 weeks

If in Doubt About Intrauterine Pregnancy

- hCG levels double every 58 hours in an IUP
  - Must have at least 1500 mIU to use as marker, so keep performing test every 2 days until reach that level

Reproduction 8

Pregnancy Poison
(teratogens and others)
nasty memorization

Know the Category Examples

- Category A = no risk during pregnancy
  - **thyroxine**
- Category B = no risk to animals (& probably humans)
  - **PCN**, cephalosporins, methyldopa, **SSRI**, Prozac
- Category C = risk not ruled out
  - codeine, Bactrim, cipro, AZT, β B, heparin
- Category D = bad
  - ASN, valium

Know the Category Examples

- Safe for the pregnant women
  - hypothyroidism: You can give thyroxine.
  - infection that's sensitive to PCN or cephalosporin? Good. Either will work
  - HTN: Give her methyldopa
  - OCD, anxiety, or depression: SSRI's are fine
- We will, but prefer not to
  - opiods for pain
  - infections: Bactrim, cipro
  - cipro, AZT, β B, heparin
- Don't mess with aspirin and valium

Common Ones: Stated Different

- Phenytoin (Dilantin)
  - fetal hydantion syndrome: craniofacial dysmorphism (epicanthal folds, oral clefts, ...)
- Trimethadione
  - facial dysmorphism
- Thalidomide
  - phocomelia (deformed limbs)
- Warfarin
  - chondrodysplasia

Common Ones: Stated Different

- In other words, phenytoin, trimethadione, thalidomide, and warfarin all cause skeletal or cartilage deformations.
  - phenytion & trimethadione: face
    - Phen Phen tried meth and done screwed up his face
  - thalidomide: phocomelia (deformed limbs)
    - How you remember that word is up to you. Yeesh!
  - warfarin: cartilage
    - interesting because cartilage doesn't get much blood flow, and warfarin is all about blood flow (sort of)

Common Ones: Stated Different

- DES:
  - we all know clear cell carcinoma in the female children of mothers who took it but did you know
  - T-shaped uterus, vaginal adenosis
    - vaginal adenosis → vaginal clear cell carcinoma
- Isotretinoin (Accutane)
  - microtia (deaf), pinna (external ear underdeveloped)
    - *Your baby is deaf w/ funky ears, but your skin looks great!*
- Streptomycin
  - CNVIII damage → hearing impairment
    - Like strept throat for Viking ears
      - (Viking ~ vestibulocochlear nerve in the mnemonic)

Immunizations

- Safe
  - Flu, hepA & B (aka HAV, HBV)
  - Pneumococcus, meningococcus
  - Typhoid
- Unsafe
  - MMR, Varicella
  - Polio
  - Yellow Fever

Reproduction 9

Pregnancy Infections

GBS

- <u>Lifelong</u> colonization
  - So, if you have a positive urine culture or have previously delivered a baby with GBS sepsis, you get treated
  - Screen: vaginal & rectum culture, 35-37w
  - If preterm (<37w) with membrane rupture > 18h, or maternal fever
- Tx: PCN
  - 2nd line: clindamycin or vancomycin

CMV (a herpes virus)

- Small-headed deaf blueberry corn muffin baby
- **PeriVentricular calcifications**
  - the 'V' is for CMV
- CMV, big liver and spleen
  - it rhymes
- Tx: Ganciclovir
  - *CMV the gang's all got it*
    - Tx is Ganciclover and this is the most common congenital viral syndrome

Rubella (RNA virus)

- Deaf blueberry muffin baby wearing glasses and holding his chest
  - Deaf, cataracts, ventriculoseptal defect
- 90% chance of infection in 1st tri, 5% in 3rd

Varicella

- Zigzag skin lesions
- Blueberry muffin baby with binoculars
  - mulberry skin spots
  - optic atrophy, cataracts, chorioretinitis
- Communicable 2 days before vesicle appear and until vesicles crust over
- Prophylaxis: VZIG w/in 96hrs of exposure
  - zigzag, Very near sighted, Varicella, VZIG

Review

- GBS – if you got it, you keep it
  - Tx clinda & vanc
- CMV
  - small-headed deaf blueberry corn muffin baby
  - periVentricular calcifications
  - Ganciclovir (the gang's all got it)
- Rubella
  - deaf blueberry muffin baby wearing glasses and holding his chest
  - RUBella: R is for RNA, RUB is for heart rub
- VeryZella Very near sighted, ZigZag pattern, VZIG

Toxoplasmosis

- Small head, big tummied baby with sunglasses and intracranial calcifications
    - chorioretinitis, intracranial calcifcations
    - microcephaly, hepatomegaly, thrombocytopenia
- Tx
    - pyrimethamine + sulfadizaine
    - Spiramycin to avoid vertical transmission

Reproduction 10

Things that are early for $1000

Multiple Gestations

- < 3d: Di-Di Di or Mono-Di-Di: separation at **morula** stage
  - twins, gender same or unknown, 2 placentas
- 4-8d: Mono-Mono-Di: separation at **blastocyst** stage
  - twins, gender always same, one placenta, 2 sacs
  - possible twin-twin transfusion
- 9-12d: Mono-Mono-Mono: at **embryonic disk**
  - twins, gender same, one placenta, one sac
  - possible twin-twin transfusion
  - umbilical cord entanglement may lead to fetal death
- > 12d conjoined twins w/ probable lethal

Review: Multiple Gestations

- < 3: DDD or MDD → 2 placentas
- 4-8: MMD → 1 placenta, 2 sacs
- 9-12: MMM → 1 placenta, 1 sac
- > 12 conjoined twins

Preterm

- 20w < preterm < 37w
  - 2 contractions in 30 min, cervical dilation > 2cm

Prevent **Pre**T**erm** **B**irth

- Cervical length > 25mm w/ prior PTB
  - weekly intramuscular 17-HO-P *(17 HOPe)*
- Cervical length < 25mm w/ prior PTB < 24w
  - weekly intramuscular 17-HO-P + cerciage

- Nothing seems to work for twins

Fetal Fibronectin (fFN)

- Biological glue binding trophoblast to maternal decidua
- If leaks into vagina, PTB is likely
- If negative test, chance of PTB w/in two weeks is < 1%

IV Mg SO4

- PTB anticipated < 32w
  - 4hr infusion
  - Check deep tendon reflexes
    - SE: respiratory depression and pulmonary edema
- O/D: treat w/ calcium gluconate

- Contraindications:
  - renal insufficiency and myasthenia gravis

Betamethasone

- < 34 weeks, lungs need to mature
  - may need to give tocolytic to prolong pregnancy
- Two IM 12mg doses, 24 hrs apart
  or
- Four IM 6mg doses, 12 hrs apart

- Decreased respiratory distress, intracranial hemorrhage, necrotizing entercolitis

ONCOLOGY CENTRIC

Breast Cancer 1

Fibrous Breast

Rule Out the Mastitis

- Lactating women may develop abscesses
  - They are not masses
- Do an I&D
- If option to perform a biopsy of the wall is offered, do it

Don't Worry

- 19yo w/ firm, rubbery, mobile mass
  - **Fibroadenoma**
  - Dx FNA or core needle biopsy or U/S
    - no mammograms in young women
      - breast is too dense

It's All About the Looks

- 13yo w/ firm, rubbery, mobile mass which has grown to 6cm
  - **Giant juvenile fibroadenoma**
  - Tx: resect for cosmetic reasons
    - not a cancer risk

Be Concerned, But Not Worried

- 27yo w/ firm, <u>maybe</u> rubbery, mobile mass that has been growing for years
  - **Cystosarcoma phyllodes**
  - Dx: biopsy – its benign, but it can turn malignant
  - Tx: margin-free resection
    - It's benign, so you don't have to control for possible invasion

Start Off Worrying (and then calm down)

- 35yo w/ 10y Hx of tenderness in both breasts associated with <u>menstrual cycle</u>. Multiple firm, maybe rubbery, mobile masses that "come and go" at different time in the <u>menstrual cycle</u>. This 2cm one <u>didn't change with the menstrual cycle</u>.
  - **palpable cyst in fibrocystic disease**
    = cystic mastitis = mammary dysplasia

Palpable Cyst in Fibrocystic Disease

- Dx: mammogram – looking for other non-palpable lesions
- Tx: aspirate the cyst (not FNA) until empty
  - If mass goes away **and** fluid is clear → done
  - If fluid is bloody → cytology
  - If mass doesn't go away → biopsy

Benign Fibrous Summary

- Firm, rubbery, mobile mass
  1. 18yo: **fibroadenoma**
     - FNA or core needle biopsy or U/S
  2. 13yo & 6cm: **giant juvenile fibroadenoma**
     - Resect for cosmetic reasons
  3. 27yo growing for years: **cystosarcoma phyllodes**
     - Biopsy → margin-free resection
  4. 35yo, B/L that come and go w/ menstrual cycle, but this one doesn't: **palpable cyst in fibrocystic disease**
     =cystic mastitis = mammary dysplasia
     - mammogram → aspirate → evaluate

Breast Cancer 2

Overall Management

Benign Fibrous Review

- Firm, rubbery, mobile mass
    1. 18yo: **fibroadenoma**
        - FNA or core needle biopsy or U/S
    2. 13yo & 6cm: **giant juvenile fibroadenoma**
        - Resect for cosmetic reasons
    3. 27yo growing for years: **cystosarcoma phyllodes**
        - Biopsy → margin-free resection
    4. 35yo, B/L that come and go w/ menstrual cycle, but this one doesn't: **palpable cyst in fibrocystic disease**
        =cystic mastitis = mammary dysplasia
        - mammogram → aspirate → evaluate

Vs. More Serious Cancer Risk

- All get mammograms → multi-core biopsies
  - May get U/S
  - Exception: lobular cancers get MRI
    - don't show up on mammogram or U/S

Resection vs. Mastectomy

- Based on closeness to nipple or disproportionate to breast size
  - Segmental resect = **lumpectomy**
  - Total mastectomy = simple mastectomy
  - Both followed by radiation
- SLNB (sentinel lymph node biopsy)
  - If mets positive → biopsy level I and II lymph nodes
  - If confined to one quadrant, no axillary sampling needed
    - ductal carcinoma in situ

Invasive Cancer

- Tx: surgery/radiation → chemo/hormonal
  - Post-menopausal, tumor < 1cm, node neg, hormone receptor positive → can skip chemo

  - <u>If pregnant, do all the above but skip the radiation</u>

Hormone Treatment

- Young women get **<u>tamoxifen</u>**
  - Young women still wear <u>tam</u>pons
- Post-menopausal women get **anastrazole**

Summary

- More serious cancer risks get a mammogram followed by multi-core biopsies
  - Except lobular cancers which get an MRI
- Resections/mastectomies + SLNB + radiation → chemo/hormonal
  - If resected mass was confined to one quadrant (ductal carcinoma n situ), no axillary sampling is needed
  - Pregnant women don't get the radiation
  - Post-menopausal, < 1cm, node-, HR+ → skip chemo
  - Hormone Tx:
    - young woman get **tamoxifen** (they still wear <u>tampons</u>)
    - post-menopausal get **anastrazole**

Breast Cancer 3

Worrisome Tumors

Review Basic Management

- More serious cancer risks get a mammogram followed by multi-core biopsies
  - Except lobular cancers which get an MRI
- Resections/mastectomies + SLNB + radiation → chemo/hormonal
  - If resected mass was confined to one quadrant (ductal carcinoma in situ), no axillary sampling is needed
  - Pregnant women don't get the radiation
  - Post-menopausal, < 1cm, node-, HR+ → skip chemo
  - Hormone Tx:
    - young woman get **tamoxifen**
    - post-menopausal get **anastrazole**

General Masses

- Hard masses ~ invasive breast adenocarcinoma
- Orange-peel skin ~ inflammatory breast CA
  - inflammatory is terrible
- Eczematoid areolar lesion ~ Paget's Disease

- All get mammography → multi-core biopsy
  - Orange-peel and eczematous → dermal punch biopsy

Intraductal Papilloma

- Bloody nipple discharge and no mass
- Dx: r/o cancer w/ mammogram
- Tx: optional resection w/ guided **galactogram**, U/S, or retroareolar exploration

Invasive Lobular Carcinoma

- Thickening of the tissue or **fullness** in one part of the breast.
  - **Doesn't form a lump**
1. Begins in the milk-producing glands (lobules)
2. Invades surroundings
  - may spread further

Special Case

- Pt w/ breast cancer 2 years ago and stopped chemo. She now presents with neurological signs.
- Suspect brain mets
- Dx/Tx
  - MRI + high-dose steroids + radiation

SHORTHAND USED

pt = patient
Hx = history
≅ : roughly the same as
≈ : approximately equal to
~ : similar to; associated with
!= : not equal to; not the same as
>> : much greater than
→ : leads to
→ → → : multiple steps later
➜ : results in

ABOUT THE AUTHOR

Ellis Myers received his Doctor of Medicine from Chicago Medical School, a master's degree in Medicinal Science from Loyola University of Chicago, and a bachelor's degree in computer systems engineering from Arizona State University.

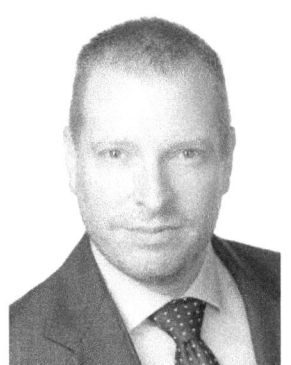

Dr. Myers built a distinguished career in the technology and engineering field. First, as an engineer and designer at IBM, then building several companies and corporations. He left his positions as CEO of Secure Salon and Senior Applications Specialist at Cyberitas Technologies to pursue his dream of becoming a physician.